Nu

D1394160

WITHDRAWN

P010197

Nursing the Acutely Ill Adult

Priorities in Assessment and Management

Edited By

David Clarke

&

Alison Ketchell

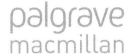

© Selection & Editorial Matter: David Clarke & Alison Ketchell 2011
Individual chapters © contributors 2011

All rights reserved. No reproduction, copy or transmission of this
publication may be made without written permission.

No portion of this publication may be reproduced, copied or transmitted
save with written permission or in accordance with the provisions of the
Copyright, Designs and Patents Act 1988, or under the terms of any licence
permitting limited copying issued by the Copyright Licensing Agency,
Saffron House, 6–10 Kirby Street, London EC1N 8TS.

Any person who does any unauthorized act in relation to this publication
may be liable to criminal prosecution and civil claims for damages.

The authors have asserted their rights to be identified as the authors of this
work in accordance with the Copyright, Designs and Patents Act 1988.

First published 2011 by
PALGRAVE MACMILLAN

Palgrave Macmillan in the UK is an imprint of Macmillan Publishers Limited,
registered in England, company number 785998, of Houndmills, Basingstoke,
Hampshire RG21 6XS.

Palgrave Macmillan in the US is a division of St Martin's Press LLC,
175 Fifth Avenue, New York, NY 10010.

Palgrave Macmillan is the global academic imprint of the above companies
and has companies and representatives throughout the world.

Palgrave® and Macmillan® are registered trademarks in the United States,
the United Kingdom, Europe and other countries

ISBN 978–0–230–58470–9

This book is printed on paper suitable for recycling and made from fully
managed and sustained forest sources. Logging, pulping and manufacturing
processes are expected to conform to the environmental regulations of the
country of origin.

A catalogue record for this book is available from the British Library.

A catalog record for this book is available from the Library of Congress.

10   9   8   7   6   5   4   3   2
20   19   18   17   16   15   14   13   12

Printed and bound in Great Britain by CPI Antony Rowe, Chippenham
and Eastbourne

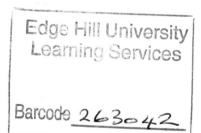

Edge Hill University
Learning Services

Barcode 263042

Contents

Tables

Figures

Preface

As we reach the end of the first decade of the new millennium it is apparent that nurses will continue to play a key role in providing modern, effective and patient-centred health services. The profession is entering an exciting new era and from 2011 nursing will go forward as a graduate entry profession. The challenge for all nurses will be to ensure that the care they and their colleagues provide is both compassionate and competent; so at one and the same time, nursing care must be sensitive to the needs of individuals and families but also demonstrate a high level of skill, knowledge and understanding. While there have been significant improvements in population health in most developed countries, the burden of ill health remains. The majority of individuals and families will at some time come into contact with and be dependent upon nurses and other health professionals to provide assessment, intervention and ongoing care during periods of acute and critical illness. Nursing roles have changed and developed substantially in recent times as nurses have responded to calls to work more flexibly, in more patient-centred ways and more collaboratively with colleagues in medicine. Investigation and treatment of common diseases has also become increasingly sophisticated and this means that individuals will require intensive monitoring and support during often shorter periods of hospitalisation. We have seen the introduction of a range of technologies to support patient assessment and monitoring; however, it remains the case that all nurses working with acutely ill adults must have a sound knowledge and understanding of normal physiology and also the pathophysiology associated with common disease processes. This knowledge and understanding is a fundamental prerequisite to competent nursing assessment and management of the acutely ill individual. It is essential that nurses can competently undertake observations of vital signs and monitor patients' physiological responses to treatment. However, it is clear that competence in vital signs recording alone is insufficient. In acute care settings, nurses must have and be able to utilise knowledge of pathophysiology and disease to underpin their technical skills; that is, apply theory in their everyday practice. All nurses working in these settings must be able to undertake a structured assessment of the acutely ill individual and prioritise the patient's needs accordingly. As part of ongoing monitoring, it is essential that nurses can recognise subtle changes in the patient's condition and understand and interpret the significance of such changes. Closely linked to this understanding and interpretation is the ability to recognise the actions that must follow in order that the changes identified do not lead to rapid deterioration and unnecessary loss of life.

This text adopts a case study approach to understanding and managing common presentations in adults with acute illness. This approach has been used to provide nurses with the knowledge, understanding and skills required to systematically assess acutely ill individuals, and correctly interpret the physiological data from initial and ongoing patient assessment. In writing this text we want to challenge nurses to develop a critical thinking approach to prioritising the nursing and medical interventions required to effectively manage a range of commonly presenting acute illnesses. We are confident that nurses working in acute and critical care settings can rise to that challenge.

David Clarke and Alison Ketchell

Notes on Contributors

Mark Bevan PhD RN
Mark is a senior lecturer and has been involved in renal patient care for over 20 years. He is involved in teaching postgraduate and post-registration education in nephrology and acute care. Mark is also involved in developing advanced assessment and diagnostic reasoning skills in advanced practitioners.

David Clarke PhD RN
David is an experienced lecturer with a clinical background in adult nursing. His teaching is now primarily focused on research methods. As a researcher David has focused on interdisciplinary team working in stroke care; his current research includes a process evaluation of a training programme for caregivers after stroke and an examination of nursing roles in stroke care.

Michelle Clayton MSc RN
Michelle has been involved in caring for liver patients for nearly 20 years. She balances clinical work with teaching a successful liver course for registered nurses. Michelle is the Lead Committee Member of the British Liver Nurses' Forum and is passionate about improving care for liver patients.

Elizabeth Cleave MSc RN
Elizabeth has been a lecturer in cardio-respiratory and acute care since 1992. Her clinical background and research interests are within acute cardio-respiratory care. She has also held a clinical liaison role in cardio-respiratory areas.

Beverley Gallacher MSc RN
Beverley has been teaching biological science and pathophysiology to healthcare students since 1995. Prior to this she was a Registered General Nurse on a variety of surgical wards for 9 years. Before entering nursing she obtained an undergraduate degree in biology at the University of York, UK.

Ian Goulden PG Dip RN
Ian is an adult critical care nurse by background and has been employed as a lecturer in higher education since 1995. His subject expertise and research

interests include adult acute and critical care, adult neuroscience and end of life in critical care.

Paula Holt MA RN

A registered nurse, Paula became a lecturer 20 years ago to share her commitment with others and to enhance practice with students, colleagues and wider communities. She has spent the last 12 years developing a professional interest in diabetes and is highly motivated and committed to improving the lives of people with diabetes.

Julie Jackson MSc RN

Julie's clinical experience includes renal medicine and critical care, in both this country and overseas. She has worked in the University of Leeds, UK as a lecturer practitioner and now works solely as a lecturer.

Alison Ketchell MSc RN

Alison has been a lecturer since 1994 and both her subject expertise and research interests are in acute and cardiac care. She is involved in teaching postgraduate and post-registration education in cardiology and acute care. Alison's clinical background was as senior sister in cardiology and coronary care and she has continued to maintain close links with clinical practice throughout her teaching career.

Robert McMaster MSc RN

Bob has worked in emergency care since qualifying as a nurse in 1983. Along the way he has gained a BSc in nursing and an MSc in education. He was appointed as one of two nurse consultants for Accident and Emergency in Leeds in 2001, and this role has provided opportunities to shape the development of services at local and national level.

Julia Maz D.Med.Sci RN

Julia is a lecturer in Adult Nursing and has worked in higher education since 1995 and has recently gained a Professional Doctorate from the University of Sheffield. Her research interests lie predominantly around both the acute and chronic sequelae which follow spinal injuries. Julia continues to maintain close practice links with musculoskeletal injuries and spinal trauma.

Acknowledgements

The authors and publishers are grateful to the following publishers and organisations for granting permission to reproduce copyright material in the main body of this book: the Department of Health for Tables 1.2, 1.3 and 6.1, all reproduced under the Open Government Licence v1.0; the National Patient Safety Agency for Table 1.4, reproduced under the Open Government Licence v1.0; the Office for National Statistics for Table 5.1, reproduced under the Open Government Licence v1.0; the National Heart, Lung, and Blood Institute, part of the National Institutes of Health and the U.S. Department of Health and Human Services for Figure 5.15; The McGraw-Hill Companies, Inc for Figures 8.2 and 8.3, originally from Seeley, R. et al.: *Essentials of Anatomy and Physiology 4th Edition* (New York: McGraw Hill, 2002); Wolters Kluwer Health for Figure 8.5, originally from Porth, C.: *Pathophysiology 7th Edition* (Philadelphia: Lippincott, Williams and Wilkins, 2004).

Every effort has been made to trace and contact all the copyright holders but if any have been inadvertently overlooked, the publishers will be pleased to make the necessary arrangements at the first opportunity.

1

The Importance of Nursing Assessment in Acute Care

David Clarke

Introduction

> Observation tells us the fact, reflection the meaning of the fact. ... The trained power of attending to one's own impressions made by one's own senses, so that these should tell the nurse how the patient is, is the sine qua non of being a nurse. (Nightingale, 1907, pp. 254–5)

In the above quotation Nightingale made the important point that observation of patients and interpretation of the observations made required skills which were an essential part of what it was to be a nurse. Although the range and type of patient observations made today has increased in number and sophistication, largely due to advanced technologies, skilled observations as part of initial and ongoing patient assessment remain central to effective nursing practice. Providing prompt and appropriate assessment, treatment and management for the acutely ill adult represents a very large part of the day-to-day activity of nursing and medical staff within hospitals in the United Kingdom (Jevon and Ewens, 2007). In addition, with the development of primary care services many acutely ill adults will be initially assessed and treated by rapid response or outreach teams, or by an advanced nurse practitioner in their own homes. While patient assessment is a fundamental part of nursing practice it is by no means a basic skill and requires integration of knowledge and understanding in clinical practice. The purpose of this book is to identify priorities in patient assessment and management in acute care situations and, through detailed discussion of these, to develop knowledge and understanding of the meaning and significance of the signs and symptoms seen in a range of commonly occurring acute illness presentations.

This introductory chapter will:

1. Define key terms: including acute illness and critical illness.
2. Briefly review factors that have influenced the development of acute and critical care services and highlighted the need for nurses to develop skills in assessment and management of the acutely ill patient.
3. Outline the guidance available to support and inform nursing assessment and management of the acutely ill adult.

Table 1.1 Glossary of terms

Acute care	The care provided to patients experiencing serious acute illness, which is often accompanied by a rapid and progressive deterioration in their condition, and which requires urgent assessment to determine the level of care required. This will normally require frequent monitoring and reassessment of need. Acute illness can complicate existing chronic illness.
Assessment	Assessment requires systematic observation and targeted questioning in order to gather and interpret physical, physiological, psychological and social data that will contribute directly to establishing a clinical diagnosis and determining the level of care required by an individual. A number of guided systems used in acute assessment, including ABCDE, ATLS, primary and secondary surveys, are reviewed in Chapter 2.
Care bundles	'A "care bundle" refers to a collection of processes used to care effectively for patients and involves putting together several evidence-based elements of care (approximately three to five practices) that are essential to improving outcomes' (DH 2005: 30).
Collaboration	Collaboration means to work together: that is, to act jointly to define and achieve a common purpose. In the context of acute and critical care this means to work alongside colleagues from medicine and other health professions in gathering, interpreting and acting upon assessment data, monitoring responses to interventions and, importantly, reporting changes in a timely manner.
Competence	Competence is more than the ability to perform specific tasks; it includes capability, which incorporates the acquisition and use of core skills in acute and critical care, the ability to assimilate underpinning knowledge and understanding, and development of the critical thinking skills needed to apply this knowledge and understanding to clinical practice (adapted from Eraut 1994).
Critical care	The care provided to patients who require intensive monitoring and/or the support of failing organs. These patients are found throughout the hospital, many in general wards, but the sickest are cared for in dedicated areas such as intensive care and high dependency units (DH 2005).

The terms acute and critical care will be used throughout this text. Table 1.1 provides definitions of these and some other commonly used terms.

Background

The importance of skilled assessment and monitoring of acutely ill patients in hospital has long been recognised but has gained increasing attention following the publication of the key policy documents *Comprehensive Critical Care* (Department of Health, (DH), 2000a) and *Quality Critical Care: Beyond Comprehensive Critical Care* (Critical Care Stakeholder Forum (CCSF), 2005). These reports highlighted the fact that in the absence of comprehensive services, early recognition of change or deterioration in health status may not occur and opportunities to prevent avoidable deaths may be lost (McQuillan et al., 1998; DH, 2000a). Later research and reports from the National Patient Safety Agency (NPSA) confirmed these claims and provided continuing evidence that identification of acutely ill patients who were at risk and in need of urgent intervention or referral to critical care services patients was frequently delayed and sometimes missed altogether (Seward et al., 2003; Young et al., 2003; NPSA, 2007).

Acute and Critical Care Service Provision

These publications identified considerable variability in the quality of service provision across the United Kingdom and established the principle that patient care should be based on the level of need identified rather than which speciality or part of the service the patient might be admitted to. The *Comprehensive Critical Care* report (DH, 2000a) mirrored other NHS policy documents published at that time in seeking to increase the quality and effectiveness of care and shift the focus from organisation of care based on professionally determined speciality services to focus on recognising and responding to the needs of patients (DH, 1999, 2000b). The policy requirement was for a 'whole systems' approach to modernisation of services to ensure acute and critical care provision was not bound by location, but was comprehensive and spanned all specialities (DH, 2000a). The report recognised the simple fact that acute and critically ill patients were not only to be found in intensive care and high dependency units. If signs of deterioration in acute and critically ill individuals are to be recognised and acted upon appropriately, it is essential that nursing and medical staff in all settings have the necessary knowledge and skills to accurately monitor vital signs, interpret the findings of this monitoring and then provide, or seek early assistance to access, the level of intervention and care required. This included establishing

Table 1.2   Description of need

Level	
0	Patients whose needs can be met through normal ward care in an acute hospital.
1	Patients at risk of their condition deteriorating, or those recently relocated from higher levels of care, whose needs can be met on an acute ward with additional advice and support from the critical care team.
2	Patients requiring more detailed observation or intervention, including support for a single failing organ system or post-operative care, and those 'stepping down' from higher levels of care.
3	Patients requiring advanced respiratory support alone or basic respiratory support together with support of at least two organ systems. This level includes all complex patients requiring support for multi-organ failure.

Source: Department of Health (2000a).
Reproduced under the Open Government Licence v1.0.

critical care outreach and support services and introducing changes in training to share critical care skills, and ensure direct care staff had the competence and knowledge to recognise and act appropriately upon signs and symptoms of deterioration or of increasing dependency and level of need. To aid health professionals in providing effective care and the right level of monitoring, the *Comprehensive Critical Care* report recommended a simple four-level system to classify patients according to need (Table 1.2).

The *Quality Critical Care* report (CCSF, 2005) confirmed that between 2000 and 2004 significant development of comprehensive critical care services occurred. However, the report also noted that service improvements were not uniform: for example, some hospitals had well established outreach teams and others had not set up such teams. In addition, while the overall number of critical care beds had increased by 35 per cent since 2000, critically ill patients were still being transferred between hospitals and the number of urgent operations being cancelled due to lack of critical care capacity was not being reduced. At the same time as critical care beds had increased in number, the overall number of hospital beds had fallen and the number of inpatients defined as acutely ill had increased (National Confidential Inquiry into Patient Outcomes and Death (NCEPOD), 2005). The *Quality Critical Care* report (CCSF, 2005) made a series of recommendations to ensure that comprehensive critical care services continued to develop and improve; these were aimed at commissioners, service providers, education providers and individual professionals. The key features that have particular relevance for this book are identified in Table 1.3.

Table 1.3   Features of a high quality critical care service relating to assessment and management of acutely ill individuals

Key feature	*Explanation*
Patient-centred care	Treating patients as individuals is fundamental and requires that they are the focus of care and that their identified needs should dictate the care provided. Keeping the patient at the centre of the care pathway requires flexible service provision.
Evidence-based care, monitoring and evaluation	Regular monitoring and evaluation of care informs clinical decision making. Where good evidence of effectiveness of specific clinical interventions exists, care should be informed by such evidence. One key area of use of best evidence identified to support comprehensive critical care was the introduction of 'care bundles'. This approach was also identified as a central element of service improvement by the NHS Modernisation Agency (2004).
Early warning systems and outreach systems	The widespread introduction and use of 'track and trigger' systems on general wards, together with intervention tools, was identified as necessary. For example, see Chapter 2, the modified early warning scoring system (Morgan et al. 1997; Goldhill and McNarry 2004).
An appropriately trained and competent workforce and staff empowerment, support and development	The report noted the importance of ensuring that staff working outside of critical care areas were competent in the recognition of critical illness. However, despite many other recommendations the report provided no specific guidance in this area. The discussion of the need for standardised programmes focused only on work-based training and did not comment on the need for changes in pre-registration undergraduate nursing education programmes, or on the level of preparation required for post registration or continuing professional development (CPD) programmes in acute and critical care.
Twenty-four hour access to multi-disciplinary teams	The report noted the obvious importance of having access to a multidisciplinary team with the right skills, knowledge and experience in acute and critical care. However, it also emphasised the need for team members to develop a culture of respect for all disciplines, for the team to engage in shared learning and be prepared to both challenge and support colleagues in order to enhance the effectiveness of patient care.

Source: Department of Health (2005).
Reproduced under the Open Government Licence v1.0.

The main aim of the *Quality Critical Care* report was to encourage organisations to build on the successes achieved since 2000 and maintain the momentum in order to ensure that critical care services continued to improve and became firmly integrated into primary and secondary care services. The successful implementation of all of the features of high quality services identified in Table 1.3 depend on skilled nursing staff being able to coordinate assessment activity with medical and other health professional colleagues and being able to undertake appropriate ongoing monitoring, including using track and trigger systems. This relies upon nurses and healthcare professionals developing a sound knowledge and understanding of the pathophysiology underlying common disease presentations and being able to competently apply that understanding when working with individual patients in clinical practice.

Education and Training

The Department of Health (2000a) recommendations for training of qualified nursing and medical staff were fairly clear, but the report did not comment on the fact that nurses in pre-registration and specialist post-registration training also needed more focused preparation to work in modernised health services where staff at all levels would be expected to be competent in assessment of the level of need. A later report from the Department of Health's Modernisation Agency (2003) did identify that education being provided at that time did not adequately prepare nurses and other healthcare providers to assess and manage the critically ill; this was particularly the case where care was being provided outside of designated critical care departments.

Two subsequent important documents from the National Institute for Health and Clinical Excellence (NICE, 2007) and the National Patient Safety Agency (NPSA, 2007) further highlighted the fact that despite significant improvements in the organisation of acute and critical care services since 2000, concerns remained about the knowledge, understanding and competence of nurses and other health professionals in recognising early and developing signs that a patient is 'at risk'. Where health professionals are enabled to develop the required competence the evidence shows that morbidity and mortality can be reduced (Bellomo et al., 2004; Priestley et al., 2004; NICE, 2007). The NPSA (2007) report clearly identified the detrimental effects that can result when such competence has not been acquired. Such knowledge and skills deficits have been shown to have a direct negative relationship on the effectiveness of comprehensive physical and physiological assessment, the use of early warning scoring systems to detect those at risk of deterioration and the usefulness of regular physiological monitoring. The NPSA (2007) analysed 1,804 serious incidents included in the national reporting learning system that had resulted in death of patients. The analysis indicated that as many as 576 of these deaths could be regarded as potentially avoidable. The majority of the 576 deaths occurred within acute and/or general hospitals. The NPSA (2007) conducted an in-depth analysis of 107 patients' deaths reported to the agency because of concerns related to the safety of the care provided for these patients during their hospitalisation. In the majority of cases (64) health professionals either took too long to notice or did not recognise signs of deterioration that may have prevented these deaths. The remaining cases related to either a failure

Table 1.4   Key recommendations to improve the care of patients who were considered to be at risk of deterioration or who were deteriorating

There needs to be	*Rationale*
Better recognition of patients who are at risk of or who have experienced deterioration and appropriate monitoring of vital signs	In the cases reviewed, formal or visual observations, including colour, or consciousness, temperature, pulse, blood pressure and oxygen saturations, were either completely or partially omitted. The most common omission was observation of the respiratory rate.
Accurate interpretation of clinical findings	In the cases reviewed, early warning scores were not calculated correctly and health professionals did not always recognise when observations gave cause for concern, which may require more intensive monitoring.
Calling for help early and ensuring that it arrives. A related recommendation was made in relation to ensuring that appropriate drugs and equipment were available to facilitate appropriate and early interventions	In the cases reviewed, there was a lack of communication and health professionals did not act on concerns identified during handovers or transfer of information between professional groups.
Training and skills development	In the cases reviewed, analysis of specific incidents resulting in death suggested that medical and nursing staff did not have the depth of knowledge and skills required to recognise deterioration and call for appropriate help.

Source: National Patient Safety Agency (2007).
Reproduced under the Open Government Licence v1.0.

to recognise cardiac arrest or not instigating early interventions and calling the cardiac arrest team once the arrest had been recognised. The NPSA (2007) also highlighted the existence of good practice in the NHS but, importantly, the report made a series of recommendations (Table 1.4) designed to improve the care of patients who were considered to be at risk of deterioration or who were deteriorating; all these issues will be considered in the context of case studies in later chapters of this book. The report also made a number of recommendations in relation to the resuscitation of the acutely ill individual. Recognising and responding to the importance of these issues, NICE (2007) developed detailed clinical guidelines (CG 50) designed to improve the recognition and response to adults presenting with acute illnesses in hospital. The NICE (2007) guidelines will be examined in more detail in Chapter 2 and subsequent chapters in this book. An important feature of both these documents is the recognition of the need for training to improve skills, knowledge and understanding for all staff involved in assessing, treating and managing the acutely ill adult. It is also clear that, although these documents focus primarily on caring for acutely ill patients in hospital, the skills required to systematically assess the acutely ill adult are transferable to the majority of settings where patients present seeking assistance from health professionals, including primary care settings, outreach services, walk-in centres and polyclinics.

Collaboration in Acute and Critical Care Provision

There is increasing acceptance by policy makers and health professionals that collaborative multidisciplinary working not only makes good sense but also results in improved patient outcomes, including reductions in morbidity and mortality (NICE, 2007; Stroke Unit Trialists' Collaboration, 2007; Massey et al., 2008). Multidisciplinary teams also include allied health professionals and an important contribution will be made by assistant critical care practitioners, traditional healthcare assistants and other support workers. In most healthcare settings there are overlapping areas of clinical work but in acute and critical care settings in particular there is a high degree of interdependence between nursing and medical work and that of other professionals (Figure 1.1).

This interdependence is in part based on the traditional roles occupied by nurses and physicians. With few exceptions, nurses spend more time in direct contact with patients than almost all other health professional groups. As a result nurses are more likely to observe subtle changes in a patient's condition even if the signs that alert the nurse to a change are not always objective and may be based on an intuitive grasp that the patient needs close observation (Benner et al., 1996; Cioffi, 2002). However, while

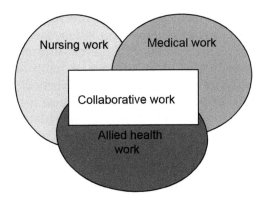

Figure 1.1   Overlapping areas of work in acute and critical care.

nurses are normally responsible for comprehensive assessment of patient need and monitor vital signs and response to treatment, determining the need for investigations and making a diagnosis is still (with the exception of some advanced practice roles) most commonly a medical activity. However, it is not difficult to comprehend how important nursing assessment and reporting of patient data is in terms of making an early diagnosis and introducing appropriate interventions for acute and critically ill patients in a timely manner; increasingly this requires collaborative decision making. In order for there to be effective collaboration, the communication between multidisciplinary team members has to be frequent and requires the use of a common, often technical, language (Andrews and Waterman, 2005; Clarke, 2009). This impacts in turn on the educational preparation of health professionals in pre-registration and continuing education programmes as it is within multidisciplinary or interprofessional programmes that shared understanding of roles, practice in joint problem solving and understanding and use of a common language are most likely to flourish (Kilminster et al., 2004; Young et al., 2007; Bandali et al., 2008).

The Organisation of This Book

This chapter has established the necessity for nurses to develop knowledge understanding and competence in assessment, early recognition and appropriate management of patients in acute and critical care settings. This is based on both the professional imperative to develop the core skill of nursing assessment and the recognition that the evidence suggests that unless nurses and other health professionals develop these competencies, patients who experience acute deterioration and/or cardiac arrest will continue to receive suboptimal care, which can lead to deaths that are largely preventable. Early recognition of acute deterioration is dependent on skilled assessment but it also requires understanding of normal anatomy, physiology and the ways in which pathophysiology and disease result in changes in and disruption in normal physiological processes. Throughout the book a series of case studies will be presented; the purpose of these is to help the reader to develop an understanding of the important interrelationship of presenting signs and symptoms, recognition of the underlying pathophysiology and the required nursing and medical assessment, investigations and interventions required in acute and critical illness. The case scenarios will pose a series of questions to provoke the reader to reflect and think critically about their current knowledge, experience and understanding. Answers to the questions posed and further explanation will be provided in the subsequent text.

Chapter 2 of this book provides a detailed examination of the purpose and conduct of systematic history taking, physical assessment, including application of the ABCDE approach, and the purpose of monitoring of vital signs using track and trigger systems, and establishes the principles underpinning interpretation of clinical data. The information contained in Chapter 2 is designed to apply to all clinical settings where acutely ill adults are seen. Chapter 3 focuses on the key problem of shock and draws on common acute care scenarios to explain the nature and causation of shock. This chapter also introduces key principles related to disturbances in acid–base balance and outlines the place of oxygen therapy in supporting acutely ill adults. These two chapters focus on essential aspects of assessment that are applied and developed in each of the subsequent chapters of the book. In the remaining chapters the authors present case studies that illustrate commonly encountered problems related to a range of acute illness situations. The authors of each chapter identify key learning and action points and links to important resources (both online and paper-based), and, because no single text can cover all the information that might be useful in acute and critical care, each chapter also includes suggestions for further reading. We believe this approach ensures that this book provides more than narrowly focused anatomy and physiology or nursing care texts can, and captures the interest of readers keen to develop their understanding of priorities in assessing and managing the acutely ill adult.

Note

All the case studies used in this book represent composites drawn from the common presenting signs and symptoms seen in acute and critical care patients; the names chosen for case study patients are fictitious.

Further Reading: Key Resources for Assessment and Management of Acute and Critical Illness

Clinical Guideline 50: *Acutely Ill Patients in Hospital: Recognition of and Response to Acute Illness in Adults in Hospital*. Prepared by the National Institute for Health and Clinical Excellence (2007). Available from: http://guidance.nice.org.uk/CG50

'Resources and Good Practice Examples', in National Patient Safety Agency, *Safer Care for the Acutely Ill Patient: Learning from Serious Incidents. Fifth Report from the Patient Safety Observatory* (London: NHS National Patient Safety Agency, 2007), pp. 26–36. Available from: http://www.npsa.nhs.uk/nrls/alerts-and-directives/directives-guidance/acutely-ill-patient/

Resuscitation Council Guidelines (2010) Available from http://www.resus.org.uk/pages/guide.htm

References

Andrews, T. and H. Waterman. 'Packaging: A Grounded Theory of How to Report Physiological Deterioration Effectively', *Journal of Advanced Nursing*, **52**(5) (2005), 473–81.

Armitage, M. E., T. Stokes and Guideline Development Group. 'Recognising and Responding to Acute Illness in Adults in Hospital: Summary of NICE Guidance', *British Medical Journal*, **335** (2007), 258–9.

Bandali, K., K. Parker, M. Mummery and M. Preece. 'Skills Integration in a Simulated and Interprofessional Environment: An Innovative Undergraduate Applied Health Curriculum', *Journal of Interprofessional Care*, **22**(2) (2008), 179–89.

Bellomo, R., D. Goldsmith, S. Uchino, J. Buckmaster, G. Hart, H. Opdam, W. Silvester, L. Doolan and G. Gutteridge. 'Prospective Controlled Trial of the Effect of the Emergency Team on Morbidity and Mortality Rates', *Critical Care Medicine*, **32**(4) (2004), 916–21.

Benner, P., C. A. Tanner and C. A. Chesla. *Expertise in Nursing Practice: Caring Clinical Judgment and Ethics* (New York: Springer, 1996).

Cioffi, J. 'Nurses' Experiences of Making Decisions to Call Emergency Assistance to Their Patients', *Journal of Advanced Nursing*, **32**(1) (2000), 108–14.

Cioffi, J. 'What Are Clinical Judgements?', in C. Thompson and D. Dowding (eds), *Clinical Decision Making and Judgement in Nursing* (Edinburgh: Churchill Livingstone, 2002).

Clarke, D. J. 'Achieving Teamwork in Stroke Units: The Contribution of Opportunistic Dialogue', *Journal of Interprofessional Care*, 8 December (2009), 1–13. Available at: http://informahealthcare.com/doi/abs/10.3109/13561820903163645

Critical Care Stakeholder Forum. *Quality Critical Care: Beyond Comprehensive Critical Care*. A Report by the Critical Care Stakeholder Forum (London: Critical Care Stakeholder Forum, 2005).

Department of Health. *Making a Difference: Strengthening the Nursing, Midwifery and Health Visiting Contribution to Health and Healthcare* (London: Department of Health, 1999).

Department of Health. *Comprehensive Critical Care* (London: Department of Health, 2000a).

Department of Health. *The NHS Plan: A Plan for Investment, a Plan for Reform* (London: Department of Health, 2000b).

Department of Health Modernisation Agency. *Critical Care Outreach: Progress in Developing Services* (London: Department of Health, 2003).

Department of Health. *The National Education and Competence Framework for Advance Critical Care Practitioners* (London: Department of Health, 2008a).

Department of Health. *The National Education and Competence Framework for Assistant Critical Care Practitioners* (London: Department of Health, 2008b).

Eraut, M. *Developing Professional Knowledge and Competence* (London: Falmer, 1994).

Goldhill, D. and A. McNarry. 'Physiological Abnormalities in Early Warning Scores Are Related to Mortality in Adult Inpatients', *British Journal of Anaesthesia*, **92**(6) (2004), 882–4.

Jevon, P. and B. Ewens. *Monitoring the Critically Ill Patient*, 2nd edn (Oxford: Blackwell, 2007).

Kilminster, S., C. A. Hale, M. A. Lascelles, P. Morris, T. Roberts, P. Stark, J. R. Sowter and J. Thistlethwaite, J. 'Learning for Real Life: Patient-focused Interprofessional Workshops Offer Added Value', *Medical Education*, **38**(7) (2004), 717–26.

McQuillan, P., S. Pilkington, A. Allan, B. Taylor, A. Short, G. Morgan, M. Nielsen, G. Barrett and G. Smith. 'Confidential Inquiry into Quality of Care before Admission to Intensive Care', *British Medical Journal*, **316** (1998), 1853–.8

Massey, D., L. M. Aitken and C. Wendy. 'What Factors Influence Suboptimal Ward Care in the Acutely Ill Ward Patient?', *Australian Critical Care*, **21**(3) (2008) 127–40.

Morgan R. J. M., F. Williams and M. M. Wright. 'An Early Warning Scoring System for Detecting Developing Critical Illness', *Clinical Intensive Care*, **8** (1997), 100.

National Confidential Enquiry into Patient Outcomes and Death. *An Acute Problem? A Report of the National Confidential Enquiry into Patient Outcome and Death (NCEPOD)* (London: NCEPOD, 2005).

National Institute for Health and Clinical Excellence. *Acutely Ill Patients in Hospital: Recognition of and Response to Acute Illness in Adults in Hospital*. NICE Clinical Guideline 50 (London: National Institute for Health and Clinical Excellence, 2007).

National Patient Safety Agency. *Safer Care for the Acutely Ill Patient: Learning from Serious Incidents*. Fifth Report from the Patient Safety Observatory (London: NHS National Patient Safety Agency, 2007).

Nightingale, F. 'Training of Nurses', in M. A. Nutting and L. Dock (eds), *A History of Nursing: The Evolution of Nursing Systems from the Earliest Times to the Foundation of the First English and American Training Schools for Nurses, Volume 2* (New York: Putman & Sons, 1907).

Priestley, G., W. Watson, A. Rashidian, C. Mozeley, D. Russell, J. Wilson, J. Cope, D. Hart, D. Kay, K. Cowley and J. Pateraki. 'Introducing Critical Care Outreach: A Ward-randomised Trial of Phased Introduction in a General Hospital', *Intensive Care Medicine*, **30**(7) (2004), 1398–404.

Seward, E., E. Greig, S. Preston, R. A. Harris, Z. Borrill, T. D. Wardle, R. Burnham, P. Driscoll, B. D. W. Harrison, D. C. Lowe and M. G. Pearson. 'A Confidential Study of Deaths after Emergency Medical Admission: Issues Relating to Quality of Care', *Clinical Medicine*, **3**(5) (2003), 425–34.

Stroke Unit Trialists' Collaboration. *Organised Inpatient (Stroke Unit) Care for Stroke* (Cochrane Database of Systematic Reviews, 3, 2007), CD000197.

Young, M. P., V. J., Gooder, K., McBride, B. James and E. S. Fisher. 'Inpatient Transfers to the Intensive Care Unit: Delays Are Associated with Increased Mortality and Morbidity', *Journal of General Internal Medicine*, **18**(2) (2003), 77–83.

2

Principles of Assessment

Julie Jackson

Introduction

The assessment and management of the acutely ill adult is an essential part of the role of the nurse. It was established in Chapter 1 that a consistent body of evidence shows that patients may be at risk of acute deterioration in clinical condition due to delayed recognition, the institution of inappropriate therapy and poor communication between clinical staff (Goldhill et al., 1999; NCEPOD, 2005; NPSA, 2007). For example, most cardio-respiratory arrests are predictable, in approximately 80 per cent of cases there is a deterioration in clinical signs prior to an event. These patients often experience physiological deterioration that is unnoticed by staff or poorly treated, leading to suboptimal clinical outcome (Resuscitation Council UK, 2006). NICE guideline CG:50 *Acutely Ill Patients in Hospital: Recognition of and Response to Acute Illness in Adults in Hospital* (NICE, 2007) and the Department of Health's (2008) *Competencies for Recognising and Responding to Acutely Ill Patients in Hospital* were developed in direct response to concerns about the care of the acutely ill adult. These guidelines recognise that staff caring for acutely ill adults should have competencies in monitoring, measurement, interpretation and prompt response appropriate to the level of care they are providing; this chapter focuses on these important issues. Assessment is essentially a practical activity but knowledge application is essential for systematic, prioritised assessment. The theoretical and practical knowledge discussed in this chapter is applicable to primary, secondary and tertiary care in equal measures. A patient may present with acute illness in any care setting and optimal clinical outcome is dependent upon early detection and management of deterioration.

Aim and Learning Outcomes

The Aim

The aim of this chapter is to explore the priorities in early assessment and management of the individual presenting with an acute event or a deteriorating clinical condition.

Learning Outcomes

At the end of this chapter the reader will be able to:

1. Discuss prioritisation of assessment and intervention.
2. Assess and monitor an acutely ill patient.
3. State the normal values of key physiological markers.
4. Identify a prioritised management plan appropriate to their own role.
5. Recognise the importance of multidisciplinary team working in acute care.

Assessment: Skills and Definitions

All patients in acute hospital settings should have a full assessment recorded at the time of admission (NICE, 2007). The preliminary assessment includes simultaneous measurement of the patient's vital signs, collection of essential biographical data, a brief accurate history of presenting signs and symptoms and specific investigation in order that life saving intervention and symptom relief can be administered immediately. The secondary assessment includes a full clinical examination and provides more detailed information on past medical history, family, social and drug history, further diagnostic investigation and bio-psychosocial aspects of activities of daily living. The focus of this book is on the preliminary assessment for the acutely ill adult.

The aim of the preliminary assessment is threefold:

1. To collect a series of clues required to translate a provisional diagnosis into a definitive one that will inform prompt, appropriate and effective management.
2. To provide a baseline against which future measures can be compared to enable the early detection of improvement or deterioration in symptoms.
3. To determine current physiological status and inform the frequency and manner of ongoing assessment and investigation.

Table 2.1 Prerequisite skills for assessment

- Observation skills
- Application of knowledge and understanding of normal and abnormal
  physiological parameters
- Interpretation skills
- Critical thinking and decision making skills
- Prioritisation of patient needs
- Communication skills and collaboration with the multidisciplinary team

---

Source: adapted from Dougherty and Lister (2008) and Alfaro-Lefevre (2006).

Nursing assessment involves gathering and synthesising clinical data, recording this information and recognising and communicating abnormalities. It is an ongoing dynamic process that requires a range of prerequisite skills (Table 2.1). Monitoring of vital signs is a fundamental aspect of care that may be considered a basic, routine activity that simply requires a practical awareness of how to perform and record the physical assessment. However, accurate and meaningful assessment is more than the ability to operate an electronic device or count pulsation at the radial artery: it is important to contextualise the data collected. Therefore a high degree of knowledge application is required if results are to be correctly synthesised, reported and responded to. Knowledge of normal physiological parameters is essential but taken in isolation can be of limited value. It is of greater importance to know what is 'normal' for a particular patient, or, if previous observations are not available, what could be considered normal with a particular clinical presentation. There is, however, a danger that accepting recordings that are believed to be 'their normal' may obscure evidence of deterioration and it is useful to remember that grossly abnormal observations are rarely 'normal'. Two or more deteriorating observations can be an ominous sign of imminent severe clinical deterioration, and to appreciate this and other issues fully, application of knowledge to practice is vital. Furthermore, competent observation, measurement, accurate recording and application of knowledge and understanding to interpretation of data are essential prerequisites for informed decision making. Observations should therefore be recorded and acted upon by clinical staff with appropriate training and knowledge. Student nurses are often responsible for the monitoring and documentation of vital signs but they should only perform this clinical activity if they have been observed and assessed by experienced nurses and are competent to do so. Lastly, communication to and collaboration with a team of staff from varying backgrounds possessing a range of skills is essential for effective clinical intervention (DH, 2008).

The structure of an assessment will depend upon the clinical presentation, the care setting and clinical need. An acutely ill patient may be encountered in primary, secondary and tertiary care and optimal clinical outcome is dependent upon early recognition and management of a potentially life threatening problem. The health professional requires good acute assessment skills in all care settings, particularly as rapid response and outreach or other acute services are now being provided in primary care. The focus of this chapter is the theoretical and practical aspects of assessment of the acutely ill adult using the ABCDE approach in a hospital setting.

Assessing the Acutely Ill Adult

The ABCDE approach provides a systematic method of clinical assessment that can be used and understood by all members of the healthcare team (Resuscitation Council UK, 2006). It ensures that the most vital signs for life are assessed and managed in a logical manner. However, a theoretical knowledge and understanding of normal and abnormal physiological parameters is essential if data is to be appropriately interpreted and acted upon. The ABCDE assessment should then form the basis for a more detailed preliminary and secondary assessment.

Underlying Principles

- Complete an initial assessment following the ABCDE approach.
- Treat life threatening problems when encountered, before moving on to the next part of the assessment.
- Reassess regularly.
- Assess the effects of treatment and interventions.
- Recognise when additional help is required – for example, other members of the multidisciplinary team – and call for help early (Resuscitation Council UK, 2006).

Always think about personal safety before any assessment begins. Look for danger in the environment; this may be from a tripping hazard, traffic, a noxious substance, electricity or any other number of potential hazards.

The Systematic ABCDE Approach

A: Airway

Airway is assessed in order to recognise any signs of obstruction. If a patient is able to talk the airway is patent. Causes of airway obstruction include

Table 2.2   Signs of compromised airway

- Difficulty talking or unable to talk
- Choking
- Shortness of breath or difficulty breathing, use of accessory muscles
- Noisy breathing: stridor, wheeze or gurgling
- See-saw respiratory pattern

Source: Resuscitation Council UK (2006).

central nervous system depression causing loss of patency and protective reflexes, vomit, a foreign body, epiglottis, infection, allergy, laryngeal spasm or bronchial secretions and bronchospasm (Resuscitation Council UK, 2006). If there is a reason to suspect that the airway may be compromised, the look, listen and feel approach will provide confirmation and potentially identify the cause (Table 2.2).

Look:

- In the mouth for any physical obstruction.
- At chest movement and breathing pattern for symmetrical movement. See-saw breathing (paradoxical abdominal and chest movement) whereby the abdomen and chest move alternately is a sign of obstruction as the air in the lungs cannot exit via the airway.

Listen:

- To the sound of breathing. Normal breathing is not noisy and so loud gurgling, snoring, wheezing or croaking is abnormal and requires intervention.

Feel:

- For breath against the hand or cheek to establish if there is evidence of air movement.
- The chest for signs of fluid. Obstruction from secretions is suspected if gurgling is heard and can sometimes be felt by placing a hand on the upper chest.

Airway obstruction is a medical emergency and requires urgent intervention to prevent hypoxic organ damage and death. If suspected get expert help immediately (Resuscitation Council UK, 2006).

Table 2.3 Treatment of airway obstruction

- Get expert help immediately (Ring 2222 in hospital, 999 out of hospital)
- Airway opening, i.e. head tilt, chin lift or jaw thrust
- Simple airway adjuncts
- Advanced techniques, i.e. intubation or emergency tracheostomy
- Provide oxygen

Source: Resuscitation Council UK (2006).

TREATMENT OF AIRWAY OBSTRUCTION

Airway obstruction is a stressful clinical situation and speed is required to prevent rapid deterioration. However, relatively simple interventions can improve outcome (Table 2.3). Repositioning a patient on their side (lateral position) unless contraindicated and insertion of simple airway adjuncts – for example, a nasal or oropharangeal airway and suctioning – can be successful in a patient with a partially obstructed airway caused by secretions (Resuscitation Council UK, 2006).This is a common cause of airway obstruction in the clinical environment and physiotherapists are often skilled at assisting with removal of excess secretions.

OXYGEN THERAPY

If a patient is critically ill or in a peri-arrest situation then 15 L/minute of oxygen therapy should be delivered via a non-rebreathe bag and reservoir mask. Once the patient has stabilised the oxygen can be reduced to maintain a normal SpO_2 of 94 to 98 per cent. Patients with COPD and other risk factors for hypercapnia (high carbon dioxide) who develop critical illness should have the same target saturations of 94 to 98 per cent as other critically ill patients, until the results of blood gas analysis are available and there is a clinical indication to reduce the target saturation and therefore the oxygen concentration (British Thoracic Society, 2008).

B: Breathing

Breathing is often the first vital sign to alter in a patient with a deteriorating condition and respiratory dysfunction can be predictive of an adverse clinical event (NICE, 2007; NPSA, 2007). Respiration is a complex process that incorporates four distinct events. Pulmonary ventilation (breathing) promotes air movement in and out of the lungs. External respiration is gas exchange at the alveoli and pulmonary capillary interface (oxygen loading and carbon dioxide unloading). Respiratory gas transport requires oxygen and carbon dioxide to be transported to and from the lungs and cells of the body via the blood

Table 2.4 Common causes of respiratory compromise

- Airway obstruction
- Underlying respiratory illness: chronic obstructive pulmonary disease (COPD), asthma
- Lung pathology: pulmonary oedema, pneumothorax, carcinoma, infection such as TB or pneumonia, pulmonary embolus, pulmonary hypertension
- Drugs: opiates, sedatives
- Central nervous system depression: disease or injury
- Shock: sepsis, cardiogenic, anaphylaxis
- Cardiac: left ventricular failure
- Chest trauma: flail chest

---

stream. Internal respiration is gas exchange at the interface between systemic capillaries and tissue cells (Marieb, 2009). All four processes must be fully functioning for effective respiration. Respiration may not only be affected by disease or injury of the respiratory system (bronchi, alveoli, chest wall etc.) but many other disorders (cerebral, neurological, cardiac, sepsis or anaphylaxis etc.) may initially present with tachypnoea (Table 2.4).

Assessment of breathing should include look, listen and feel.

Look for:

- difficulty breathing;
- sweating;
- tachypnoea (respiratory rate > 20 breaths per minute);
- accessory muscle use;
- skin colour – central cyanosis is notable as a blue tinge to mucosal membranes;
- abnormal physiology, i.e. deviated trachea or uneven chest movement;
- altered consciousness level;
- a measure of SpO_2;
- sputum production and expectoration.

Listen for:

- noisy breathing – wheeze, gurgling, stridor, cough;
- breath sounds (auscultation) for bilateral air entry.

Feel for:

- lung expansion;
- presence of secretions or surgical emphysema;
- chest percussion (Resuscitation Council UK, 2006).

RESPIRATORY RATE

Respiratory rate is measured over one minute and each count includes the rise and fall of the chest which equates to one breath (Dougherty and Lister, 2008). Opinion on normal values varies slightly but 12 to 20 breaths per minute is generally accepted as normal (Resuscitation Council UK, 2006). Tachypnoea is an early sign of respiratory distress and a deteriorating clinical condition (Table 2.5). Respiratory depth, pattern and sound such as wheezing, stridor, obstruction or coughing should also be documented (Woodrow, 2005). Cheyne Stokes respiration describes an irregular breathing pattern interrupted by periods of apnoea and is associated with brain stem ischaemia and end of life (Kennedy, 2007). Deep, rapid respirations or Kussmaul's breathing (air hunger) is associated with metabolic acidosis (Jevon and Ewens, 2007) caused by sepsis, uraemia or diabetic ketoacidosis (see Chapter 9). A period of tachypnoea followed by a slower rate of less than 12 breaths per minute may be a sign of impending respiratory arrest that could be misconstrued as an improvement when in fact the reverse could be true. Normal breathing should be effortless whereas the use of accessory muscles, seen in the shoulders and neck, will give the appearance of difficult and laboured breathing (dyspnoea). A bluish tinge to the skin and mucous membranes combined with clammy skin may indicate hypoxia.

It is important to check the central position of the trachea in the suprasternal notch as deviation to one side suggests mediastinal shift and requires urgent intervention (Resuscitation Council UK, 2006). A chest X-ray will provide detailed anatomical information such as the presence of a pneumothorax, pleural fluid, pulmonary oedema, infection or lung fibrosis.

Table 2.5 Glossary of respiratory terms

- Tachypnoea: a respiratory rate above 20
- Bradypnoea: a respiratory rate below 12
- Apnoea: an absence of respiration
- Cyanosis: a bluish discolouration of the skin and mucous membranes caused by lack of oxygen in the blood
- Hypoxia: inadequate oxygen supply is available to the tissues
- Dyspnoea: laboured difficult breathing
- Hypoxaemia: reduced arterial blood oxygen ($PaO_2 < 8$ kPa). Can be with or without increased arterial carbon dioxide.
- Hypercapnia: increased arterial carbon dioxide ($PaCO_2 > 6$ kPa)

Source: Marieb (2009).

OXYGEN SATURATION

During respiration oxygen crosses the alveolar capillary interface of the lungs and enters the circulation. Up to four oxygen atoms can attach to the haemoglobin of each red blood cell, forming oxyhaemoglobin, which is then transported to the tissues in the blood stream. The percentage of haemoglobin saturated with oxygen is known as the oxygen saturation (SaO_2) (Booker, 2008). Arterial blood gas saturations (SaO_2) are very similar to peripheral (capillary) saturation (SpO_2) and so differences are considered insignificant for practice (Woodrow, 2006). Pulse oximetry is an inexpensive and non-invasive method of continuous measurement of arterial oxygen saturation (Jevon and Ewens, 2007). A pulse oximeter consists of a peripheral probe, attached to a patient's finger, and a processing unit, which measures SpO_2 by calculating the amount of haemoglobin saturated with oxygen (Cooper et al., 2006). The relationship between SaO_2 and the partial pressure of oxygen in the arterial system (PaO_2) is shown by the S shaped haemoglobin oxygen dissociation curve (Figure 2.1).

A saturation of 93 per cent equates approximately to a PaO_2 of 8 kPa. Figure 2.1 demonstrates that as the saturation falls below 90 per cent the PaO_2 falls rapidly below 8 kPa following the steep decline of the S shaped curve. The body at this point would become critically short of oxygen with severe hypoxaemia. Conversely, at normal levels of PaO_2 (11 to 13 kPa) the SaO_2 will be above 95 per cent. As the curve flattens an increase in SaO_2 has very little effect upon PaO_2. Recent national guidelines suggest aiming for an SpO_2 of 94 to 98 per cent or 88 to 92 per cent in patients with type 2

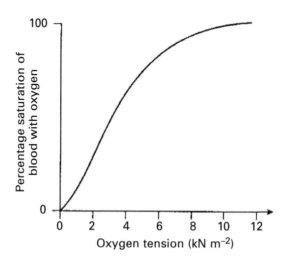

Figure 2.1   The oxygen dissociation curve.

Table 2.6 Treatment of breathing problems

- Open airway
- Position patient appropriately
- Administer oxygen (BTS 2008 Guidelines)
- Get expert help
- Treat underlying cause
- Support breathing if inadequate i.e. pocket mask ventilation or bag-valve and mask

---

Source: Resuscitation Council UK (2006).

respiratory failure (see Chapter 6) until blood gas results are available (British Thoracic Society, 2008). Pulse oximetry is extremely useful but care must be taken to ensure an accurate reading. A regular waveform trace should correspond to pulse rate to ensure accuracy (Jevon and Ewens, 2007). The probe should be positioned in an area that is warm and well perfused with blood and it should be repositioned regularly to avoid pressure sore development. Dark nail polish may interfere with the signal, causing inaccuracy (Booker, 2008) and anaemia can lead to an underestimate of oxygen saturation. A haemoglobin (Hb) level of 8.0 g/dL can underestimate SaO_2 by 10 to 15 per cent (Cooper et al., 2006) and pulse oximetry is not reliable if carbon monoxide poisoning is suspected (Woodrow, 2006). A pulse oximeter is not a replacement for observation of the patient and should be interpreted alongside other vital signs and clinical signs and symptoms. It is very important to be aware that SpO_2 is only a measure of oxygenation and not ventilation (Jevon and Ewens, 2007). It provides no information regarding arterial carbon dioxide tensions ($PaCO_2$) or abnormalities such as carbon dioxide retention or blood pH; arterial blood gas (ABG) analysis provides more detailed information. The blood pH must be maintained between 7.35 and 7.45 for the cells of the body to function effectively (Marieb, 2009). A rise in arterial carbon dioxide levels above the normal range (4.6 to 6.0 kPa) will cause the blood pH to fall below 7.35 causing a respiratory acidosis in the absence of metabolic compensation (Resusitation Council UK, 2006) (see Chapters 3 and 6).

PATIENT POSITIONING

Patient positioning will depend upon the clinical presentation. If a patient is conscious and struggling to breathe, sitting upright is the optimal position for lung expansion. If, however, they have an altered consciousness level and are unable to maintain an open airway, a supine position is required to facilitate airway management and breathing support. The patient can be managed in the lateral position when stabilised. Expert help will be required during the assessment of breathing to establish the underlying cause of compromise, and life threatening conditions must be diagnosed and treated immediately: for example, acute severe asthma, tension pneumothorax and pulmonary oedema (Resuscitation Council UK, 2006).

C: Circulation

Circulatory assessment includes a general observation of the patient while recording a number of vital signs. Table 2.7 lists some of the common causes of cardiovascular compromise; however, almost all pathophysiological organ dysfunction will manifest in changes to circulatory status. The look, listen and feel approach can also be used.

- Look at the patient – peripheries may be pale or cyanosed.
- Feel the pulse for rate, rhythm and depth.
- Assess peripheral perfusion – capillary refill time.
- Assess the state of the veins – collapsed could be a sign of hypovolaemia.
- Measure blood pressure.
- Assess organ perfusion – urine output, chest pain, consciousness level (AVPU).
- Perform an ECG.
- Look for haemorrhage or fluid loss
  (Resuscitation Council UK, 2006).

HEART RATE

The expansion and recoil of an artery that occurs with each beat of the left ventricle creates a wave of pressure that travels through the arterial system. This pressure wave can be palpated when an artery passes over a bone as the pulse. In a healthy individual heart rate will equate to pulse rate (Marieb, 2009). The normal range is generally regarded to be 60 to 100 beats per minute, though the average heart rate is slightly faster in adult females (72 to 80 beats per minute) than in males (64 to 72 beats per minute) (Marieb, 2009). Common causes of abnormal heart rate are listed in Table 2.9.

Table 2.7   Common causes of cardiovascular compromise

- Acute coronary syndromes
- Heart failure
- Cardiac arrhythmias
- Shock (hypovolaemic, septic, cardiogenic, neurogenic, anaphylactic)
- Pulmonary embolism

Table 2.8 Glossary of cardiovascular terms

- Tachycardia: An excessive heart rate above 100 beats per minute
- Bradycardia: A slow heart beat below 60 beats per minute
- Normotensive: a blood pressure that is within a normal range 100/60–140/90 mmHg
- Hypotension: generally considered to be a systolic blood pressure below 100 mmHg (potential causes are physiological shock, acute coronary syndromes, heart failure)
- Hypertension: a condition of sustained elevated arterial pressure of 140/90 mmHg or higher

---

Source: Marieb (2009).

Table 2.9 Common causes of abnormal heart rate

Increased rate	*Decreased rate*
• Exercise • Pain, anxiety • Pyrexia • Cardiac arrhythmia • Compensatory response to low BP, e.g. myocardial infarction, left ventricular failure, hypovolaemia • Chronotropic drugs, e.g. atropine®, isoprenaline® • Inotropic drugs, e.g. dobutamine®	• Increased vagal activity, e.g. carotid sinus massage • Athletic heart • Cardiac conduction defects • Raised intracranial pressure • Drugs: beta blockers, e.g. atenolol®; calcium channel blockers, e.g. verapamil®

When assessing the pulse it is also important to assess rhythm and amplitude (Dougherty and Lister, 2008). The pause between pulsations provides information about the heart rhythm, which should be smooth and regular. An irregular heart rate could have many causes such as ectopic (extra) beats, atrial fibrillation (AF) or conduction defects, and should be reported immediately. Application of a sound knowledge base to practice is an essential part of assessment if relevant clinical signs and symptoms are to be synthesised and communicated. The amplitude reflects the pulse strength and elasticity of the arterial wall. A pulse may be 'weak', 'strong', 'faint' or 'bounding' (Dougherty and Lister, 2008); however, assessment of amplitude is by its nature reliant upon a degree of subjectivity and there-fore tends to be reported by more experienced nurses or physicians. Both peripheral and central pulses should be assessed for rate, rhythm and amplitude. A bounding pulse may indicate sepsis and a barely palpable central pulse can be caused by low cardiac output (Resuscitation Council UK, 2006). Amplitude and rhythm are rarely detected by any electronic monitoring device, so a pulse must be palpated manually for accurate assessment, usually using the radial artery for convenience and counted over one minute. The sole reliance in some clinical areas upon electronic monitoring devices may be detrimental to the assessment process and lead to some inaccuracies or incomplete data collection, and could also deskill healthcare professionals.

SYSTOLIC BLOOD PRESSURE

Blood pressure (BP) is the pressure exerted by the blood against the inner walls of arteries and is responsible for maintaining blood circulation between heartbeats. It is directly related to cardiac output (CO) (amount of blood ejected from the left ventricle in one minute) and systemic vascular resistance (SVR) (the diameter of the vessel) (Marieb, 2009):

$$BP = CO \times SVR$$

Arterial blood pressure has two measurements. Systolic pressure is the pressure in the arteries at the peak of left ventricular (LV) contraction and diastolic pressure is the pressure exerted when the ventricles relax. Blood pressure is usually expressed in terms of millimetres of mercury (mmHg). In a normal adult at rest systolic blood pressure varies between 110 and 140 mmHg but blood pressure varies with age, weight, race, mood and physical activity (Marieb, 2009). In track and trigger systems, a comparable numerical figure is required, which is usually the systolic pressure as it is regarded as a more reliable marker of health status than diastolic pressure. Diastolic pressure usually varies in a normal adult at rest between 60 and 90 mmHg. BP may initially be recorded within normal limits despite underlying pathophysiological abnormality as it is maintained by stimulation of a number of compensatory mechanisms and increased peripheral resistance in response to an initial fall in BP (see Chapter 3). However, the pulse pressure may be narrowed (the difference between systolic and diastolic pressure, normally 35 to 45 mmHg). Other signs of poor cardiac output, such as altered consciousness level and oliguria (urine volume less than 0.5 mL/kg/hour), should also be noted (Resuscitation Council UK, 2006). An increase in BP may be associated with anxiety or pain associated with the situation or may indicate underlying hypertension. The cause of essential (primary) hypertension is multifactorial, often associated with lifestyle characteristics such as obesity, physical inactivity, high salt intake and stress; it can also be hereditary. Secondary hypertension is associated with anatomical or pathophysiological disorders: for example, raised intracranial pressure (ICP), renal, adrenal or aortic disease. Many conditions may cause low BP, such as myocardial dysfunction, low ICP, antihypertensive medication or hypovolaemia. Low BP caused by haemorrhage is not always immediately obvious. External bleeding may be visible from wounds and drains, but internal haemorrhage is less visible but is often characterised by localised pain and swelling. There are manual, electronic and invasive methods of recording blood pressure but the most reliable and accurate method is often regarded as the manual technique, so it is an essential skill for all healthcare professionals assessing acutely ill patients.

MEAN ARTERIAL PRESSURE

In the critical care environment mean arterial pressure is often used as a marker of clinical status but this is more difficult to calculate as it requires an intra-arterial catheter or a mathematical calculation (Dougherty and Lister, 2008):

$$\text{Mean arterial pressure (MAP)} = 1/3 \text{ systolic pressure} + 2/3 \text{ diastolic pressure}$$

CAPILLARY REFILL TIME

Peripheries are often pale and cool in cardiovascular compromise and capillary refill time (CRT) can be prolonged. CRT can be measured by applying pressure to a fingertip held at heart level for five seconds to cause blanching (loss of colour). CRT is measured as the time it takes to return to normal colour. A CRT greater than two seconds is considered abnormal although older age and low environmental temperature can have the same effect (Resuscitation Council UK, 2006). CRT may also be misleading in pyrexial septic patients due to an inflammatory response causing peripheral vasodilation, characterised by very warm peripheries. Pale, cool peripheries can be due to poor perfusion caused by arterial vasoconstriction, suggestive of hypovolaemic shock or cardiac failure.

In almost all medical and surgical emergencies, until proven otherwise, hypovolaemia should be considered as the primary cause of shock. Unless a cardiac problem is suspected intravenous fluids should be given to any patients with cool peripheries and tachycardia (Table 2.10). Important additional evaluation of haematological, biochemical, coagulation and microbiological investigations and crossmatching should aid diagnosis if haemorrhage is suspected. A fluid challenge of 500 ml of warmed intravenous crystalloid for a normotensive patient, or one litre if the patient is hypotensive, can be prescribed by a suitably qualified health professional (Resuscitation Council UK, 2006). Some clinicians may prefer to give colloid (see Chapter 3). The heart rate and blood pressure should be checked every

Table 2.10 Treatment of circulatory problems

- Seek expert help
- Treat cause if known (cardiac tamponade, haemorrhage, shock)
- IV Access – take bloods
- Give fluid challenge
- Reassess and monitor
- Treat acute coronary syndromes (see Chapter 5)

---

five minutes during the acute stage of intervention to prevent fluid overload and cardiac failure (Resusciation Council UK, 2006). A raised jugular venous pressure (JVP) or central venous pressure (CVP) (right atrial pressure, measurable if a central line is present) could indicate fluid overload and inotropes or vasopressors may be prescribed (see Chapter 3).

D: Disability

Assessment to establish the cause of an altered state of consciousness is imperative.

LEVEL OF CONSCIOUSNESS

A reduced consciousness level is associated with potentially life threatening complications, including airway obstruction, hypoxaemia and aspiration (Cooper et al., 2006) and so is a very important element of the assessment process. AVPU is a rapid method of neurological assessment and is particularly useful in an emergency situation where speed is required (Resuscitation Council UK, 2006).

AVPU stands for:

- Alert;
- Responsive to verbal stimuli;
- Responsive to painful stimuli;
- Unresponsive.

A normal level of consciousness would include an alert patient and one who could respond to verbal stimuli from a state of sleep. A patient who requires painful stimuli to achieve a response (see Chapter 4) or who is unresponsive would be classed as having an altered level of consciousness (Table 2.11). If greater depth of neurological assessment is required the Glasgow Coma Score provides a numerical score and so a more quantifiable and comparable figure (see Chapter 4). If a patient is alert then their airway will be patent but if they present with an altered level of consciousness then their airway

Table 2.11 Common causes of neurological compromise

- Hypoxia
- Poor cerebral perfusion
- Cerebral pathology (disease or injury)
- Drugs (opiates, sedatives) and alcohol
- Hypercapnia
- Hypoglycaemia or hyperglycaemia
- Uraemia
- Hypovolaemia
- Cardiac arrhythmia
- Peri/post cardiac arrest

may be compromised and so it is essential that assessment returns to ABC to establish if the situation is a medical emergency.

Examine and assess:

- review and treat ABCs (treat hypoxia and hypotension);
- assess consciousness using AVPU and/or GCS (and check pupil, size, equality and reaction to light);
- check drug chart (naloxone® can be given for opioid toxicity);
- measure blood glucose (exclude hypoglycaemia: if less than 3 mmol, give 50 ml of 10 per cent glucose IV) or diabetic ketoacidosis (see Chapter 9);
- nurse unconscious patients in the lateral position if possible (Resuscitation Council UK, 2006).

E: Exposure

Full exposure of the patient's body may be required to gain a complete clinical picture, maintaining privacy and dignity and preventing heat loss. An initial examination can exclude any obvious external haemorrhage and note any skin rash, redness or oedema.

- Take a full clinical history.
- Review the case notes and charts.
- Note vital sign trends.
- Give prescribed medications.
- Review the results of investigations (laboratory and radiological).
- Consider the level of care required by the patient (i.e. ward, HDU or ICU) (Table 1.2).
- Record in the patient notes details of assessment, treatment and response to therapy (Resuscitation Council UK, 2006).

TEMPERATURE

In a healthy individual core body temperature is relatively constant, with a normal range of 35 to 37 °C (Woodrow, 2006), though opinion varies and 37.5 °C is accepted by some physicians as the upper end of the normal range. Higgins (2008) defines pyrexia as a temperature above 37.5 °C and hypothermia as a temperature below 35.0 °C (Table 2.12). A temperature above 41 °C (hyperpyrexia) is dangerous and may cause convulsions and be fatal (Table 2.13). A temperature below 32 °C is similarly dangerous and can cause cardiac arrythmias (Woodrow, 2005). Through autonomic nervous system pathways the hypothalamus regulates body temperature. In a pyrexial illness macrophages, white blood cells and injured tissue cells release pyrogens that act directly on the hypothalamus, altering the internal thermostat to a higher temperature. The body initiates heat conserving mechanisms, vasoconstriction redirects blood away from the skin surface preventing heat loss from radiation and convection, and shivering creates heat (Marieb, 2009).

A patient who is pale, shivering and complaining of the cold may well have a high temperature. Once the thermostat is reset due to the administration of medication or an improvement in the clinical condition, the patient will begin to sweat and the skin may appear flushed. A fever can actually speed up the healing process and inhibit bacterial growth by

Table 2.12   Glossary of temperature terms

Pyrexia	Temperature above 37.5 °C
Febrile	Temperature above 37.5 °C
Apyrexial	Temperature between 36–37.5 °C
Afebrile	Temperature between 36–37.5 °C
Hypothermia	Temperature below 35 °C

Source: Marieb 2009.

Table 2.13   Causes of hypothermia and hyperthermia

Causes of hypothermia	*Causes of hyperthermia (pyrexia)*
• Exposure	• Infection (commonly)
• Metabolic derangement	• Central nervous system problem
• Medication	• Systemic inflammatory response
• Alcohol	syndrome (Sirs)
• Septic shock	• Medication

Source: adapted from Higgins (2008).

increasing the metabolic rate; however, if the thermostat is set too high body proteins may be denatured and permanent brain damage can occur (Marieb, 2009). When devising a management plan for a pyrexial patient it is important to consider the comfort of the patient, the dangers associated with an elevated temperature and the protective nature of fever.

Body temperature can be recorded orally, per axilla, rectally, via the ear canal (tympanic) or via a skin probe. There are a wide range of thermometers available and the choice will depend upon the availability of the equipment and the condition of the patient, though oral and tympanic thermometers are commonly used. If a patient is to have an oral reading taken they must not have had a hot or cold drink or smoked in the 15 minutes prior to assessment in order to ascertain accurate data (Trim, 2007). As with any equipment, training and competency will be required before use and with any multi-use equipment it should be clean in line with infection control policies.

Oxygen consumption will be elevated in a pyrexial patient so SpO_2 will often decrease as temperature rises. A pyrexia will shift the oxygen dissociation curve to the right (Figure 2.1) so the affinity of haemoglobin for oxygen decreases, causing unloading of oxygen at the tissues and increased tissue oxygenation. Conversely, hypothermia shifts the curve to the left and the haemoglobin affinity for oxygen increases (Woodrow, 2006). An increase in body temperature will have a marked effect upon other vital signs. Heart rate and respiratory rate will rise as the metabolic rate increases, so as with all vital sign interpretation assessment must be comprehensive to be accurate.

Additional Assessment Data

In addition to the physiological observations required NICE (2007) suggests monitoring:

- biochemistry (Table 2.14);
- haematology (Table 2.15);
- arterial blood gases (ABGs) (see Chapter 3, Table 3.5);
- microbiology if infection is suspected;
- liver function tests (LFT) (see Chapter 10, Table 10.3);
- hourly urine output;
- pain.

Nurses are often responsible for accepting blood and urine results so it is essential to have a good working knowledge of 'normal values'.

Table 2.14 Blood biochemistry normal values (mmol/L)

Urea and electrolytes (U&E)	
Sodium (Na⁺)	135–145
Potassium (K⁺)	3.5–5.0
Chloride (Cl)	95–105
Urea	2.2–7.7
Creatinine	50–120
Bicarbonate (HCO_3)	22–32
Glucose	3.0–5.0
Calcium	2.1–2.6
Magnesium	0.7–1
Cholesterol	3.0–5.0
Triglyceride	0.0–2.3

Note: Normal values differ between men and women and local laboratory test procedures.

Table 2.15 Haematology normal values

Full blood count (FBC)	
Haemaglobin (Hb)	11.5–16 g/dL
Mean cell volume (MCV)	70–100 fL
Red blood cells (RBC)	$3.7–5.5 \times 10^{12}$/L
White blood cells (WBC)	$4–11 \times 10^9$/L
Platelets	$130–400 \times 10^9$/L
Clotting	
Prothrombin time (PT)	12–16 seconds
International normalised ratio (INR)	1
Fibrinogen	1.5–4.0 g/L

Note: Normal values differ between men and women and local laboratory test procedures.

Hourly Urine Output

A fluid balance chart collated over a 24-hour period will provide valuable information regarding a patient's fluid status. In health, intake will largely equal output, with a degree of insensible loss. The amount of urine produced will depend upon intake but a healthy individual can be expected to produce 1 ml/kg/hr (Scales and Pilsworth, 2008). A urine output of less than 30 ml/hr in an adult patient suggests the kidneys are underperfused and requires further investigation and intervention (see Chapter 7). Fluid resuscitation for hypovolaemia should result in a positive fluid balance over 24 hours, whereas diuretic or renal therapy should culminate in a negative balance.

Pain

Pain assessment and control is required to ensure patient comfort and a variety of pain assessment tools exist to aid this process. The choice of tool will depend upon patient presentation. There are also important physiological reasons for good pain control as the effects of severe pain include:

- tachycardia, hypertension and increased myocardial oxygen demand;
- nausea and vomiting;
- inadequate lung expansion and inability to cough – basal atelectasis and chest infections;
- urinary retention;
- thromboembolism due to inactivity;
- pressure sores due to immobility
  (adapted from Cooper et al., 2006).

Physiological Track and Trigger Systems

Physiological track and trigger systems should be used to monitor all patients in acute hospitals (NCEPOD, 2005; NICE, 2007). Track and trigger systems are also known as early warning scoring systems (EWSS). They emerged from the review of adult critical care services (DH, 2000) and were designed to recognise early signs of deterioration in level 0 and 1 patients (Oakey and Slade, 2006). There are a wide variety of systems in use but they all rely on observation of selected basic physiological signs (tracking) with predetermined calling criteria (triggers) for requesting the attendance of staff who have competencies in the management of acute illness (NICE, 2007). Figure 2.2 shows an example of an adult modified early warning scoring (MEWS) system. It aims to help both nursing and medical staff to identify patients who are acutely ill or at risk of deterioration. The tracking signs are heart rate, systolic blood pressure, respiratory rate, oxygen saturations, respiratory support, urine output in four hours and AVPU, relating to conscious level. Each tracking sign receives a score depending upon patient presentation and scores are added together to provide a final score. The final MEWS score triggers a response, shown in Figure 2.2. A low MEWS score (0 to 1) suggests the patient is stable and at low risk of deterioration, which is reflected by the trigger response for 12-hourly observations in line with NICE guidelines (NICE, 2007). A high MEWS of 5 or above suggests immediate registrar review, hourly observations for at least six hours, strict fluid balance, consultant discussion and outreach involvement.

Score	3	2	1	0	1	2	3
Heart Rate		<40	40 - 50	51 – 100	101-110	111-130	>130
Systolic BP	<70	71 – 80	81 - 100	101 - 179	180 - 199	200-220	>220
Resp Rate		<8	8-11	12 - 20	21 - 25	26-30	>30
Oxygen Saturations	<85%	85-89%	90-94%	>94%			
Respiratory Support	BIPAP/ CPAP	Hi-Flow Non-re-breathe mask	Oxygen Therapy				
Urine Output in Last 4 Hrs/mls	<80	80-119	120-200 Dialysis	201-799 New admission	>800		
AVPU			New Confusion	Alert and responsive	Responds to Voice	Responds to Pain	Unresponsive

Figure 2.2   Adult modified early warning scoring (MEWS) system.
Source: Critical Care Outreach Team at Leeds Teaching Hospitals Trust (2010).

The NICE (2007) guideline suggests that the frequency of monitoring should increase if abnormal physiology is detected. Track and trigger systems are objective and provide direct guidance to clinical staff when faced with an acutely ill patient, and anecdotal evidence suggests they are generally regarded as useful tools. However, there is little evaluative evidence to suggest that early warning score systems actually improve

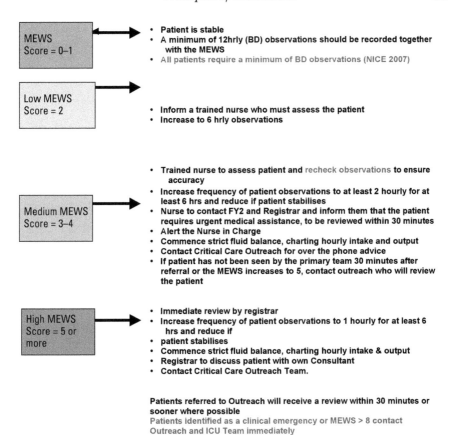

Figure 2.2   *continued*

clinical outcome and so more high quality research is recommended (McGaughey et al., 2008).

Assessment and Communication

Good communication skills are essential to high quality nursing care and nurses are required to develop their use of appropriate communication and interpersonal skills in order to achieve therapeutic relationships with patients (NMC, 2008). Some nurses, however, find communicating with other health professionals more difficult than communicating with patients. This can have a negative effect on the assessment process. The use of ABCDE and track and trigger systems relies upon communication with team members who have specific expertise. Cooper et al. (2006) suggest that a good attitude, focused communication, teamwork and situation awareness are as important as a good management plan when managing an acutely ill patient. A simple structure is suggested when communicating concerns to a colleague:

1. State where you are and your request.
2. Give a brief history.
3. Describe the vital signs. (These may include consciousness level, pulse, blood pressure, respiratory rate, oxygen therapy and saturations and urine output if appropriate.)

Providing a summary of deranged vital signs is the fastest way of communicating a deteriorating clinical condition. A high MEWS score is effectively a summary of deranged vital signs that triggers a required response.

Summary

Inadequate monitoring of basic vital signs and an inability to act upon documented abnormal results are, it seems, not uncommon in clinical practice (NPSA, 2007). Hypoxaemia with increased respiratory rate and hypotension leading to hypoperfusion, metabolic acidosis and tissue hypoxia are the most common abnormalities prior to cardiac arrest (Cooper et al., 2006). If undetected and untreated a patient will rapidly and often irretrievably deteriorate. In order to prevent this it is crucial for front line nursing staff in all clinical settings to have good assessment skills, the ability to accurately record, interpret and document vital signs and prioritise assessment, intervention and care. Knowledge and understanding of normal and abnormal physiology is essential for prompt recognition and interpretation of data collected. A structured, systematic approach based on Airway, Breathing, Circulation, Disability and Exposure (ABCDE), as recommended by the Resuscitation Council UK (2006), will ensure that assessment is prioritised and any abnormalities are responded to before moving on to the next stage, and track and trigger systems can provide guidance and direction for less experienced healthcare staff. Lastly, effective communication and collaborative team working are more likely to result in successful clinical outcomes.

Useful Websites

ALERT (Acute Life-threatening Events Recognition and Treatment) is a multi-professional acute care course: http://web.port.ac.uk/alert/intro.htm

Useful Websites *continued*

British Thoracic Society: http://www.brit-thoracic.org.uk

Cochrane Collaboration: http://www.cochrane.org

Resuscitation Council UK: http://www.resus.org.uk. Information regarding the ALS (Advanced Life Support) and ILS (Intermediate Life Support) courses is available

The National Patient Safety Agency (UK): http://www.npsa.nhs.uk

References

Booker, R. 'Pulse Oximetry', *Nursing Standard*, **22**(30) (2008), 39–41.

British Thoracic Society. *Guideline for Emergency Oxygen Use in Adult Patients: Executive Summary* (London: British Thoracic Society, 2008). Available from www.brit-thoracic.org.uk (accessed 8 January 2009).

Cooper, N., K. Forrest and P. Cramp. *Essential Guide to Acute Care*, 2nd edn (Oxford: Blackwell, 2006).

Department of Health. *Comprehensive Critical Care: A Review of Adult Critical Care Services* (London: The Stationery Office, 2000).

Department of Health. *Competencies for Recognising and Responding to Acutely Ill Patients in Hospital* (London: The Stationery Office, 2008). Available from www.dh.gov.uk/en/consultations/closedconsultations/DH_083630 (accessed 8 December 2008).

Dougherty, L. and S. Lister. *The Royal Marsden Manual of Clinical Nursing Procedures*, 7th student edn (Oxford: Wiley-Blackwell, 2008).

Goldhill, D. R., L. Worthington, A. Mulcahy, M. Tarling and A. Sumner. 'The Patient at Risk Team: Identifying and Managing Seriously Ill Patients', *Anaesthesia*, **54** (1999), 853–60.

Higgins, D. 'Patient Assessment: Part 2 – Measuring Oral Temperature', *Nursing Times*, **104**(8) (2008). Available from http://www.nursingtimes.net (accessed 8 December 2008).

Kennedy, S. 'Detecting Changes in the Respiratory Status of Ward Patients', *Nursing Standard*, **21**(49) (2007), 42–6.

Jevon, P. and B. Ewens. *Monitoring the Critically Ill Patient*, 2nd edn (Oxford: Blackwell, 2007).

McGaughey, J., F. Alderdice, R. Fowler, A. Kapila, A. Mayhew and M. Moutray. *The Cochrane Database of Systematic Reviews. Outreach and Early Warning Systems (EWS) for the Prevention of Intensive Care Admission and Death of Critically Ill Adult Patients on General Hospital Wards* (2008). Available from http://0-ovidsp.uk.ovid.com.wam.leeds.ac.uk/spa/ovidweb.cgi?&S=CDEAPDBEPDH (accessed 21 November 2008).

Marieb, E. N. *Essentials of Human Anatomy and Physiology*, 9th edn (San Francisco: Pearson Benjamin Cummings, 2009).

National Confidential Enquiry into Patient Outcome and Death. *An Acute Problem?* (London: National Confidential Enquiry into Patient Outcome and Death, 2005).

National Institute for Health and Clinical Excellence. *Acutely Ill Patients in Hospital: Recognition of and Response to Acute Illness in Adults in Hospital. Clinical Guideline 50* (London: NICE, 2007).

National Patient Safety Agency. *Safer Care for the Acutely Ill Patient: Learning from Serious Incidents* (London: NPSA, 2007).

Nursing Midwifery Council. *The Code: Standards of Conduct, Performance and Ethics for Nurses and Midwives* (London: Nursing Midwifery Council, 2008).

Oakey, R, J. and V. Slade. 'Physiological observation track and trigger system', *Nursing Standard*, **20**(27) (2006), 48–54.

Redmond, A. and M. McDevitt. 'Acute Renal Failure: Recognition and Treatment in Ward Patients', *Nursing Standard*, **18**(22) (2004), 46–53.

Resuscitation Council (UK). *Advanced Life Support*, 5th edn (London: Resuscitation Council, 2006).

Scales, K. and J. Pilsworth. 'The Importance of Fluid Balance in Clinical Practice', *Nursing Standard*, **22**(47) (2008), 50–7.

Trim, J. 'Monitoring Temperature', *Nursing Times*, **101**(20) (2007), 30–1. Available from http://www.nursingtimes.net/ntclinical/monitoring-temperature.html (accessed 16 March 2009).

Woodrow, P. 'Practice Update: Clinical Skills with Older People. Recognising Acute Deterioration', *Nursing Older People*, **17**(5) (2005), 31–2.

Woodrow, P. *Intensive Care Nursing*, 2nd edn (Abingdon: Routledge, 2006).

3

Shock Presentation

Ian Goulden

Introduction

Shock is never a primary diagnosis but is a physiological consequence of a range of pathophysiological problems. It can be broadly classified into cardiogenic, neurogenic, anaphylactic, septic or hypovolaemic shock. Regardless of the underlying cause of shock, without prompt assessment and intervention it will almost certainly lead to death. Yet shock is a common presentation and it is therefore crucial that nurses understand the causes, physiological responses, assessment strategies and management priorities in order to provide optimum care for the patient.

Aim and Learning Outcomes

The Aim

The aim of this chapter is to outline the various classifications of shock and to explore by use of a case study the priorities of early accurate assessment and management of the individual presenting with hypovolaemic shock.

Learning Outcomes

At the end of this chapter the reader will be able to:

- Describe the main causes of shock.
- Identify and explain the pathophysiological basis of the presenting signs and symptoms observed in the patient with shock.
- Prioritise the immediate assessment, specific monitoring and key investigations required to enable an accurate and timely diagnosis.

- Outline the main aspects in the management of the patient with shock.
- Recognise indicators of patient deterioration.

The Definition of Shock

Fundamental Physiological Concepts

Body cells require an adequate supply of oxygen (O_2) to enable them to produce energy from food fuels and to function correctly. This is known as aerobic metabolism. The cardiovascular and respiratory systems work together to transport oxygen from the environment to the cells. Inspired oxygen in the lungs is transported into the blood stream at the alveolar capillary membrane, where it binds to haemoglobin for circulation around the body to the tissues. On arrival at the cells haemoglobin releases the oxygen, which enters the cells by a process of diffusion, i.e. from an area of high concentration to an area of lower concentration. Adequate perfusion of body cells is therefore dependent upon:

1. Efficient respiration – inspiration of oxygen and expiration of carbon dioxide.
2. An efficient cardiac pump to maintain cardiac output (Table 3.1).
3. Adequate blood pressure (Table 3.2).
4. A vascular system that transports oxygenated blood from the left heart via arteries to the tissues, permits release of O_2 from capillaries to

Table 3.1   Determinants of cardiac output (CO)

- Cardiac output = heart rate × stroke volume (normal range 4–8 L/min)
- Average CO at rest = 75 × 70 ml = 5.25 L/min
- Heart rate (Hr) is influenced by the autonomic nervous system:
  - Sympathetic nervous stimulation = increased heart rate, atrioventricular (AV) conduction and myocardial contractility
  - Parasympathetic nervous stimulation = decreased heart rate and atrioventricular conduction (no effect upon myocardial contractility)
- Stoke volume (SV) is influenced by:
  - Preload = the volume of blood in the ventricle at the end of diastole (filling)
  - Afterload = the resistance against which the ventricle must eject blood volume (equates to blood pressure)
  - Contractility = myocardial contractile strength to enable complete ventricular emptying
  - Distensibility = myocardial relaxation to enable complete ventricular filling

Table 3.2 Determinants of systemic blood pressure (BP)

- Blood pressure is defined as the force which the blood exerts on the walls of the vessels in which it is contained. It is composed of systole and diastole. Systolic pressure reflects the force of ventricular contraction, degree of systemic vascular resistance and compliance of the arteries. Diastolic pressure reflects the velocity of run-off of blood from the aorta, the elasticity of the arterial walls and the degree of vasoconstriction.
- Blood pressure (BP) = cardiac output (CO) × systemic vascular resistance (SVR).
- Blood pressure is determined by:
  - cardiac output
  - circulating blood volume
  - systemic vascular resistance
  - venous return
  - elasticity of arterial walls
  - blood viscosity.

---

cells and returns deoxygenated blood via veins to the right heart and lungs.
5. Sufficient blood volume to fill the vascular system.
6. Cells that are able to use and extract oxygen from the blood.

When one or more of these factors is compromised there may be *inadequate oxygen delivery to the cells*. When oxygen delivery to the cells is reduced, they use a less effective energy production process known as anaerobic metabolism. Anaerobic metabolism does not rely upon oxygen for energy production but does result in a severe reduction in the level of energy produced within the cells and the formation of lactic acid as a metabolic waste product. An increase in cellular lactic acid leads to a fall in blood pH. This is potentially harmful to the cells and is known as metabolic acidosis.

Metabolic acidosis has a detrimental effect upon intracellular and cell membrane function. As cell function deteriorates, the cell membrane becomes more permeable and allows abnormal leakage of electrolytes and fluids in and out of the cells. If this process is not rapidly reversed, cell structures are damaged and cell necrosis will ensue, leading to potential organ failure. Failure of organ systems increases the likelihood of death.

The Classification of Shock

Shock is the term used to describe a 'clinical syndrome characterised by inadequate tissue perfusion that results in impaired cellular metabolism' (McKinley, 2005). Shock is an unstable and dynamic state of great complexity. It is *never* a primary diagnosis, but is always a physiological adaptation to a

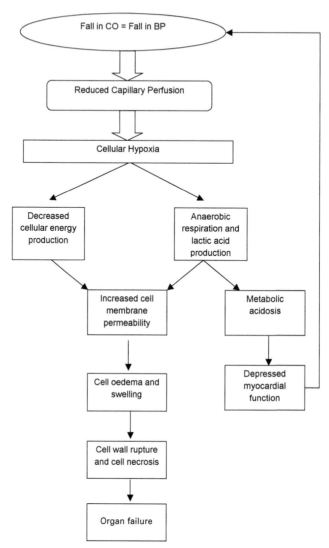

Figure 3.1   The hypoxic sequence in shock.

potentially life threatening situation. The most consistent clinical features in all forms of shock are a reduced BP, diminished capillary blood flow (hypoperfusion), widespread tissue hypoxia and abnormalities in cell metabolism (Figure 3.1).

The primary goal of resuscitation is to restore adequate tissue oxygen delivery, to treat the underlying pathology and to prevent further deterioration.

Although sharing much of the underlying physiology, shock has traditionally been classified according to its cause or to reflect the failing organ.

Cardiogenic Shock

Cardiogenic shock occurs when the heart's ability to pump effectively is impaired, causing cardiac output and blood pressure to fall.It may be caused by open heart surgery or trauma to the heart, but it is seen most commonly after a large myocardial infarction (MI). The prognosis for patients with cardiogenic shock is poor and it is the most common cause of death in patients hospitalised with an acute MI (Topalian et al., 2008). Treatment includes restoration of blood supply to the damaged myocardium and the use of drugs to support the damaged heart and circulation. New techniques to revascularise or restore blood flow to the heart muscle may improve survival rates (see Chapter 5).

Neurogenic Shock

The autonomic nervous system controls involuntary muscles within blood vessel walls that maintain the squeeze (vascular tone) so that the volume within the vessels stays constant even if the body changes position against gravity. Neurogenic shock results from a loss of vasomotor tone. It can occur following anaesthesia (both general and spinal), in patients with spinal cord injury, at times of profound emotional distress and in those with severe pain. Impulses from the sympathetic autonomic nervous system are lost, allowing unopposed parasympathetic activity. Massive vasodilatation results and the patient's blood pressure falls. This situation looks like hypovolaemic shock, although there is no absolute loss of blood volume. As a consequence of the unopposed parasympathetic activity, in contrast to other types of shock the heart rate may be slower than normal. Management includes treating the cause, fluid resuscitation and occasionally the use of drugs such as adrenaline (epinephrine) to increase vascular tone.

Anaphylactic Shock

This represents an exaggerated, violent and systemic allergic response to a drug or substance. Common triggers include bee and wasp stings, nuts, shellfish, eggs, latex and certain drugs such as penicillin. There is sudden profound vasodilatation, pooling of blood in the peripheries and increased capillary permeability. This is again a type of hypovolaemic shock, but in this case the loss of blood volume is real. An urticarial rash is common and there may be obvious oedema in the face. Bronchospasm may result in a pronounced wheeze and laryngeal oedema can obstruct the upper airway. Untreated severe anaphylaxis may be life threatening. Treatment is by airway management, fluid resuscitation and drugs such as adrenaline (epinephrine), antihistamines and steroids (for example, hydrocortisone).

Septic Shock

Septic shock results from an overwhelming infection commonly caused by gram negative organisms such as *E. coli*, *Proteus*, *Klebsiella* and *Pseudomonas*, although gram positive organisms and fungi are also implicated. There is widespread peripheral vasodilatation and increased capillary wall permeability. As with anaphylactic shock this is a subset of hypovolaemic shock and again the loss of blood volume is real. Septic shock is further compounded by sepsis-related depression of the myocardium and by a range of life threatening complications such as disseminated intravascular coagulation (DIC) and multiple organ dysfunction syndrome. Septic shock is fatal in nearly 50 per cent of cases and warrants admission to an intensive care unit. Treatment is based on support of organ perfusion with fluids and vasoactive agents while attempts are made to interrupt the septic cascade. The 'Sepsis Care Bundle' (June 2005) has guided doctors in the management of sepsis and septic shock (see http://www.library.nhs.uk/EMERGENCY/ViewResource.aspx?resID=269247 for further details). Since the observed pathophysiology seen in neurogenic, anaphylactic and septic shock states relates to abnormal fluid distribution they are often referred to by the collective term distributive shock.

Hypovolaemic Shock

In health, fluid intake and urine output are the most important mechanisms for regulating blood volume. Table 3.3 lists the pathological conditions that promote or reflect fluid loss and may lead to hypovolaemic shock. Hypovolaemic shock is the most common type of shock seen in practice.

It is characterised by diminished circulating volume such that there is inadequate filling of the blood vessels and the body's metabolic needs cannot be met. This loss can be either visible (external) or invisible (internal) and can result from actual blood loss due to haemorrhage or from the excessive loss of plasma or water (Table 3.3).

The degree of shock is determined not only by the volume of fluid lost,

Table 3.3   Pathological causes of fluid loss

- Haemorrahage: loss of whole blood, e.g. fractured femur, trauma injury
- Dehydration: fluid, e.g. excessive diaphoresis (sweating)
- Severe vomiting and diarrhoea
- Excessive urine output, e.g. diabetes mellitus, diabetes insipidus, diuretic overdose
- Burns injury: loss of plasma
- Sepsis

---

but also by the rate of loss. A loss of 10 per cent of normal blood volume can be tolerated without any significant effects if the rate of loss is controlled, such as in blood donation. Rapid loss of a lesser volume may result in significant symptoms and as haemorrhage may not always be immediately evident, the amount of blood loss after blunt trauma is often underestimated. A simple rib fracture can account for up to 125 mL, a closed fracture of the femur can result in loss of up to 2 litres of blood (40 per cent of circulating volume) and a pelvic fracture may cause the loss of 3 to 4 litres (60 to 80 per cent) of circulating blood volume. The abdominal cavity may contain a large amount of blood or fluid without any obvious distension. All causes of shock including hypovolaemia can lead to cardiac arrest and death, and therefore early accurate assessment, monitoring and diagnosis is imperative if appropriate management is to be instigated and death avoided. The acute assessment and management of hypovolaemic shock is the focus of the remainder of this chapter.

The Case Scenario: The Presenting Complaint

Billy is a 34-year-old, previously fit and well man who is brought to the accident and emergency department after feeling unwell while playing rugby. He is complaining of left sided upper quadrant abdominal pain and feels lightheaded. Billy is communicating with members of the healthcare team but he appears to be restless and a little confused. He is complaining of nausea, but has not vomited. His initial observations are:

Temperature: 36.5 °C
Heart rate: 105 beats per minute
BP: 110/70 mmHg
Respiratory rate: 16 breaths per minute

Billy's skin is cool to touch and clammy, and he looks pale.

Blood is taken for full blood count, urea and electrolytes, lactate, glucose, blood group cross match and save. A 12 lead ECG is performed. Billy has a 14 gauge cannula inserted and is commenced a 0.9 per cent sodium chloride IV infusion. Oxygen is administered at 40 per cent via face mask.

A provisional diagnosis of ruptured spleen is made. Doctors decide to manage the condition conservatively.

Consider the following:

1. With reference to his current observations, what might be your first impression?
2. What pathophysiological mechanisms might account for the vital signs recorded so far?
3. What would be your immediate assessment priorities?

The Compensatory Stage of Shock

Shock represents a severe disturbance in homeostasis and no matter what the cause the body will initially respond with the same compensatory mechanisms. In hypovolaemic shock, compensatory mechanisms come into play when the loss of circulating volume reaches 10 to 15 per cent (loss of about 750 mL). A reduction in blood volume causes a fall in venous return (preload), leading to a fall in stroke volume (SV), cardiac output (CO) and blood pressure (BP) (Tables 3.1 and 3.2):

$\downarrow SV \times HR = \downarrow CO$. This in turn leads to $\downarrow CO \times SVR = \downarrow BP$

Compensatory mechanisms are induced in an effort to increase stroke volume and cardiac output and so restore BP. In the elderly and in those with chronic disease compensatory mechanisms may be less effective, and in cardiogenic shock, as a consequence of damage to the myocardium, compensatory mechanisms are counterproductive and progression through the stages of shock is much more rapid.

The Compensatory Mechanisms

$$HR \times SV = CO$$

There is a direct relationship between heart rate, stroke volume and cardiac output whereby an increase in either heart rate or stroke volume will result in an increase in cardiac output and conversely a decrease in either of the factors will result in a fall in cardiac output. In the event of a sudden fall in SV, a compensatory increase in HR will normally occur in an effort to maintain CO. The increase in Billy's heart rate to 105 beats per minute may be evidence of this mechanism.

Sympathetic Nervous Activation

A fall in BP caused by fluid loss will be detected by sensory receptors to stretch, known as baroreceptors, located in the aortic arch and carotid sinus. The detection of a fall in sensory stretch will be transmitted to the medulla oblongata in the brain, which houses the cardiac vasomotor (acceleratory and inhibitory) centre. In response to the fall in BP the acceleratory centre will increase sympathetic nervous stimulation with the following consequences:

1. Noradrenaline (norepinephrine) release at the beta 1 (β_1) receptors located at the sinus node will stimulate a further increase in heart rate.

2. Noradrenaline release at the beta 1 (β_1) receptors located at the atrioventricular (AV) node will increase electrical impulse conduction from atria to ventricles.
3. Noradrenaline release at the beta 1 (β_1) receptors located within the myocardium will enhance the force of contraction.
4. Noradrenaline release at the beta 1 (β_1) receptors located within the arterial walls will cause arterial vasoconstriction and lead to an increase in BP.
5. Adrenaline (epinephrine) and noradrenaline (norepinephrine) release will cause selective vasoconstriction and a redistribution of blood flow. Blood is diverted away from less vital centres such as the gut, skin and kidneys to vital centres such as the brain, heart and lungs. This may explain why Billy looks pale and his skin is cool and clammy to touch. Reduced peripheral perfusion will increase capillary refill time beyond the normal two second period and diversion of blood flow away from the gut may explain Billy's feeling of nausea. Increased levels of circulating adrenaline are associated with a feeling of impending doom and this should be seen as a significant sign in patients expressing such thoughts (Sheppard and Wright, 2006). Catecholamines stimulate the liver's conversion of glycogen to glucose, resulting in hyperglycaemia.

Renin–Angiotensin–Aldosterone Activation

A fall in BP and subsequent selective vasoconstriction may reduce renal artery perfusion and glomerular filtration rate (GFR) to approximately 25 per

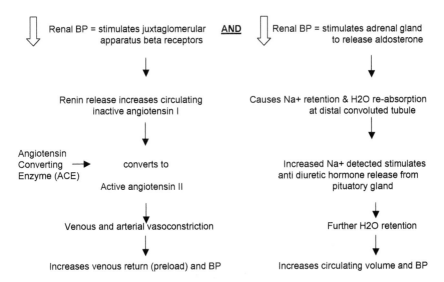

Figure 3.2   Renin–angiotensin–aldosterone release.

cent of the normal rate, causing a fall in diuresis. The kidneys are highly sensitive to a fall in renal perfusion pressure and will activate the renin–angiotensin–aldosterone compensatory mechanism (Figure 3.2).

Vasoconstriction and increased circulating volume may initially maintain Billy's blood pressure within the normal range. A satisfactory blood pressure may be maintained with as much as 1500 mL of blood loss (Sheppard and Wright, 2006) and clinicians may well not recognise the signs of shock until there is a dramatic fall in blood pressure (Tippins, 2005). Therefore monitoring of blood pressure alone in this early or compensatory stage may not be a good indicator of the patient's actual condition. Observations of heart rate, skin temperature, skin colour and capillary refill time are all essential additions to the monitoring regime. Billy may experience a small increase in respiratory rate as the body tries to increase the amount of oxygen in the blood and any reduction in blood flow to the brain may manifest as mild confusion.

The Case Scenario: Assessment and Diagnosis

Since admission two hours previously Billy appears to be becoming increasingly difficult to arouse and is less responsive to commands. A more recent set of observations reveals:

Temperature: 36.2 °C
Heart rate: 132 beats per minute
BP: 80/55 mmHg
Respiratory rate: 28 breaths per minute
SpO_2: 95 per cent
Billy has not passed urine since admission.
He is receiving oxygen 40% via a facemask.
Arterial blood gas (ABG) results are as follows:

- pH: 7.25
- PaO_2: 12.5 kPa
- $PaCO_2$: 4.8 kPa
- HCO_3: 20 mmol/L
- SaO_2: 96 per cent
- BE: −2

Immediate Assessment
1. What are the immediate assessment priorities in Billy's case and what is the rationale for each measure?
2. Identify the common characteristics that help to distinguish the different causes of shock.
3. What is the most likely cause of Billy's sudden deterioration?

The Progressive Stage of Shock

Once 30 to 40 per cent of the circulating blood volume has been lost the ability to compensate diminishes, leading to the progressive stage of shock. The blood pressure will fall, tissues become hypoxic and continued cellular anaerobic metabolism leads to a worsening metabolic acidosis. Metabolic acidosis leads to depression of myocardial function and then to vasodilatation and pooling of blood in the peripheries, which will in turn lead to a further fall in blood pressure. The heart rate and respiratory rate will increase in an attempt to increase the delivery of oxygen to the tissues, but any sustained period of cellular hypoxia will compromise the function of vital organs. The brain is affected, leading to altered consciousness, and decreased kidney function results in low urine output (less than 30 mL/hour). If interventions are unsuccessful the patient will enter a decompensation (or refractory) phase.

Assessment and Reaching a Diagnosis

In practice, a full systematic preliminary assessment should have commenced on admission. However, in order to demonstrate the importance of early, accurate recognition of potential signs of deterioration and to highlight the potential to miss important clues if the practitioner lacks sufficient knowledge and awareness, the detailed assessment will be discussed here. Assessment must include simultaneous measurement of the patient's vital signs, a brief accurate history of presenting signs and symptoms and specific investigations in order that life saving intervention and symptom relief can be administered immediately. For the sake of narrative fluency each aspect will be discussed separately; however, in practice it is the integration of assessment information that is essential for an accurate and prompt definitive diagnosis. Table 3.4 identifies the key signs and symptoms to be aware of.

The Preliminary Assessment

Airway

Initially Billy was conscious and talking so his airway was clearly patent, but constant observation and assessment of his airway is imperative (see Chapter 1). The sequence of shock events can cause rapid deterioration and loss of consciousness, which can lead to airway problems requiring prompt intervention. This may require the use of adjuncts, such as an oral airway,

Table 3.4   Signs and symptoms of shock

Compensatory stage	*Progressive stage*
• Tachycardia	• Increasing tachycardia.
• Possible weak thready pulse	• Weak, rapid, thready pulse
• Blood pressure may be normal.	• Hypotension
• Increased respiratory rate: tachypnoea	• Tachypnoea with shallow respirations
• Cool, pale skin	• Cold and cyanotic skin
• Reduced urine output/concentrated urine	• Further reduction in urine output
• Confusion/anxiety	• Further deterioration in level of consciousness
• Nausea	
• Sweating	• Signs of hypoxaemia
• Increased blood sugar	• Hyperkalaemia

Note: This typical picture may show some variation. For example, in the early stages of septic shock the skin may be warm and dry and the pulse bounding, and in neurogenic shock the heart rate may be low.

or in the seriously ill patient endotracheal intubation and mechanical ventilation may be required.

Breathing

On admission Billy's respiratory rate is slightly elevated; however, there was no other information about the effectiveness of his respiratory system. It is imperative that Billy's respiratory rate, depth and pattern should be monitored and documented at least every 30 minutes to reveal a trend and draw attention to any potential changes. A chest X-ray may be requested. A pulse oximeter should be applied to measure Billy's peripheral oxygen saturation (SpO_2). Peripheral vasoconstriction can cause problems with the quality of the signal and therefore SpO_2 may not provide a completely accurate picture. Since a pulse oximeter assesses the amount of haemoglobin saturated with oxygen, if large amounts of blood have been lost the value of SpO_2 displayed may be inappropriately high (Casey, 2001). An arterial blood gas will provide a more accurate measure of Billy's respiratory status.

Initially Billy was showing signs of the compensatory stage of shock and was prescribed supplemental oxygen. The amount of oxygen prescribed would depend upon his respiratory rate, SpO_2, skin colour, ABG results and co-morbid history. Although unlikely in Billy's case, should there be a history of chronic obstructive pulmonary disease (COPD) he would need to be given oxygen with caution, with close monitoring for any reduction in his respiratory rate (see

Chapter 6). The second set of observations reveals an elevated respiratory rate. Low oxygen and rising carbon dioxide levels in the blood will stimulate the respiratory centre to increase the rate of oxygen inspiration and expiration to 'blow off' excess carbon dioxide. At this stage Billy requires continued monitoring and unless contraindicated he should receive 100 per cent oxygen via a non-rebreathe mask at 10 to15 litres per minute (British Thoracic Society, 2008). Humidification is recommended to minimise the risk of sputum retention and chest infection, which are associated with the drying effect of the oxygen (Pilkington, 2004). If Billy's blood pressure will allow he should be nursed with a degree of head elevation to aid his breathing. Supine positioning (lying flat on his back) increases the risk of respiratory infection and should be avoided whenever possible. Arterial blood gas measurement will guide the management of Billy's respiratory system and involves the use of a needle and syringe to withdraw a small amount of arterial blood. The radial artery in the wrist is the most common site, but other arteries such as the femoral artery in the groin can be used. Billy's blood sample is tested and results compared with normal values (Table 3.5).

Billy's low pH indicates that his blood is more acidotic than normal. The pH of arterial blood can fall for a number of reasons: for example, retention of respiratory acid carbon dioxide (see Chapter 6), retention of normal metabolic acids as a consequence of acute kidney injury (see Chapter 7) or the overproduction of metabolic acids in diabetic ketoacidosis (see Chapter 9). In Billy's case the fall in arterial pH is a consequence of excess production of lactic acid associated with impaired tissue perfusion (anaerobic metabolism). Base excess (BE) provides a numerical value of the degree of acid–base imbalance. The level of bicarbonate, an alkali (or base), has fallen as the body attempts to buffer the rising level of acid with a base. The level of arterial carbon dioxide ($PaCO_2$) has fallen to the low side of normal as a consequence of Billy's increased respiratory rate. The amount of oxygen in the blood (PaO_2) and the

Table 3.5   ABG: normal range and Billy's results

	Normal range of ABG values on air	*Billy's ABG results 2 hours after admission on 40% oxygen*
pH	7.35–7.45	7.25
PaO_2	11–13.3	12.5
$PaCO_2$ (kPa)	4.8–6.0	4.8
HCO_3 (mmol/L)	21–28	20
BE	–2 to +2	–2
SaO_2 (%)	95–100	96

Note: Normal values differ between men and women and local laboratory test procedures oxygen saturation are initially maintained; however, the normal limits shown are for a patient breathing atmospheric air (oxygen content 21 per cent). Billy is receiving supplemental oxygen so the measured values must be seen with some caution and continued monitoring of respiratory parameters is vital.

Circulation

On admisssion Billy's blood pressure was within the normal range and the changes to his peripheral circulation (cool and pale skin) and the increase in his heart rate suggested that compensatory mechanisms had been activated to counteract an earlier reduction in blood pressure. At this stage frequent monitoring of his pulse and blood pressure should occur and if available three or five lead cardiac monitoring should have been commenced. Billy's radial pulse should be manually palpated at least every 30 minutes to gain an indication of the volume and strength. In hypovolaemic states the pulse is likely to be fast but to lack volume and strength and may even be described as 'weak and thready'. In severe cases it may be necessary to palpate a more central artery such as the carotid pulse, although in practice this is not always easy to locate. Electronic monitoring of Billy's BP every 30 minutes may initially suffice as a means of recording and documenting a trend over time. However, as the BP begins to fall below a systolic pressure of 90 mmHg electronic monitoring may become inaccurate and necessitate manual BP recording at 10 to 15 minute intervals in the first instance. Patients who are nursed in high dependency or critical care environments may have an arterial catheter inserted, which permits a continuous display of arterial blood pressure. A 20 mmHg fall in blood pressure when moving a patient from lying to standing indicates at least a 20 per cent loss in circulating blood volume, and hypotension in the supine patient is indicative of a loss of approximately 40 per cent (Marini and Wheeler, 2006). Pulse pressure is the difference between the diastolic and systolic blood pressure and in hypovolaemia the pulse pressure is often narrow (Table 3.6). Billy's fall in skin temperature reflects poor peripheral perfusion and lack of urine output indicates low renal perfusion.

A large bore (14 to 16 gauge) intravenous cannula was inserted on admission but as Billy's condition has deteriorated he will require a second intravenous

Table 3.6   Billy's blood and pulse pressures

	On admission	*After 2 hours*
Blood pressure (mmHg)	110/70	80/55
Pulse pressure (mmHg)	40	25

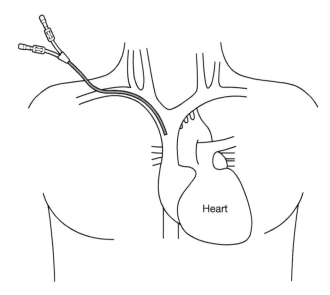

Figure 3.3   Placement of a central venous catheter.

cannula for continued fluid resuscitation. To allow closer monitoring of his central venous pressure, Billy may have a central venous line inserted into either the subclavian or internal jugular vein and advanced along the vein until its tip is close to the right atrium (Figure 3.3).

Central venous pressure (CVP) is the pressure within the right atrium of the heart. It normally reflects the volume of blood being returned to the right side of the heart, which is referred to as the venous return or preload. The normal CVP is in the range 5 to 12 cmH$_2$O (3 to 10 mmHg), although there is considerable variation as to what is considered the norm. A fall in CVP is often associated with hypovolaemia. A single reading of CVP is less important than the monitoring of trends over time and the measurement of its change following fluid replacement therapy. If Billy's CVP does not change after a fluid challenge with 500 mL of crystalloid fluid such as 0.9 per cent sodium chloride given over 30 minutes, then he is still volume depleted and will require more fluid. If the CVP rises slightly, but falls after 10 minutes, again he will require additional fluid. If, however, following a fluid challenge Billy's CVP rises above 10 cmH$_2$O and does not fall then he has been adequately resuscitated. It is important to remember, however, that monitoring of CVP alone is not a reliable measure of fluid balance, but when used in conjunction with continuous measurement and documentation of blood pressure, pulse, cardiac rhythm, urine output and conscious level will give a more complete picture of Billy's physiological status. Central venous catheters are not ideal for rapid fluid volume resuscitation as a consequence of their length and narrow diameter.

Disability

Although initially awake and communicating Billy was a little confused, which may be indicative of reduced blood flow to the brain. Billy's confusional state and level of consciousness should be monitored at least hourly using the AVPU system (see Chapter 2) and if there is further cause for concern or should his condition deteriorate the Glasgow Coma Scale (GCS) will provide a more detailed evaluation of Billy's neurological status (see Chapter 4). Billy reported abdominal pain, which can lead to further physiological as well as psychological complications (Woodrow 2006) and he will therefore need a thorough assessment of the site, character and intensity of his pain and administration of analgesia as prescribed. Billy describes his pain as being in the upper left part of his abdomen with radiation to the left shoulder when he lies down. Referred pain such as this is common in many situations, but coupled with his left sided abdominal pain, the history of trauma and the signs of hypovolaemia tend to support the diagnosis of ruptured spleen. Opioids such as IV morphine remain at the forefront of acute pain management and will be prescribed according to Billy's age, body mass and pain response.

Exposure

As the body redirects blood flow to the vital centres it reduces blood flow to the kidneys. When the kidneys have reduced perfusion their function is impaired and urine output declines. An accurate measure of urine output can provide further evidence of the function of the cardiovascular system. Normal urine output is 0.5 mL/kg/hr or approximately 30 mL/hour for a patient weighing 65 kg. Reduced urine output (oliguria) is a key sign of a shocked presentation. On admission it would not be appropriate to insert a self-retaining urinary catheter to monitor Billy's urine output, but as his condition deteriorated this option would be considered to ensure accuracy of measurement. As a consequence of the reduced renal perfusion and the renal retention of water any urine passed will be dark and concentrated and have a higher then normal specific gravity. Billy will be kept nil by mouth until the potential for emergency surgery is excluded. Gastric distension may increase pressure on the spleen and so a nasogastric tube will be passed to enable gastric decompression.

Billy is now tachycardic, hypotensive, cool, pale and clammy and these and the lack of diuresis are all indications that he is in the progressive stage of hypovolaemic shock. However, although Billy's condition may be as a result of internal blood loss following a ruptured spleen, there are many causes of a shocked presentation and assessment of signs and symptoms and further investigations are necessary to determine the primary cause.

Specific Investigations

Full blood count (FBC), urea and electrolytes (U and E), serum lactate, blood group, save and cross-matching for potential blood transfusion, coagulation studies, blood glucose, liver function tests and a 12 lead ECG will be adequate to determine the type of shock. For example, blood loss may be reflected in a low Hb and haematocrit but if the blood test was taken after aggressive fluid resuscitation, haemodilution may have occurred, so the results must be reviewed with some caution. Early stage sepsis should be suspected if there is a raised temperature, warm, dry skin, a bounding pulse, a raised white cell count and a raised C-reactive protein (CRP), and should be confirmed with positive blood cultures. As a consequence of the stress response patients with shock often present with a raised blood glucose level and elevated serum lactate confirms the presence of anaerobic metabolism. Chest pain, palpitations, changes on a 12 lead ECG and raised troponin may indicate an underlying MI or arrhythmia induced cardiogenic shock. A detailed history of current events may reveal sources of anaphylaxis or spinal cord injury. A rash and signs of peripheral oedema are more common with anaphylaxis. Billy describes receiving a blow to his abdomen during a rugby match, which would be classed as a blunt trauma injury, and is complaining of abdominal pain, so imaging including plain X-rays, abdominal ultrasound and an abdominal CT scan may be indicated.

Medical Management Strategies

Management strategies must focus upon:

- restoring circulating blood volume;
- control of fluid loss/treatment of cause;
- restoration of the oxygen carrying capacity of the blood.

Fluid Resuscitation

The average adult requires a fluid intake of about 3 litres a day to maintain homeostasis; however, in illness this may change dramatically in terms of both the volume and the composition of the fluid required. For example, when a patient has a high temperature they will require an additional 500

The Case Scenario: Management and Care Issues

Billy's condition has not yet shown any signs of recovery. He remains increasingly difficult to arouse and is less responsive to commands. He has been commenced on 500 mL of IV gelofusine® to infuse over 20 minutes via a wide bore peripheral cannula and has a CVP line inserted into the subclavian vein attached to 1 litre of IV 0.9 per cent sodium chloride solution. He has had IV morphine 5 mg for pain relief with some effect. A more recent set of observations reveals:

AVPU: V
GCS: 12 (E3, V4, M5)
Temperature: 36.0 °C
Heart rate: 130 beats per minute
BP: 80/55 mmHg
CVP: 2 cmH$_2$O
Respiratory rate: 28 breaths per minute
SpO$_2$: 98 per cent
Billy has a urinary catheter in situ and has passed a total of 35 mL of dark coloured urine in the past two hours.
He is receiving oxygen 100 per cent via a facemask.
Arterial blood gas (ABG) results are as follows:

- pH 7.15
- PaO$_2$ 14.5 kPa
- PaCO$_2$ 5.2 kPa
- HCO$_3$ 18 mol/L
- SaO$_2$ 98 per cent
- BE −2

Billy's Hb level is reported as 9.5 g/dL with a PCV (haematocrit) of 25 per cent.

Consider the following:

1. What are Billy's management priorities now?
2. Describe the rationale for the treatment interventions given.
3. What are Billy's main care issues?

mL of maintenance fluid for every degree above 37 °C. To fully appreciate the importance of fluid replacement therapy it is necessary to understand about body fluid compartments. About 60 per cent of the total body weight of an adult is fluid (almost entirely water). This fluid is distributed either within the cells (intracellular fluid) or outside of the cells (extracellular fluid) in a ratio of about 2/3 to 1/3 (Figure 3.4). When considering fluid volume replacement the key components of the extracellular fluid are the fluid contained within the blood vessels (the intravascular compartment) and the

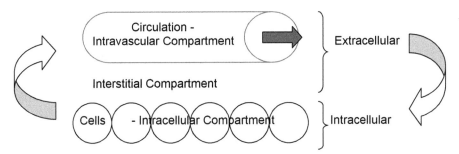

Figure 3.4 Body fluid compartments.

fluid contained in the spaces between the blood capillaries and the cells, the interstitium or interstitial compartment. Fluid is constantly moving between the compartments and loss should largely equal gain. The interstitial compartment gains a small amount of fluid and this is drained away as lymph.

Circulating blood volume is approximately 5 litres and at any given time about 65 per cent of this volume is contained within the intravascular compartment. When fluid moves out of or is lost from the intravascular compartment, blood pressure will fall and tissue perfusion will be compromised. To compensate for this fluid is drawn out of the cells and the interstitium. The rapid loss of about 1 litre of blood will be compensated within about 10 minutes by the movement of approximately 600 mL of fluid from the cells and the interstitium into the vascular compartment. This has been referred to as an 'internal transfusion' (Noble et al., 2005). When fluid shifts out of the intracellular compartment, cells can become dehydrated and cellular processes become less efficient. Depletion of the interstitial compartment is not in itself life threatening.

The importance of fluid volume replacement is proven but the type, amount and speed of infusion remains a focus of debate. Crystalloids such as 0.9 per cent sodium chloride solution and Hartmann's solution and colloids such as Haemaccel® and Gelofusine® are capable of restoring blood volume, but each has a different impact upon physiological systems. Crystal fluids temporarily replace fluid lost in the circulatory volume but the majority of the fluid is absorbed from the circulation into the extracellular fluid and then into the cells. In the case of 0.9 per cent sodium chloride solution, 750 mL of each litre given is rapidly lost from the vascular compartment to the extracellular and cellular compartments (Jordan, 2000). It will therefore replace not only the fluid lost from the blood stream, but also that lost from the cells. The Resuscitation Council UK (2005) recommends that a 1litre fluid challenge is given over 5 to 10 minutes for the management of hypotension, as in Billy's case. Alternatively, though less commonly adopted in the UK, 1 to 2 litres of Hartmann's solution may be given for shock-related fluid resuscitation because when metabolised in the liver and kidneys bicarbonate is produced, which will act to buffer the lactic acid produced from anaerobic metabolism (Evans and Tippins, 2007). In addition, the increased chloride load associated with the infusion of large volumes of 0.9 per cent sodium chloride solution may produce a hyperchloraemic acidosis, which will result in renal vasoconstriction and reduced GFR. For this reason Powell-Tuck et al. (2009) recommend that Ringer's lactate or Hartmann's solution should replace 0.9 per cent sodium chloride solution.

Colloids are much larger molecules that do not readily cross capillary membranes like crystalloids and therefore provide a more sustained expansion of circulating blood volume. They are, however, associated with an increased risk of complications such as cellular dehydration, and so large volumes of colloid for resuscitation and volume expansion should be used with caution, though small volumes are still used in practice (Alderson et al., 2004; Roberts et al., 2004; Perel and Roberts, 2009). Bunn et al. (2009) suggest that no colloid has any advantage over another. The rapid infusion of small amounts of colloid will provide for a more sustained improvement in blood volume and will increase the amount of oxygen available to the cells. Billy was commenced a fluid challenge of 500 mL of Gelofusine® over 10 to 20 minutes at the first sign of fluid volume depletion. Because of the way crystal fluid moves out of the vascular compartment, much greater volumes of crystalloid than colloid will be needed. Two to four litres of crystal fluid will provide the same level of vascular expansion as one litre of colloid. The use of such large volumes of crystal fluid is not without complications and patients must be observed for the development of pulmonary oedema and adult respiratory distress syndrome.

Crystal and colloid fluids increase the volume but not the oxygen carrying capacity of the blood and when blood loss is suspected or proved a blood transfusion may be required. There is no advantage in using blood for fluid volume resuscitation when blood has not been lost (Marini and Wheeler, 2006). Whole blood contains red and white cells, platelets, plasma and electrolytes and provides for the best volume expansion in the haemorrhaging hypovolaemic patient. Packed red cells contain the same volume of red blood cells, but have a smaller volume of plasma and as such produce less volume expansion (Kneale, 2003). Although the normal Hb is in the range 12 to 18 g/dL the optimal Hb value following blood transfusion is patient- and circumstance-dependent. A balance needs to be drawn between the value of Hb required to ensure adequate oxygen carrying capacity and a lower Hb, which will decrease blood viscosity and promote organ perfusion

(Woodrow, 2006). A consequence of the 'internal transfusion' described earlier is haemodilution and a fall in haematocrit. Sheppard and Wright (2006) suggest that a blood transfusion should be given if the measured haematocrit or packed cell volume (PCV) is less than 30 per cent or if the Hb is less than 10 g/dL. As Billy's Hb was 9.5 g/dL and his PCV was 25 per cent the need for a blood transfusion became more evident. The amount of blood transfused will depend upon repeat haematological results. If large volumes of blood are required it is common also to give regular transfusions of platelets and fresh frozen plasma to minimise the risk of blood clotting problems. The infusion of mismatched blood or blood products can lead to a potentially life threatening transfusion reaction and vigilance and checking are required to ensure that the patient receives the correct blood. Once a transfusion is in progress frequent observations of temperature, pulse, respirations and blood pressure plus observation of the skin for flushing or the development of a rash will enable early detection of a transfusion anaphylaxis. Complications can occur during any form of fluid resuscitation and it is important to continue monitoring of pulse, blood pressure, CVP, respirations and temperature. In addition the patient's jugular veins can be assessed, as fluid overload may result in jugular vein distension. The infusion of large volumes of fluid at room temperature, or much cooler if blood (usually about 4 °C), can cause a rapid reduction in the patient's body temperature and the use of fluid warming devices is recommended. When treating haemorrhage a rapid increase in blood pressure is contraindicated due to the risk of dislodging any clot formation and producing a worsening of the blood loss. Therapy to aim for a systolic blood pressure of 90 mmHg is recommended (Evans and Tippins, 2007).

Oxygen Therapy

It is essential to increase the arterial oxygen concentration and as such the amount of oxygen delivered to the tissues. All shocked patients should receive high flow oxygen via a non-rebreathe face mask. Billy's PaO_2 and $PaCO_2$ are within normal parameters, but he will continue to receive 100 per cent oxygen via the non-rebreathe mask until his overall condition improves. Where the required level of tissue oxygenation is not achieved, non-invasive respiratory support (see Chapter 6) or intubation and mechanical ventilation is indicated.

Vasoactive and Inotropic Drugs

Pharmacological support is rarely needed in hypovolaemic shock except when it is severe or when surgical intervention is delayed (McLukie, 2003).

If, however, after volume loading the blood pressure is still too low, drugs such as positive inotropes (dobutamine®) or vasopressors (adrenaline/epinephrine®, noradrenaline/norepinephrine®) might be considered to optimise cardiac output and to increase blood pressure. Positive inotropes will act to increase myocardial contractility, whereas drugs with vasopressor properties act upon the tone of blood vessels and tend to increase venous return (preload). Patients with septic or cardiogenic shock are most likely to need vasoactive or inotropic drugs, but in all cases patients needing these drugs should be transferred to a high dependency or intensive care environment.

Electrolyte Management

When a patient has a major haemorrhage there is a total loss of electrolyte volume relative to each other and before the body's compensatory mechanisms begin blood biochemistry would appear largely unchanged (O'Shea, 2005). However, the developing altered physiology, renal impairment and fluid replacement therapy will all disrupt Billy's normal electrolyte balance, requiring regular monitoring of serum electrolytes (see Chapter 2, Table 2.14). Abnormalities in the levels of sodium, potassium, calcium and magnesium affect myocardial and smooth muscle contractility and elevated potassium (hyperkalaemia) or a low level of calcium (hypocalcaemia) is a frequent cause of cardiac dysrhythmias. Elevated levels of chloride (hyperchloraemia) and sodium (hypernatraemia) may occur following the infusion of large quantities of 0.9 per cent sodium chloride solution and this may cause or worsen a metabolic acidosis (Marini and Wheeler, 2006). Monitoring of acid–base balance via arterial blood gas analysis is essential.

Acid–Base Balance

The body is very intolerant of an arterial blood pH outside of the normal range (7.35 to 7.45). All causes of shock lead to a metabolic acidosis, which if untreated will lead to cardiac dysrhythmias, impaired cardiac conduction, a further decline in cardiac output and blood pressure and depression of the central nervous system. A pH of 7.0 or below may lead to disorientation and coma, and a pH of less than 6.8 is usually incompatible with life. In Billy's case the cause of his metabolic acidosis is the increased production of lactic acid from cellular anaerobic metabolism. The treatment aimed at improving cell perfusion will in many cases result in the normalisation of acid–base balance. Should this not occur then small amounts of sodium bicarbonate may be given intravenously. Metabolic acidosis related to acute kidney injury will require renal replacement therapy (see Chapter 7).

Surgical Intervention

If conservative management is unsuccessful in managing Billy's underlying cause of a ruptured spleen, he will be transferred to the operating theatre for surgery once he is haemodynamically stable. If the damage is limited it may be possible to repair the spleen; however, a splenectomy to remove the entire spleen is more likely. The spleen plays a major role in filtering foreign organisms from the blood and in the production of protective antibodies, so when it is removed the body's ability to fight infection is impaired. Billy should be made aware of the need to take extra care to protect himself against infection and he should be vaccinated against pneumococcal infection. Annual vaccination against influenza is recommended and some people take prophylactic antibiotics to try to prevent infections.

Ongoing Care Issues and the Role of the Nurse

In addition to care in support of the management strategies, patients in shock require a broad range of nursing care interventions. Close observation, frequent monitoring and location within the ward should be considered and transfer to a high dependency or intensive care unit may be required. There is a direct relationship between the stress response and the manifestation of anxiety, and expressions of fear and anxiety are common in shock. Information giving, psychosocial support, communication and the development of trusting, supportive relationships with Billy and his close family and friends are essential aspects of shock management (Bench, 2004). An impaired level of consciousness will impact upon Billy's ability to meet his own personal hygiene needs. This, coupled with fluid loss, a restricted oral intake and ongoing oxygen therapy, makes assistance with oral hygiene of vital importance. Failure to meet Billy's oral hygiene needs will increase discomfort and the incidence of oral and systemic infection (Woodrow, 2006). Skin integrity may also be compromised by reduced tissue perfusion and immobility, and regular position changes coupled with frequent assessment and the use of pressure relieving aids or mattresses is indicated.

The Refractory Stage of Shock: What if the Interventions Don't Work?

When 40 per cent (2 litres) or more of the circulating blood volume is lost the body is no longer able to compensate and death is assured with blood loss of 50 per cent (Evans and Tippins, 2007). In this decompensated stage there is a persistent tachycardia and severe hypotension. Poor coronary artery blood flow results in reduced myocardial contraction, a predisposition to arrhythmias and an increased risk of myocardial infarction. Ischaemia of alveolar cells leads to rapidly worsening respiratory function, with hypoxaemia, CO_2 retention and rapid irregular respirations. Acute respiratory distress syndrome with severe hypoxaemia and bilateral pulmonary infiltrates may supervene. As brain cell ischaemia progresses the patient will become unconscious, and the pupils dilate and become slow to react to light. A prolonged reduction in renal blood flow will lead to renal failure and liver failure will lead to jaundice and the accumulation of waste products in the blood. Poor perfusion of the gastrointestinal tract may promote gastric ulceration, haemorrhage and the movement (translocation) of bacteria from the gut into the bloodstream, leading to sepsis. A multiple organ dysfunction syndrome (MODS) will exist, reflecting irreversible dysfunction of more than one organ system. Organ systems commonly associated with MODS are cardiovascular, respiratory, hepatic, renal and gastrointestinal, although there are no universal criteria. Mortality is in the region of 50 per cent and this worsens as more organ systems become involved. Treatment is largely organ-specific and supportive, and may include mechanical ventilation, optimised fluid resuscitation, renal replacement therapy and pharmacological interventions to support the failing heart.

Summary

Shock is a life threatening presentation that arises from the body's inability to maintain its own internal homeostasis. Inadequate treatment or delay in the recognition and treatment of shock can lead to an increase in morbidity and mortality. Assessment and monitoring of the patient in shock are crucial and nurses must ensure that they have the necessary knowledge and skills. Treatment of the underlying cause and management of the pathophysiological sequelae of hypovolaemic shock with appropriate, timely fluid and electrolyte resuscitation can reverse the shock pattern and lead to a successful outcome.

Further Reading

Higgins, C. *Understanding Laboratory Investigations: For Nurses and Health Professionals*, 2nd edn (Oxford: Blackwell, 2007).

Jevon, P. and B. Ewens (eds). *Monitoring the Critically Ill Patient*, 2nd edn (Oxford: Blackwell Science, 2007).

Scott, W. *Fluids and Electrolytes Made Incredibly Easy!* (London: Lippincott, Williams and Wilkins, 2010).

References

Alderson P., F. Bunn, A. Li Wan Po, L. Li, I. Roberts and G. Schierhout. 'Human Albumin Solution for Resuscitation and Volume Expansion in Critically Ill Patients', in *Cochrane Database of Systematic Reviews*, issue 4 (Chichester: John Wiley and Sons, 2004).

Bench, S. 'Clinical Skills: Assessing and Treating Shock. A Nursing Perspective', *British Journal of Nursing*, **13**(12) (2004), 715–21.

Bunn, F., D. Trivedi and S. Ashraf. 'Colloid Solutions for Fluid Resuscitation (Review)', in *Cochrane Database of Systematic Reviews*, issue 2 (Chichester: John Wiley and Sons, 2009).

British Thoracic Society. 'BTS Guideline for Emergency Oxygen Use in Adult Patients', *Thorax*, **63**(suppl. VI) (2008), 1–68.

Casey, G. 'Oxygen Transport and the Use of the Pulse Oximeter', *Nursing Standard*, **15**(47) (2001), 46–53.

Evans, C. and E. Tippins. *The Foundations of Emergency Care* (Maidenhead: Open University Press, 2007).

Kneale, J. 'Understanding Hypovolaemic Shock', *Journal of Orthopaedic Nursing*, **7** (2003), 207–13.

Jordan, K. S. 'Fluid Resuscitation in Acutely Injured Patients', *Journal of Intravenous Nursing*, **23**(2) (2000), 81–7.

McKinley, M. G. 'Shock and Sepsis', in M. L. Sole, D. G. Klein and M. J. Moseley (eds), *Introduction to Critical Care* (St Louis: Elsevier Saunders, 2005).

McLukie, A. 'Shock: An Overview', in A. D. Bernsten, N. Soni and T. E. Oh (eds), *Oh's Intensive Care Manual*, 5th edn (Philadelphia: Butterworth Heinemann, 2003).

Marini, J. J. and A. P. Wheeler. *Critical Care Medicine: The Essentials*, 3rd edn (Philadelphia: Lippincott, Williams and Wilkins, 2006).

Noble, A., R. Johnson, A. Thomas and P. Bass. *The Cardiovascular System. Basic Science and Clinical Conditions* (London: Elsevier, 2005).

O'Shea, A. '*Principles and Practice of Trauma Nursing*' (Edinburgh: Churchill Livingstone, 2005).

Perel, P. and I. G. Roberts. 'Colloids versus Crystalloids for Fluid Resuscitation in Critically Ill Patients', in *Cochrane Database of Systematic Reviews*, issue 2. (Chichester: John Wiley and Sons, 2009).

Pilkington, P. 'Humidification for Oxygen Therapy in Non-ventilated Patients', *British Journal of Nursing*, **13** (2004), 111–15.

Powell-Tuck, J., P. Gosling, D. Lobo, S. Allison, G. Carlson, M. Gore, A. Lewington, R. Pearse and M. Mythen. 'Summary of the British Consensus Guidelines on Intravenous Fluid Therapy for Adult Surgical Patients (GIFTASUP)', *Journal of the Intensive Care Society*, **10**(1) (2009), 13–15.

Resuscitation Council UK. *Resuscitation Guidelines 2005* (London: Resuscitation Council UK, 2005).

Roberts, I., P. Alderson, F. Bunn, P. Chinnock and G. Schierhout. 'Colloids versus Crystalloids for Fluid Resuscitation in Critically Ill Patients', in *Cochrane Database of Systematic Reviews*, issue 4 (Chichester: John Wiley and Sons, 2004).

Sheppard, M. and M. Wright. *Principles and Practice of High Dependency Nursing*, 2nd edn (London: Bailliere Tindall, 2006).

Tippins E. 'How Emergency Department Nurses Identify and Respond to Critical Illness', *Emergency Nurse*, **13**(3) (2005), 24–33.

Topalian, S., F. Ginsberg and J. E. Parrillo. 'Cardiogenic Shock', *Critical Care Medicine*, **36**(1) (2008), S66–S74.

Woodrow, P. *Intensive Care Nursing: A Framework for Practice*, 2nd edn (London: Routledge, 2006).

4

Traumatic Brain Injury

Ian Goulden

Introduction

Head injury is a broad term that can refer to any injury of the scalp, the skull or the brain and may be associated with widely varying levels of morbidity and mortality. In the under 45s traumatic brain injury (TBI) is the leading cause of death and severe life-long disability worldwide (Werner and Engelhard, 2007). In the UK, over 700,000 people attend accident and emergency departments every year following a head injury and half of these are under 16 years of age (National Institute for Clinical Health and Excellence (NICE), 2007). Although only 10 per cent of head injuries are classed as moderate (Glasgow Coma Score (GCS) 9–12) or severe (GCS 3–8), approximately 5,000 people die in the UK each year as a result of head injury. In excess of 30 per cent of those that survive severe TBI will be left with a long-term disability (Bader and Arbour, 2005). Management of the patient with an acute severe head injury is complex and challenging. Damage at the time of injury (primary damage) is largely irreversible; however, the effects of secondary damage can be reduced by rapid accurate assessment and intervention. Guidelines for the assessment and management of head injured patients were published by NICE in 2007, and the Scottish Intercollegiate Guidelines Network (SIGN) in 2009.

Aim and Learning Outcomes

The Aim

The aim of this chapter is to explore the priorities of early accurate assessment and management of the individual presenting with elevated intracranial pressure following a head injury that has resulted in traumatic brain injury. A case scenario will be used to provide the template for application of evidence-based decision making to clinical practice.

Learning Outcomes

At the end of this chapter the reader will be able to:

1. Describe the main causes of altered consciousness.
2. Describe the main mechanisms of TBI.
3. Identify and explain the pathophysiological basis of a range of presenting neurological signs and symptoms.
4. Consider the immediate assessment, specific monitoring and key investigations required to enable an accurate and timely diagnosis in the patient with neurological dysfunction.
5. Outline the priorities in the management of the patient with raised intracranial pressure.
6. Appreciate the potential long-term impact of TBI.

The Case Scenario: The Presenting Complaint

Louise is a previously fit and well 28-year-old. She is brought to the accident and emergency (A&E) department complaining of headache and nausea. She appears somewhat restless and confused. Louise's husband tells you that she fell down a flight of stairs yesterday while out shopping, but that she had refused to attend A&E as 'she was alright'. Her initial observations are:

> Temperature: 36.7 °C
> Heart rate: 90 beats per minute
> BP: 130/70 mmHg
> Respiratory rate: 14 breaths per minute
> She is moving all limbs equally
> AVPU score is A
> SpO_2: 97 per cent (on air)
> A bruise is noted to the right side of her forehead

Consider the following:

1. With reference to the underlying pathophysiology explain Louise's signs and symptoms.
2. What do the initial observations reveal?
3. How might the head injury affect Louise's behaviour?

Fundamental Physiological Concepts

'The human brain is by far the most complex structure in the known universe' (Thompson, 1993, in Sheppard and Wright, 2005, p. 159) and it is beyond the scope of this chapter to discuss complex brain function. However, a basic understanding of brain structure (Figure 4.1), function (Table 4.1) and a number of fundamental physiological principles is an essential prerequisite for accurate assessment and management of TBI.

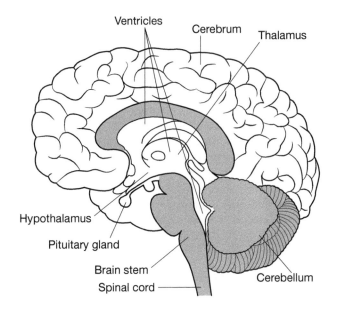

Figure 4.1   Brain structure.

There are multiple potential diseases and disorders (Table 4.2) that will affect the structure and function of one or more parts of the brain. The manifestation of common clinical signs and symptoms will be dependent upon the type of disease or disorder and the affected part of the brain. Louise may have suffered cerebral trauma as a result of her fall and the associated changes in pressure within the brain may give rise to a number of specific clinical signs and symptoms.

Table 4.1   Brain structure and function

Cerebrum	Consists of the two cerebral hemispheres. Multiple roles including the direction of conscious movement, sensory processing, speech and language, learning and memory and the sense of smell.
Cerebellum	Processing centre for coordination of muscular movement and balance.
Ventricles	Four connected ventricles contain cerebrospinal fluid (CSF). The main function of CSF is to cushion the brain from injury.
Hypothalamus	Responsible for autonomic regulation via the sympathetic and parasympathetic nervous system.
Thalamus	Relay and processing centre for all sensory information other than smell.
Pituitary Gland	Complex two-lobed endocrine gland secreting multiple hormones, including thyroid stimulating hormone, growth hormone and antidiuretic hormone.
Brain Stem	Connection between the brain and spinal cord. Contains cardiac, respiratory and vasomotor centres and the reflex centres of coughing, swallowing, vomiting and sneezing. Contains the reticular activating system. Site of origin of 10 of the 12 pairs of cranial nerves.
Meninges	The meninges cover the brain and spinal cord. There are three layers. The outer dura mater lines the inside of the skull. The middle arachnoid mater loosely encloses the brain and the inner pia mater covers the entire surface of the brain.

The Monro–Kellie Doctrine

The Monro–Kellie doctrine (Figure 4.2) describes the relationship between the intracranial contents and the pressure within the skull, termed the intracranial pressure (ICP). The intracranial contents are brain and intracellular water (80 to 85 per cent), cerebral blood volume (3 to 7 per cent) and cerebrospinal fluid (5 to 12 per cent). These are contained within a structure (the skull) the volume of which is for all practical purposes fixed. As pressure is related to volume, any increase in the volume of one of the compartments will have to be buffered by a decrease in the volume of the others. Should such compensation not occur or be inadequate the intracranial pressure will become elevated.

Intracranial Pressure (ICP)

Intracranial pressure (ICP) is a normal phenomenon that can be measured and is a reflection of the total intracranial volume against the rigid skull. The normal value is less than 15 mmHg. A number of homeostatic mechanisms

Table 4.2   Diseases and disorders of the brain

Problem	*Examples*
Trauma	Concussion, contusion, extra-/sub-dural haematoma, sub-arachnoid haemorrhage
Vascular	Transient ischaemic attack (TIA), stroke due to cerebral bleed or infarction (thrombus)
Infection	Meningitis: bacterial, e.g. meningococcal, tuberculosis (TB) Encephalitis: viral, e.g. herpes simplex
Neoplasm	Primary benign or malignant tumour Secondary metastases
Endocrine	Pituitary problems
Auto-immune	Systemic lupus erythematosus
Congenital	Cerebral palsy, hydrocephalus
Degenerative	Alzheimer's disease
Metabolic	Glycogen storage disorder
Iatrogenic	Drug toxicity
Idiopathic	No known cause
Psychological	Psychological, e.g. anxiety, depression Psychiatric, e.g. schizophrenia, bipolar disorder

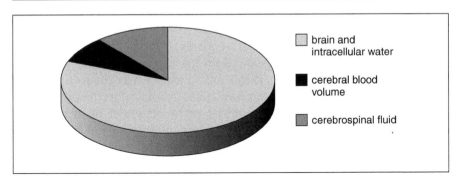

Figure 4.2   The Monro–Kellie doctrine.

work to maintain the ICP within its normal range. The most important of these is cerebrospinal fluid (CSF) displacement. This represents a process by which CSF volume is reduced by increased re-absorption, decreased production or increased displacement into the subarachnoid space. The large cerebral veins are readily compressed and will expel some of their blood into the extracranial veins; however, this option is limited by available volume and by adequate venous drainage pathways and is therefore not a major player. Brain volume displacement refers to displacement of the brain tissue itself, e.g. by brain tumour, but this can only occur to a very slight degree. If the tumour increases above this displaceable volume then the ICP will begin to rise. Normal fluctuations in ICP occur with respect to respiration and blood pressure and transient rises are associated with activities such as coughing, straining at stool and sneezing. However, a persistent increase in ICP will give rise to symptoms such as headache and nausea and may be detected as changes in consciousness level, heart rate, BP and respiratory status, though this is not yet evident in Louise's case.

Cerebral Perfusion Pressure (CPP)

CPP is the pressure required to maintain an adequate cerebral blood flow. It is the difference between mean cerebral arterial and cerebral venous blood flow and as such reflects the blood pressure gradient across the brain. Cerebral perfusion pressure can be calculated as:

CPP = mean arterial pressure − ICP

An acceptable CPP is above 60 mmHg. A CPP below 30 mmHg may lead to cessation of the cerebral blood flow.

Cerebral Blood Flow

The brain is only 2 per cent of the total body mass, yet it requires 750 mL of oxygenated blood each minute, which equates to 15 per cent of the cardiac output. Cerebral blood flow is essential for the supply of oxygen and nutrients to the cerebral tissues. A critical relationship exists between cerebral blood flow and ICP. Cerebral blood flow is disadvantaged in the presence of elevated ICP. The automatic adjustment of blood vessel diameter is an important factor involved in maintaining a constant cerebral blood flow. Homeostatic processes can maintain cerebral blood flow within normal limits using mechanisms of vasodilatation and vasoconstriction. However this mechanism is impaired by ischaemia, hypoxia or hypercapnia and begins to fail when the CPP is below 60 mmHg or above 160 mmHg.

Traumatic Brain Injury

At a basic level the brain can be traumatically injured by one or more of the four following mechanisms:

1. Stretching of nerve fibres.
2. Shearing, which is damage caused by the movement of nerve fibres over each other.

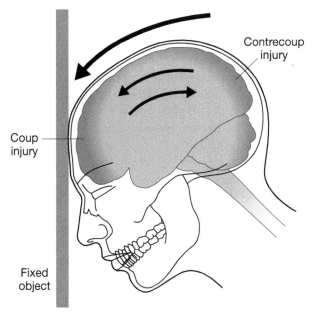

Figure 4.3 Contrecoup injury.

The Case Scenario: The Immediate Assessment Priorities

Louise appears to be becoming increasingly drowsy and though she makes some attempt to answer questions when prompted she is not always clear or coherent. A further set of observations reveals:

Temperature: 36.7 °C
Heart rate: 80 beats per minute
BP: 140/75 mmHg
Respiratory rate: 12 breaths per minute
SpO$_2$: 95 per cent (on air)
She is moving all limbs equally.
AVPU score is A
GCS is 12/15 (E3, V4, M5)
PERLA

Consider the following:

1. What are the immediate assessment priorities for Louise and what is the rationale for each measure?
2. What do the observations indicate in Louise's case?
3. How would a definitive cause and diagnosis be established in Louise's case?

3. Contusion, which is bruising of brain tissue.
4. Haemorrhage.

When the brain is injured by deceleration such as from a fall in Louise's case or following a road traffic accident a concept called coup/contrecoup must be considered (Figure 4.3). The brain strikes the inside of the skull at one point and if the force of impact is great enough the brain tissue will rebound and strike the skull again at the opposite point. As such the brain may receive two distinct points of damage.

Assessment and Reaching a Diagnosis

As per NICE (2007) guidelines for the management of head injured patients Louise should be seen by a doctor or nurse within 15 minutes of her arrival in A&E and the ABCDE approach to assessment should be used. Louise has a clear airway and is breathing adequately. Her vital signs are within the normal range and she is graded A on the AVPU system. In the initial assessment of consciousness, the AVPU scale (see Chapter 2) together with examination of the pupils, which is discussed in more detail later, is useful (Jevon, 2008). However, the nature of her injury and the altered level of consciousness require a more focused assessment of her neurological condition. Neurological assessment should include measurement of vital signs, an assessment of the level of consciousness, evaluation of motor function and assessment of pupillary signs (Table 4.3). Consciousness is defined as a general awareness of oneself and the surrounding environment (Hickey, 2008). When conscious, individuals are capable of responding to sensory stimuli, whereas a state of unconsciousness represents an inability to respond to sensory stimuli. Alterations in consciousness level may be slow and progressive or may be acute; loss of consciousness may be brief or prolonged. Assessment of consciousness is difficult because it cannot be measured directly, it can only be assessed by observing a person's behaviour in response to different stimuli (Hickey, 2008). There are two aspects to consciousness:

1. Arousal or wakefulness is a function of the reticular activating system (RAS) located in the brain stem,
2. Awareness or cognition is a function of the cerebral hemispheres.

Consciousness is dependent upon the cerebral hemispheres being intact and interacting with the ascending RAS. It is maintained by a constant stream of impulses that are sent from the brain stem upwards into the two cerebral

Table 4.3 Neurological assessment

Vital signs: T, P, R, BP and SpO$_2$
Level of consciousness: Glasgow Coma Score
Motor function: limb assessment
Pupillary function

Source: NICE (2007).

Table 4.4 Potential causes of altered consciousness

Cerebral hemisphere malfunction	Brain stem malfunction
Drug and alcohol intoxication	Direct damage:
Hypoxic brain injury	Brain stem infarct
Stroke	
Metabolic disorders such as hypoglycaemia	Indirect damage:
Infection	Cerebral mass (clot, tumour,
Post seizure	abscess)
	Cerebral oedema (infarct,
	hypoxia, infection, injury)

hemispheres. Changes in the level of consciousness therefore reflect two general mechanisms, which are cerebral hemisphere malfunction and brain stem malfunction. The Monro–Kellie doctrine demonstrates that the brain stem is at particular risk from elevated intracranial pressure and many causes of brain stem malfunction are secondary to cerebral hemisphere dysfunction. Louise's drowsiness and altered consciousness level suggests some brain stem malfunction, which may be indicative of raised ICP. Some potential causes of altered consciousness are given in Table 4.4.

Accurate assessment of consciousness level is one of the most important roles of the healthcare practitioner. Assessment of the patient following head injury should only be performed by professionals competent in the assessment of brain injury (NICE, 2007).

The Glasgow Coma Scale

The Glasgow Coma Scale (GCS) (Table 4.5) was introduced in 1974 (Teasdale and Jennett, 1974) as a tool for grading the severity of traumatic head injury and is the most widely used scoring system for quantifying consciousness. It assesses the two aspects of consciousness, arousal and awareness and permits standardisation of assessment. The GCS consists of three aspects of behavioural response, each of which is evaluated independently:

Table 4.5   The Glasgow Coma Scale

	6	5	4	3	2	1
Eye opening (E)			Spontaneous	To speech	To pain	None
Best verbal response (V)		Orientated speech	Confused speech	Words only	Sounds only	None
Best motor response (M)	Obeys commands	Localises to pain	Withdraws from pain	Flexion to pain	Extension to pain	None

- eye opening;
- best verbal response;
- best motor response.

A derivative of the GCS is the Glasgow Coma Score. This is an artificial index obtained by adding scores from the three categories. The highest score that can be achieved is 15, the lowest 3. The total score when recorded and communicated should be stated as a fraction of 15, such as 15/15 or 12/15, and monitoring and exchange of information about patients should clearly identify the score for each category, e.g. GCS 13/15, E4, V4, M5 (NICE 2007). One of the main criticisms of the GCS as an assessment tool is its subjectivity; however, further exploration of each of the assessment themes can minimise that risk.

Eye Opening

Eye opening assesses the arousal aspect of consciousness. A score of 4 is given when the patient is able to open their eyes without any active stimulation by the observer, 3 indicates that the patient will only open their eyes when spoken to and 2 is when a painful stimulus is required. If the patient does not open their eyes even with the application of a painful stimulus a score of 1 is given. 'C' is recorded if the patient is physically unable to open their eyes due to trauma, pre-existing disease or the presence of a dressing (Jevon and Ewens, 2007). Louise scores 3 for eye opening.

Best Verbal Response

This category assesses awareness by determining whether the patient understands what has been said and can formulate and articulate a reply (Waterhouse, 2005). First, a brief assessment of hearing, language difficulties and understanding is necessary (Adam and Osborne, 2005). Scores are given as follows:

5 = Patient can hold a normal conversation and is orientated in time and place.

4 = A degree of confusion with an inability to identify time, place, month, year, as in Louise's case.

3 = Patient responds with single words only and conversation is absent.

2 = Sounds that cannot be identified as words, such as mumbling and groaning.

1 = No verbal response at all.

It is worth noting that patients scoring 3 and below will tend to respond to physical rather than verbal stimulation and are largely unaware of their surroundings (Mooney and Comerford, 2003). A 'T' is recorded if the patient is unable to vocalise as a consequence of tracheal intubation (Jevon and Ewens, 2007).

Best Motor Response

This category is perhaps the most confusing as it introduces terms and patterns of movement that may only be seen in patients with severe neurological dysfunction. The GCS is an assessment of conscious level and not motor function so there is no need to record left and right differences and the best arm response should be recorded. Leg responses are not measured as these may be spinal rather than brain initiated. If the patient will obey commands such as lift up your arms, stick out your tongue or raise your eyebrows then they score 6. For patients who will not obey commands then a painful stimulus is applied and the response to stimulus observed. If the patient can localise to the source of the pain – that is, they move their hand towards it with purpose – then a 5 is given. If the patient moves their hand towards the pain but does not localise to the source this is graded with a 4. A 3 is given for flexion (a decorticate response). This is a slower response than above and is characterised by internal rotation of the shoulder with flexion of the elbow and wrist. If the patient extends their arm to pain, that is the elbows and wrists straighten and the hands tend to drift away from the body this is a poor neurological sign (called decerebrate posture) and is scored 2. No movement at all to a painful stimulus scores 1.

Applying a Painful Stimulus

Louise scored 6 for best motor response and therefore application of a painful stimulus is not necessary. However, in some cases a full GCS assessment may require the application of a painful stimulus to illicit a purposeful and specific response to the painful stimulus (not just a response to the

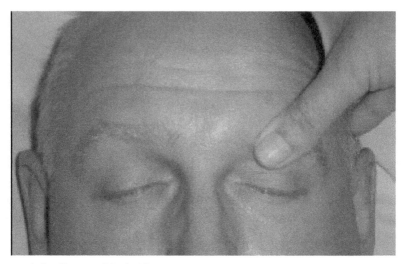

Figure 4.4   Supraorbital ridge pressure.

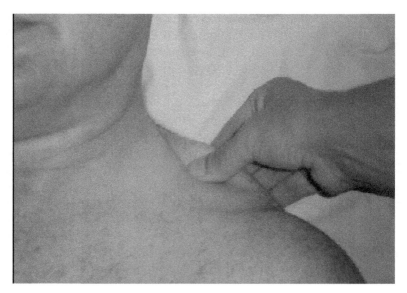

Figure 4.5   Trapezius muscle pinch.

irritation). Only a central painful stimulus will demonstrate localisation to pain. The 'normal' expected response is the patient moving their hand upwards, ideally to at least chin level (Waterhouse, 2005). Two techniques, either application of pressure to the supraorbital ridge of the eye (Figure 4.4) or pinching of the trapezius muscle (Figure 4.5), are favoured. To minimise soft tissue injury no stimulus should be applied for longer than 10 seconds

(Waterhouse, 2005). The application of pressure to the supraorbital ridge is considered to be the best approach as the patient's response is less likely to be misinterpreted (Fairley, 2005). However, pressure should not be applied to the supraorbital ridge if trauma to the face is identified or suspected. Application of a painful stimulus should start with light pressure and gradually increase. If the patient finds objects such as nasogastric tubes and oxygen masks irritating and localises spontaneously to such sources of irritation then the application of a painful stimulus is not necessary.

Pupillary Signs

Reaction of the pupil to light is dependent upon the normal functioning of two cranial nerves. The optic nerve (cranial nerve II) reacts to light entering the eye, while the occulomotor nerve (cranial nerve III) causes constriction of the pupil. Any change in pupil size and response to light potentially indicates elevated ICP and compression of the optic or occulomotor nerves. Louise's pupils will be assessed and monitored for their size, shape and reaction to light. The resting size of both pupils should be assessed and should be equal (average size 2 to 5 mm). The shape should be round; an oval shape could indicate intracranial hypertension (Fairley, 2005). To test pupil reaction, room lights should be dimmed and a pen torch or other source of bright light briefly directed towards each pupil. The normal response is a brisk constriction of the pupils. The direct response, which is the pupil response in the eye you are shining the light into, and the consensual reaction of the other eye should be noted. Pupils should react as a pair. The cranial nerves do not cross over so altered reaction in one pupil indicates a pressure build up on the same side of the brain as the affected pupil (Hickey, 2008). In the early stages of elevated ICP the pupil on the affected side will begin to gradually dilate, but is still reactive to light. As ICP continues to rise the pupil becomes more dilated and ultimately becomes unreactive (fixed). Although unlikely in this case, a range of drugs, both prescribed and recreational, can alter pupil responses (Fairley, 2005). Benzodiazepines such as diazepam can cause bilateral dilation of the pupils, whilst opioid drugs including morphine and its derivatives cause bilateral constriction.

Limb Assessment

Limb assessment is required to assess for focal damage such as stroke. Spontaneous movement of all four limbs should be observed. If movement is limited then a painful stimulus should be applied to the limb and the response noted. Comparison of one side of the body to the other is necessary, as symmetry is the most important consideration when identifying

Table 4.6   Louise's GCS on admission

Eye opening	3
Best verbal response	4
Best motor response	5
Total	12/15

focal findings. Hemiparesis or hemiplegia will usually (but not always) be seen in the limbs on the opposite side to the brain lesion.

Louise had her GCS assessed at 12/15 (Table 4.6) and her pupils were equal and reacting normally. This is often recorded as PERLA – pupils equal, reacting to light and accommodation. Her temperature, pulse, blood pressure and respirations are within normal limits but she has a reduced GCS and is complaining of headache and nausea. These coupled with her history of head injury suggest the possibility of the early stages of elevated ICP. In TBI, ICP rises globally due to cerebral oedema. Increased ICP leads to a reduction in cerebral blood flow and to brain tissue hypoxia. Brain cells when deprived of oxygen switch to anaerobic metabolism and produce acidic by-products. The pH falls locally and this promotes local vasodilatation and a further increase in the ICP. A vicious circle may develop. Brain tissue does not have pain fibres, but headache results from traction on pain sensitive structures such as the meninges and blood vessels. Headache associated with elevated ICP is generalised rather than local to one area (Lindsay and Bone, 2004). Increasing pressure on the floor of the fourth ventricle of the brain leads to nausea and vomiting, and altered consciousness may be caused by increased ICP. Further eye examination using a fundoscope to examine Louise's retina may be performed by a doctor. Increased pressure on the optic nerve results in oedema of the nerve head, which is called papilloedema. NICE (2007) guidelines state that any patient with a GCS of < 13 on admission should be referred for immediate CT scan; the scan should be performed and interpreted within one hour of the request being made. Louise will be scheduled for urgent CT scan, and vital signs monitoring and neurological assessment will continue. NICE (2007) proposes that if a patient has or is found to be at risk of developing brain injury, GCS observations should be conducted every half an hour until a GCS of 15/15 has been achieved. Once 15/15 has been achieved GCS should be recorded half hourly for a further two hours, then every hour for four hours and every two hours afterwards, providing that their GCS remains at 15/15. Should the GCS fall observations should return to half hourly. Louise will have vital signs and neurological assessment performed at least every 30 minutes and ideally would be placed on continuous cardiac monitoring.

The Case Scenario: Reaching a Diagnosis

One hour later Louise is very difficult to rouse and is unresponsive to commands. A more recent set of observations reveals:

Temperature: 36.7 °C
Heart rate: 70 beats per minute
BP: 140/80 mmHg
Respiratory rate: 10 breaths per minute
SpO$_2$: 95 per cent on 40 per cent oxygen via a facemask
GCS 8/15 (E2, V2, M4)
Left pupil is reacting, normally size 4 mm. Right pupil is now 7 mm with a sluggish response.

1. What are the immediate assessment priorities now?
2. What is the most likely cause of Louise's deterioration?
3. How will her management plan change?

Louise's GCS has fallen from 12 to 8 (Table 4.7). With a GCS of 8 and below Louise's airway is at risk so a doctor will insert an endotracheal tube to secure her airway. Intubation following head injury must be performed with caution until the risk of associated injury to the cervical spine has been eliminated by X-ray. Once the airway is protected a nasogastric or orogastric tube will be inserted to allow the stomach to be emptied. Elevated intracranial pressure (ICP) is associated with an increased risk of vomiting. Vomiting will in turn further increase the ICP. If imaging studies have not excluded the risk of a skull base fracture an orogastric tube will be used due to the danger of passing a nasogastric tube into the brain. Having secured the airway Louise will be placed on a mechanical ventilator to ensure her breathing. Louise now has abnormal pupil responses, with the right pupil being dilated and slow to respond. This indicates compression of the occulomotor nerve on the right side of the brain. Her pulse and blood pressure show her cardiovascular system to be unaffected at this time, but close monitoring would continue, as an elevated ICP may cause bradycardia and systemic hypertension. Louise would be referred to the neurosurgeons and an immediate CT scan is required to determine the cause of Louise's rapid deterioration although an intracranial bleed is highly likely. CT scanning remains the most important imaging tool for traumatic brain injury as it is better able to demonstrate fresh bleeding and bony trauma than MRI. Plain X-rays of the skull are no longer recommended for the assessment of head injury (NICE, 2007).

Table 4.7   Louise's GCS scores

	Admission	1 Hour Post Admission
Eye opening	3	2
Best verbal response	4	2
Best motor response	5	4
Total	12/15	8/15

The CT scan reveals that Louise has an extradural haematoma. Impact to the front and temporal regions of the skull can result in partial or complete rupture of the middle meningeal artery. This artery lies between the dura mater and the skull and the resultant bleeding separates the dura from the skull. The haematoma formed exerts increasing pressure within the skull (Evans and Tippins, 2007). Extradural haemorrhage is seen in approximately 10 per cent of severe head injuries and has a significant mortality. For a given severity of injury, women appear to have more brain swelling and intracranial hypertension than men (Farin et al., 2003).

Medical Management Strategies

Primary injury is damage that occurs at the time of the initial insult and cannot be avoided. Therefore the focus of attention is prevention or reduction of secondary injury. This refers to a group of physiological conditions such as hypoxia, hypotension, elevated ICP, infection and seizure activity that, if not managed, will exacerbate the primary injury and result in a poorer outcome. The principle aims of medical management are maintenance of adequate and stable cerebral perfusion, adequate oxygenation, avoidance of hyper/hypocapnia and avoidance of hyper/hypoglycaemia (Moppett, 2007).

Respiratory Interventions

Once Louise's airway is secure, through either positioning or endotracheal intubation, the aim is to maintain normal blood levels of oxygen (PaO_2) and to maintain the $PaCO_2$ towards the low side of normal (4.5 to 5.0 kPa) (Oertel et al., 2002). The cerebral arterioles are very sensitive to changes in their metabolic environment. As such cerebral blood flow 'responds' to the metabolic needs of the tissues. CO_2 is a potent vasodilator and can produce unwanted effects on both cerebral blood flow and ICP. The effect of raised levels of CO_2 is vasodilatation of the cerebral vessels, with a resultant increase in cerebral blood flow and therefore the ICP. A fall in PaO_2 produces an increase in cerebral blood flow, but only after a threshold has been reached (PaO_2 less than 6.6 kPa). In a state of hypoxaemia at or around these levels, ICP will be elevated as a direct result of an increase in cerebral blood flow. Blood flow through the brain is increased to compensate for the reduction in available oxygen. Oxygen therapy will be given as required or the patient will be mechanically ventilated, as in Louise's case. SpO_2 monitoring will be in place and ABG analysis will be performed as required. Neurogenic pulmonary oedema is a reasonably common complication of elevated ICP and represents increased blood flow to the lungs and damage to the pulmonary capillaries. The aetiology is not well understood, but it may be caused by vascular changes associated with elevated ICP. Treatment is by diuretics and respiratory support, coupled with measures to reduce the ICP

Cardiovascular Interventions and Fluid Balance

IV fluids will be prescribed to maintain normovolaemia. Infusions such as 5 per cent glucose should be avoided as they may worsen any cerebral oedema. It is essential that hypotension is avoided and drugs to support blood pressure (positive inotropes) and to control any cardiac dysrhythmias will be prescribed. Head injury results in a hypermetabolic state and enteral feeding should be commenced as soon as is possible. Early feeding has been shown to improve outcome in patients with traumatic brain injury (Härtl et al., 2008). Elevated ICP can compress the pituitary gland and cause a reduction in secretion of the anti-diuretic hormone, leading to the loss of large volumes of dilute urine and potential hypovolaemia. This is known as diabetes insipidus. Louise is likely to have a urinary catheter inserted to enable accurate hourly output monitoring and early detection of excessive diuresis. This may require the use of a drug called vasopressin, which mimics the action of ADH.

Control of ICP

Following admission to a neurosurgical intensive care unit Louise's ICP can be invasively monitored by insertion of a special catheter into her brain. When elevated ICP is proven it is common practice for it to be managed with a range of interventions including analgesia, sedation, neuromuscular blockade, control of $PaCO_2$ and diuretic therapy. Hypertonic saline is being used increasingly as a therapy to manage elevated ICP. It has been shown to produce a reduction in cerebral oedema by moving water out of the cells; the decrease in cell size reduces the intracranial volume and ICP falls (Helmy et al., 2007).

Management of Blood Glucose

Severe head injury provokes a complex sympathetic and hormonal response, with increased secretion of catecholamines such as adrenaline. This leads to hyperglycaemia with approximately 50 per cent of patients showing blood glucose levels > 11.1 mmol/L within the first 24 hours after admission. Failure to normalise blood glucose is associated with increased mortality (Laird et al., 2004), but the best approach to managing hyperglycaemia in the head injured patient is yet to be decided. Hypoglycaemia may mimic the effects of TBI (Table 4.4), but is not itself a direct result of severe head injury.

Seizure Activity

A seizure represents intermittent and abnormal neural activity within the brain. They are relatively common following TBI, with a reported incidence of between 4 and 25 per cent in the first week following injury (Moppett, 2007). They must be controlled as they increase ICP and if continuous can lead to cerebral oedema. The patient's safety must be maintained throughout the seizure and details such as type of seizure and duration should be noted. Anticonvulsants such as phenytoin or carbamazepine may be prescribed both as prophylaxis against seizure activity and to aid control should a seizure occur.

Surgical Intervention

As discussed earlier there is very little capacity for an increase in volume within the skull and a haematoma in excess of 75 mL is usually fatal (Michael-Titus et al., 2007). Surgical aspiration of the haematoma is therefore a potentially lifesaving procedure.

Ongoing Care Issues and the Role of the Nurse

Following surgical intervention Louise will be nursed on a neurosurgical ICU. She will be sedated, ventilated and will require specialist care. Texts such as Adam and Osborne (2005) and Woodrow (2006) provide detailed information on caring for the ventilated patient. Continuous neurological and cardiovascular monitoring will continue until a stable trend of measurements within normal parameters is maintained. There are, however, a number of care issues more specific to the management of head trauma and these include the following.

The Case Scenario: Ongoing Care Issues

Louise's neurological condition continued to deteriorate. The CT scan revealed a right sided extradural haematoma and so she was transferred to the ICU where she was sedated, intubated and mechanically ventilated. A nasogastric tube was inserted though enteral feeding was not commenced until a surgical opinion was obtained. Continuous cardiac and SpO_2 monitoring was commenced to assess Louise's heart rate, BP and respiratory status, an ICP measurement catheter was inserted and regular assessment of ABGs and capillary blood glucose maintained. An infusion of IV 0.9 per cent sodium chloride was commenced and Louise was prepared for neurosurgery to remove the haematoma and relieve the raised ICP.

Nursing Care Issues
1. Consider the appropriate post-operative monitoring required for Louise.
2. What specific care needs will Louise require?
3. What will happen if the interventions do not work?
4. What are the long-term implications of TBI?

Positioning

Correct positioning and careful movement can promote cerebral venous drainage and minimise spikes in ICP. The head of Louise's bed will be elevated 15 to 30° to facilitate venous outflow and her head will be maintained in neutral alignment to prevent jugular vein compression. Hip flexion will be avoided to prevent any increase in intra-abdominal pressure, which would in turn increase intrathoracic pressure, which would impede venous drainage from her brain. Uncoordinated repositioning must be avoided and to maintain neutral head and neck alignment Louise will be log rolled when turned.

Temperature Control

Elevated ICP impacts upon the ability of the hypothalamus to control body temperature and so Louise may become hyperthermic. This must be avoided as an elevated temperature is associated with an increased body demand for oxygen and with the production of increased levels of CO_2. For every 1 °C rise in body temperature, cerebral oxygen use rises by 10 per cent (Evans and Tippins, 2007). Normothermia is the goal and cooling methods such as fans, tepid sponging, ice packs and cooling blankets may be used. Anti-pyretic drugs such as paracetamol may be prescribed.

Control of Noxious Stimuli

Louise's care environment will be controlled to prevent clustering of activities and excessive stimulation. Painful and distressing procedures will be limited and unnecessary instrumental touch avoided.

What if the Interventions Don't Work?

If homeostatic compensatory mechanisms fail, a small additional change in intracranial volume results in a large increase in ICP. An ICP greater than 33 mmHg is associated with a reduction in cerebral blood flow. This causes stimulation of the vasomotor centre within the brain stem, causing a rise in systemic blood pressure, a widening pulse pressure and bradycardia. This phenomenon of rising blood pressure and falling heart rate is called Cushing's reflex and reflects a compensatory response that attempts to provide adequate CPP in the presence of markedly elevated ICP (Hickey, 2008). When hypertension and bradycardia are associated with an abnormal respiratory pattern such as bradypnoea this is called Cushing's triad and is a warning of imminent or actual brain stem herniation. The descent of the brainstem into the foramen magnum is the end point of malignant brain swelling. The brain stem becomes compressed and brain stem death is imminent. With ICP at this level both pupils are generally fixed and dilated.The diagnosis of brain stem death is governed by clinical guidelines and is rarely seen outside of an intensive care unit. Solid organ donation may be possible after brain stem death.

The Long-term Impact of Traumatic Brain Injury

Nearly half of all patients admitted to hospital following TBI are left with long-term physical or psychological problems (Whitnall et al., 2006); 65 per cent of adults with moderate injury and 85 per cent of adults with severe injury are disabled at one year. Recovery often continues for two to three years, although in many cases patients never fully recover. The potential disabling effects of TBI are multiple (Table 4.8) and include: physical problems, such as difficulty with balance and coordination; emotional and behavioural problems, such as agitation, depression and apathy; and cognitive difficulties, including loss of memory, an inability to concentrate and changes in the speed of information processing (see http://www.headway.co.uk for more information).

Patients who have had sustained TBI requiring surgery must notify the

Table 4.8 Potential long-term impact of traumatic brain injury

Physical problems	• Movement, balance and coordination • Loss of sensation • Tiredness • Headaches • Speaking and swallowing disorders • Bladder and bowel incontinence • Seizures • Sexual problems
Emotional and behavioural problems	• Agitation, anger and irritability • Lack of awareness and insight • Apathy and poor motivation • Depression • Anxiety • Inflexibility and obsessionality • Sexual problems
Cognitive problems	• Memory • Attention and concentration • Speed of information processing • Planning, organising and problem solving • Visio-spatial and perceptual difficulties • Language skills

DVLA and will lose their driving licence for a period of between six months and one year. In 2009 the brain injury charity Headway received Department of Health funding to establish an 'approved provider' scheme, which will set standards for nursing homes, residential homes, transitional living units and those providing respite for someone who has sustained a brain injury.

Summary

The past 20 years have seen major progress in our understanding of the physiology of secondary brain injury. Research as to the optimum way to manage the patient with elevated intracranial pressure goes on, but there is no doubt that patient outcome is improved when secondary problems are reduced or prevented. Accurate assessment is crucial and this chapter has focused on the nurse's role in the assessment of the patient with altered consciousness.

Further Reading

Adam, S. K. and S. Osborne. *Critical Care Nursing: Science and Practice*, 2nd edn (Oxford: Oxford Medical, 2005).

Jevon, P. 'How to Ensure Patient Observations Lead to Effective Management of Altered Consciousness', Nursing Times, 106(6) (2010), 17–18.

NICE. *Head Injury: Triage, Assessment, Investigation and Early Management of Head Injury in Infants, Children and Adults* (London: NICE, 2007).

National Collaborating Centre for Acute Care. *Head Injury: Triage, Assessment, Investigation and Early Management of Head Injury in Infants, Children and Adults* (London: Royal College of Surgeons, 2007) (commissioned by the National Institute for Health and Clinical Excellence).

Scottish Intercollegiate Guidelines Network (SIGN). *Early Management of Patients with a Head Injury: A National Clinical Guideline* (Edinburgh: Scottish Intercollegiate Guidelines Network, 2009).

References

Adam, S. K. and S. Osborne. *Critical Care Nursing: Science and Practice*, 2nd edn (Oxford: Oxford Medical, 2005).

Bader, M. K. and R. Arbour. 'Refractory Increased Intracranial Pressure in Severe Traumatic Brain Injury', *AACN Clinical Issues*, **16**(4) (2005), 526–41.

Evans, C. and E. Tippins. *The Foundations of Emergency Care* (Maidenhead: Open University Press, 2007).

Fairley, D. 'Using a Coma Scale to Assess Patient Conscious Levels', *Nursing Times*, **101** (2005), 38–47.

Farin, A., R. Deutsch, A. Biegon and L. F. Marshall. 'Sex-related Differences in Patients with Severe Head Injury: Greater Susceptibility to Brain Swelling in Female Patients 50 Years of Age and Younger', *Journal of Neurosurgery*, 98 (2003), 32–6.

Härtl, R., L. M. Gerber, Q. Ni and J. Ghajar. 'Effects of Early Nutrition on Deaths Due to Severe Traumatic Brain Injury', *Journal of Neurosurgery*, **109** (2008), 50–6.

Helmy, A., M. Vizcaychip and A. K. Gupta. 'Traumatic Brain Injury: Intensive Care Management', *British Journal of Anaesthesia*, **99**(1) (2007), 32–42.

Hickey, J. V. *The Clinical Practice of Neurological and Neurosurgical Nursing*, 6th edn. (Philadelphia: Lippincott-Raven, 2008).

Jevon, P. *Treating the Critically Ill Adult* (Oxford: Blackwell, 2008).

Jevon, P. and B. Ewens (eds). *Monitoring the Critically Ill Patient*, 2nd edn (Oxford: Blackwell Science, 2007).

Laird, A. M., P. R. Miller, P. D. Kilgo, J. W. Meredith and M. C. Chang. 'Relationship of Early Hyperglycaemia to Mortality in Trauma Patients', *Journal of Trauma: Injury, Infection and Critical Care*, 56 (2004), 1058–62.

Lindsay, K. W. and I. Bone. *Neurology and Neurosurgery Illustrated*, 4th edn. (Edinburgh: Churchill Livingstone, 2004).

Michael-Titus, A., P. Revest and P. Shortland. *The Nervous System: Basic Science and Clinical Conditions* (Edinburgh: Churchill Livingstone, 2007).

Mooney, G. P. and D. M. Comerford. 'Neurological Observations', *Nursing Times*, **99** (2003), 24–5.

Moppett, I. K. 'Traumatic Brain Injury: Assessment, Resuscitation and Early Management', *British Journal of Anaesthesia*, **99**(1) (2007), 18–31.

Oertel, M., D. F. Kelly, J. H. Lee et al. 'Efficacy of Hyperventilation, Blood Pressure Elevation, and Metabolic Suppression Therapy in Controlling Intracranial Pressure after Head Injury', *Journal of Neurosurgery*, **97** (2002), 1045–53.

Sheppard, M. and M. Wright. *Principles and Practice of High Dependency Nursing*, 2nd edn. (London: Bailliere Tindall, 2005).

Teasdale, G. and B. Jennett. 'Assessment of Coma and Impaired Consciousness, a Practical Scale', *Lancet*, **2** (1974), 81–4.

Waterhouse, C. 'The Glasgow Coma Score and Other Neurological Observations', *Nursing Standard*, **19**(33) (2005), 56–64.

Werner, C. and K. Engelhard. 'Pathophysiology of Traumatic Brain Injury', *British Journal of Anaesthesia*, **99** (2007), 4–9.

Whitnall, L., T. M. McMillan, G. D. Murray and G. M. Teasdale. 'Disability in Young People and Adults after Head Injury: 5–7 Year Follow up of a Prospective Cohort Study', *Journal of Neurology, Neurosurgery and Psychiatry*, **77**(5) (2006), 640–5.

Woodrow P. *Intensive Care Nursing: A Framework for Practice*, 2nd edn (London: Routledge, 2006).

5

Acute Coronary Syndrome

Alison Ketchell

Introduction: Coronary Heart Disease in Context

Coronary heart disease (CHD) remains the leading cause of death in men and women in England and Wales, accounting for over 80,000 deaths per year despite pharmacological and technological advances (England & Wales Office for National Statistics, 2007) (Table 5.1). In March 2000, the Department of Health published a set of targets within the National Service Framework for Coronary Heart Disease (NSF CHD), which aimed to reduce mortality and morbidity from CHD (DH, 2009). Acute coronary syndrome (ACS) is an umbrella term used to describe a range of acute cardiac events associated with CHD, ranging from unstable angina (UA) to non-ST segment elevation myocardial infarction (NSTEMI) and ST segment elevation myocardial infarction (STEMI). In response to overwhelming evidence of the survival benefit of reperfusion therapy for acute STEMI (within six hours of onset of symptoms), the National Infarct Angioplasty Project (NIAP) recommends primary percutaneous coronary intervention (PCI)

Table 5.1 UK death rates in 2006 from coronary heart disease

Men	=	46,316 (1 in 5)
Men < 75 years	=	19,480
MI all ages	=	18,845
Women	=	36,272 (1 in 6)
Women < 75 years	=	6,868
MI all ages	=	14,347
UK CHD total	=	82,588
UK MI total	=	33,192

Source: England and Wales Office for National Statistics (2007). Reproduced under the Open Government Licence v1.0.

within 120 to 150 minutes of the patient's call for help ('call-to-balloon' time) if available (DH, 2008). Alternatively, in areas where PCI is currently not available within this time frame, eligible patients presenting within 60 minutes of calling for help (60 minute call-to-needle goal) and 30 minutes of hospital arrival (door-to-needle time) should receive thrombolysis (DH, 2000). Achieving these targets necessitates prompt and accurate assessment of all chest pain patients in order that a definitive working diagnosis can be established to inform the most appropriate and timely treatment strategy. In line with NICE clinical guidance 50 (NICE, 2007a), emphasis upon the importance of a full clinical assessment, monitoring and management of a patient presenting with chest pain during the acute phase is the focus of this chapter.

Aim and Learning Outcomes

The Aim

The aim of this chapter is to explore the priorities of early accurate assessment and management of the individual presenting acutely with sudden onset of central chest pain. The main focus of the chapter is acute coronary syndrome with a specific emphasis upon acute STEMI. The case scenario provides the basis for the application of evidence-based theoretical rationale to clinical practice.

Learning Outcomes

At the end of this chapter the reader will be able to:

1. Define acute coronary syndrome and distinguish between the differing manifestations of ACS.
2. Identify and explain the pathophysiological basis of the presenting signs and symptoms of acute ST elevation myocardial infarction.
3. Recognise the immediate assessment, specific monitoring and key investigations required to enable an accurate and timely diagnosis.
4. Explore the evidence underpinning immediate priorities of management with a particular focus upon pharmacological and invasive interventions.
5. Appreciate the role of different health professionals in acute assessment and management of ACS.
6. Be aware of the common complications associated with acute MI.

The Case Scenario: The Presenting Complaint

John is a 58-year-old, previously fit and well Caucasian gentleman who was admitted to the accident and emergency department at 09.00 hours, complaining of severe crushing central chest pain, which awoke him at 07.30 hours that morning. At 08.30 hours Gaviscon® had not relieved the pain and so John called 999. The paramedic ambulance crew gave John 300 mg of soluble aspirin orally and a 3 mg suscard buccal tablet was placed between his upper lip and gum during the journey to hospital. On admission John continued to complain of pain with radiation into his left arm and neck and he looked pale, was sweaty, felt nauseous, appeared to be restless and agitated and reported never having experienced pain like this before. John is divorced and lives alone though his partner and two children, who are both married, live locally. John is an HGV driver; he smokes twenty cigarettes per day; drinks five to six units of alcohol a week; enjoys walking and swimming and has a body mass index (BMI) of 26. A provisional diagnosis of acute coronary syndrome is made.

Consider the following:

1. With reference to the underlying pathophysiology describe what is meant by ACS.
2. What are the common signs and symptoms associated with ACS?
3. List the known modifiable and non-modifiable risk factors for heart disease and identify those that appear to directly affect John.

Coronary Heart Disease

The Coronary Circulation

An explanation of normal coronary anatomy is a useful prerequisite to understanding the pathological disease process associated with coronary artery disease. The function of the heart requires a continuous supply of nutrients and oxygen to the myocardium, which is supplied via a network of coronary arteries and veins. There are two main coronary arteries – the right and left – which originate from the right and left coronary sinus of valsalva, respectively, just above the aortic valve.

The right coronary artery (RCA) follows the right atrioventricular groove, eventually dividing into two large branches: the posterior descending (PD) and marginal (M) branches (Figure 5.1). In most hearts, the RCA and its branches are responsible for supplying oxygenated blood to the right atrium, the right ventricle (RV) and the inferior surface of the left ventricle

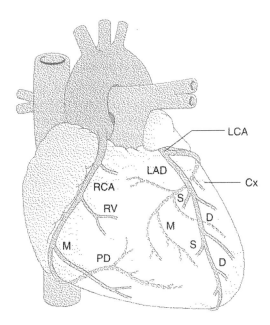

Figure 5.1   The normal coronary circulation.

(LV), the sinus node (about 70 per cent of cases), atrioventricular node (about 90 per cent of cases) and the common bundle of the conduction system. The left coronary artery (LCA) leaves the aorta as the left main stem (LMS) before almost immediately dividing into two major coronary arteries: the left anterior descending (LAD) and the circumflex (Cx) (Figure 5.1). The LAD descends along the interventricular septum, further dividing into large septal (S) and diagonal (D) branches, which supply oxygenated blood to the anterior surface of the left ventricle and most of the left and right bundle branches of the conduction system. The Cx follows the left atrioventricular groove, supplying the lateral and posterior aspects of the left ventricle, the sinus node (about 25 per cent of cases, with the RCA and Cx jointly responsible in the remaining 5 per cent) and the atrioventricular node (about 10 per cent of cases). The major vessels lie on the epicardial surface of the myocardium before further dividing to form a perfuse system of smaller branches that perforate the entire thickness of the muscle wall. The arteries then divide to form arterioles and a massive capillary network, which surrounds and supplies each muscle fibre with essential nutrients and oxygen and from which almost all the oxygen is extracted by the myocardial fibres. Collateral connections of less than 200 micrometres (µm) in diameter exist between the branches of the coronary arteries at subarteriolar level, though under normal circumstances very few collateral vessels are visible. Venules and veins join to form large venous channels, which return the deoxygenated blood, carbon dioxide and waste products of cellular metabolism to the right atrium via the anterior cardiac veins (right coronary blood) and the coronary sinus (left coronary blood).

The coronary artery lining is composed of an outer collagenous layer (tunica adventitia) for protective strength, a thicker medial layer of elastic fibres and smooth muscle (tunica media) enabling contraction and relaxation and an endothelial lining of simple squamous cells (tunica intima) to promote a laminar flow of blood along the vessel (Figure 5.2). The endothelium is normally a metabolically active barrier between circulating blood and the vessel lining which is responsible for secreting a range of protective vasoactive substances that promote a non-thrombogenic and non-adherent surface.

Coronary Artery Disease (CAD)

Coronary artery disease describes a pathological process affecting the coronary artery. The commonest cause of coronary artery disease is **atherosclerosis**, though other pathological disorders of the coronary arteries do exist (Table 5.2). CAD may exist for a number of years without affecting myocardial function and is therefore not necessarily synonymous with coronary (ischaemic) heart disease.

The Development of Coronary Atherosclerosis

CAD is largely attributed to the presence of atherosclerotic plaque between the inner (intima) and muscle (medial) linings of the walls of large and medium sized arteries (Figure 5.2). The development of atherosclerotic plaque is thought to begin with a 'fatty streak', commonly found within the

Table 5.2   Pathological disorders of the coronary arteries

- Congenital deformities, e.g. arterio-venous fistulae, anomalous origin of pulmonary artery
- Coronary embolism, e.g. arising from left atrium, left ventricle, mitral or aortic valve disorders, infective endocarditis
- Syphilitic aortitis
- Dissecting aortic aneurysm occluding coronary artery
- Connective tissue disorders, e.g. polyarteritis, pseudoxanthoma elasticum, systemic lupus erythematosus
- Coronary artery spasm of normal or diseased arteries
- Atherosclerosis is the commonest cause

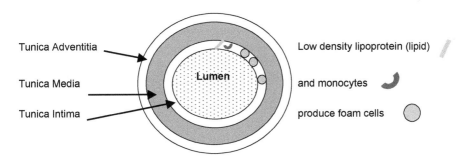

Figure 5.2   The fatty streak.

intimal lining at a very young age. Excess circulating low density lipoproteins (LDLs) infiltrate and accumulate within the inner lining of the artery
where they become oxidised and engulfed by macrophagic monocytes to
form 'foam cells'. Circulating T cell lympohocytes move into the space, activating an inflammatory response. The foam cells, macrophages and
lymphocytes form the 'fatty streak' (Figure 5.2). Fatty streaks are relatively
innocuous in themselves; however, they may increase in frequency between
8 and 18 years and exist in the aorta and coronary arteries of most individuals by the age of 20 (Lilly, 2007) and may develop into a more injurious
atherosclerotic lesion.

Progression of the fatty streak into an atherosclerotic lesion known as
'fibro-lipid plaque' is dependent upon the location within the coronary
artery and the presence of predisposing risk factors (Table 5.3). It may
develop as young as 15 years, with a propensity to progress rapidly between
15 and 35 years in susceptible individuals (Jowett and Thompson, 2003).
Risk factors, regardless of their modifiability, interact in a synergistic manner
and therefore the more risk factors that John has the more susceptible he is
to the development of coronary artery atherosclerotic disease.

John's evident risk factors are his age and gender, smoking and possible
stress related to his occupation as an HGV driver, and are sufficient to have
increased John's susceptibility to atherosclerotic development. The pathological progression of fatty streak to fibro-lipid plaque is a complex process mediated by endothelial dysfunction and foam cell activity. Increased endothelial
permeability facilitates further entry of lipid into the intima and failure to
secrete normal anti-thrombotic molecules attracts platelets to the area and
increases the potential for localised platelet aggregation and adhesion. Foam
cells, activated platelets and endothelial cells also secrete a number of factors
that stimulate the migration and proliferation of smooth muscle cells into the
intima, which then engulf lipid to form more 'foam cells'. A highly thrombo-
genic necrotic core encased within a fibrous cap develops (Figure 5.3).

Table 5.3   Predisposing risk factors associated with development of atherosclerotic plaque

Pathophysiological factors
- Epicardial section of the coronary artery especially at bends and bifurcations
- Increased C-reactive protein (CRP) (AHA 2003) or elevated homocysteine (Yusuf et al. 2001a)
- Infection, e.g. chlamydia pneumoniae, helicobacter pylori, herpes, cytomegalovirus have been implicated though their role remains unclear (Ross 1999)

Non-modifiable risk factors
- Genetic predisposition (family history of early CHD)
- Increasing age
- Gender: males are more susceptible
- Personality type D, anger, hostility (Denollet et al. 2006)
- Ethnic origin, e.g. South Asian origin (Yusuf et al. 2001b)

Modifiable risk factors
- Smoking
- High serum cholesterol levels, i.e. elevated low density lipid (LDL) and low high density lipids (HDL)
- High glucose levels, diabetes and/or insulin resistance
- High saturated fat diet
- Hypertension
- Overweight and obesity
- Physical inactivity and sedentary lifestyle
- Chronic work related stress
- Social isolation and depression (Barth et al. 2004)

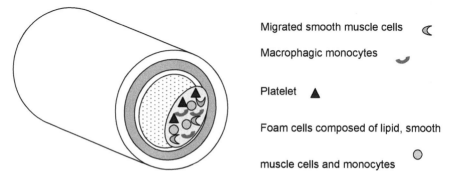

Migrated smooth muscle cells

Macrophagic monocytes

Platelet

Foam cells composed of lipid, smooth

muscle cells and monocytes

Figure 5.3   The fibro-lipid plaque.

It is thought that plaque enlargement may be further augmented by small recurrent ulcerations within the cap, which expose plaque contents to the circulation, attracting further aggregation and adhesion of activated platelets, which become incorporated into the lesion. Initially most atherosclerotic plaque expands away from the vessel lumen. However, as it increases in size plaque may begin to project inwards, causing progressive narrowing of the lumen. Many individuals live unknowingly with coronary artery disease for a number of years as the degree of narrowing is not thought to be of significance until it obstructs approximately 70 per cent of the luminal diameter. Once atherosclerotic plaque produces significant stenosis of the vessel it may impair sufficient blood flow to the serving myocardium, leading to clinical symptoms of coronary (ischaemic) heart disease.

Coronary (Ischaemic) Heart Disease

The Joint International Society and Federation of Cardiology and World Health Organisation Task Force have described CHD as myocardial impairment caused by an imbalance between coronary blood flow and myocardial demand directly associated with changes in the coronary circulation. In practice it is often referred to as ischaemic heart disease (IHD). Early symptoms are often precipitated by exercise when a narrowed coronary artery fails to increase blood supply in response to increased myocardial demand. Insufficient oxygen supply leads to myocardial cell ischaemia, which most often presents as chest pain or chest discomfort, known as 'angina'. Stable angina describes chest pain that is triggered by exercise and usually responds to rest and coronary vasodilation with rapid onset, short acting nitrate therapy in various forms such as glyceryl trinitrate (GTN) spray, a GTN tablet below the tongue or suscard buccal® between the lip and gum. A provisional diagnosis of stable angina based upon symptom presentation may be confirmed by a non-invasive exercise tolerance test demonstrating ischaemic electrocardiographic (ECG) changes or invasive coronary angiography. It is often managed by general practitioners with beta blockers (e.g. atenolol® or metoprolol®), which slow the heart rate and therefore reduce the demand for myocardial oxygen, and a daily anti-platelet agent such as aspirin 75 to 150 mg daily. Prophylactic use of GTN prior to exercise or in response to chest pain should also be advised. Stable angina is generally considered to be a warning sign of CHD rather than an acute event in itself. Some individuals presenting acutely will have a history of stable angina; however, as in John's case the acute event may be the first sign of coronary artery disease.

Acute Coronary Syndrome

The acute coronary event is now thought to be a consequence of sudden rupture or erosion of the plaque cap and thrombus formation rather than vessel occlusion caused by progressive plaque enlargement. The fate of the plaque may in part be dependent upon the composition of the plaque cap and contents. Plaque composed of a high proportion of smooth muscle cells and connective tissue and covered in a thick fibrous cap tends to be more prominent on angiography yet often appears to be relatively stable and less likely to rupture. In contrast, plaques rich in lipid with a thin fibrous cap are considered to be 'vulnerable' and much more susceptible to rupture despite their often minor appearance on angiography (Lilly, 2007). Current theory suggests that the presence of factors such as excessive smoking, hyperlipidaemia, diabetes, infection, stress and hypertension may cause sudden changes in coronary blood pressure or vascular tone, which may predispose plaque rupture leading to further plaque enlargement or an acute coronary event. The term 'acute coronary syndrome' (ACS) describes a spectrum of clinical syndromes ranging from unstable angina (UA) to myocardial infarction.

Unstable Angina

Unstable angina results from superficial fissuring of plaque and collagen exposure to the circulation, which attracts activated platelets to the area, enabling platelet aggregation, adhesion and platelet deposition, commonly known as 'white clot'. Partial occlusion of the vessel severely restricts flow of blood and oxygen to the myocardium beyond the narrowing, leading to cell ischaemia. Ischaemic myocardium classically presents as a sudden onset of chest pain at rest that is not easily resolved with nitrate therapy, a normal or abnormal ST segment and T wave on ECG and negative serum troponin at twelve hours post onset of symptoms. Approximately 10 to 20 per cent of patients diagnosed with unstable angina will progress to MI within the ensuing days or weeks if they fail to respond well to medical therapy. John's chest pain presentation could indicate unstable angina as a possible differential diagnosis; however, given his minimal response to nitrate therapy (suscard buccal®) further investigation is required before a definitive diagnosis can be made.

Myocardial Infarction

Angiographic evidence suggests that approximately 15 per cent of MIs occur as a result of severe (> 90 per cent) stenosis of the artery but the majority are

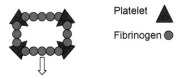

Platelet adhesion provides the platform for the clotting cascade to activate clotting factor X (CFX)

⟹ CFXa necessary for the final common pathway of clotting

⇩

CFXa converts prothrombin (CFII) to thrombin (CFIIa)

⇩

Thrombin (CFIIa) converts soluble fibrinogen to insoluble fibrin = 'red clot' formation

Figure 5.4 Clot formation.

as a direct consequence of plaque rupture and total coronary occlusion with thrombus. In most cases the site of platelet deposition facilitates the clotting mechanism, leading to the conversion of soluble prothrombin and fibrinogen into insoluble thrombus formation and fibrin deposition, known as 'red clot', at the site of rupture.

The subsequent total coronary occlusion causes abrupt cessation of blood and oxygen to the serving myocardium, resulting in patchy areas of ischaemia, injury and infarction. Myocardial injury is reversible damage caused by temporary blood and oxygen deprivation, which may be resolved if blood flow is restored within 30 to 45 minutes. If the sudden cessation of blood flow is not limited to less than 45 minutes myocardial infarction (cell necrosis) ensues from endocardium to epicardium in a time-dependent manner with permanent necrotic damage to affected cells leading to cell fibrosis, electrical inactivity and loss of contractility. The extent of necrosis and resulting size of infarction may be restricted to patchy areas of muscle or may affect the full thickness of myocardium, and is dependent upon the length of time of absent blood flow, the degree of diminution of blood flow affected by localised vasomotor changes and the extent of collateral flow. In the presence of atherosclerotic coronary artery obstruction, collateral connections may become larger and functionally capable of restoring some blood flow to a distal portion of an obstructed vessel from a non-obstructed neighbour. In some individuals the collateral coronary circulation may play a significant role in myocardial damage limitation and greatly improve long-term prognosis. MI typically manifests as a sudden onset of chest pain unrelieved by nitrate, with (STEMI) or without (NSTEMI) ST segment elevation on ECG, and is associated with elevated serum troponin levels.

The Case Scenario: The Immediate Assessment Priorities

John's chest pain was not relieved despite the suscard buccal® and he began to complain of headache. Twenty-four per cent oxygen therapy via a face mask was commenced and venous access was secured with a 14G cannula inserted into his left antecubital fossa. The suscard buccal® was removed and IV diamorphine 5 mg and IV metoclopramide 10 mg was administered.

Immediate Assessment
1. What are the immediate assessment priorities in John's case and what is the rationale for each measure?
2. Describe the common cardiac and non-cardiac causes of chest pain.
3. Identify the common characteristics that help to distinguish different causes of chest pain.
4. Describe the underlying pathophysiology of ischaemic chest pain.
5. How would a definitive cause and diagnosis for the chest pain be established?
6. Describe the rationale for the treatment received so far.

Assessment and Reaching a Diagnosis

For the sake of narrative fluency each aspect of the preliminary assessment will be discussed separately; however, in practice it is the integration of assessment information that is essential for the accurate and prompt definitive diagnosis required for appropriate symptom relief and life saving intervention. Secondary assessment involves a more detailed history, examination and further investigation once the patient is stabilised.

The Preliminary Assessment

Myocardial ischaemia, injury and infarction alters cell membrane permeability to essential ions for normal electrophysiological and contractile function and may predispose life threatening arrhythmias such as ventricular tachycardia (VT), ventricular fibrillation (VF) and atrio-ventricular (AV) node conduction defects, as well as adversely affecting contractile strength. Bennett (2006) offers further explanation and ECG interpretation of a range of common arrhythmias. Death from myocardial infarction is most likely to occur within the first hour of onset of symptoms and the usual cause is VF. The incidence of primary VF post acute MI is approximately 4.7 per cent (Dubois et al., 1986; Thompson et al., 2000; Henkel et al., 2006) and therefore the ABC approach to assessment is essential to establish John's immediate haemodynamic status.

Airway

Most patients like John are fully conscious and able to maintain a patent airway; however, the risk of cardio-respiratory arrest is sufficiently significant to warrant continuous vigilance. In the event of clinical deterioration the 'look, listen and feel' method of airway assessment should be employed (see Chapter 2) and basic life support measures including insertion of adjunct airway management must be instigated in the event of inadequate airway maintenance.

Breathing

Breathing assessment will include respiratory rate, depth, regularity and noise observed for 30 seconds and thereafter every four hours if findings fall within normal parameters (Table 5.4). The presence and characteristics of a cough and sputum should be documented and a sample of expectorant collected for microbiology if infection is suspected. Provided peripheral perfusion is adequate, continuous non-invasive oxygen saturation (SpO_2) monitoring measures the adequacy of respiration and should be maintained above 95 per cent. Adequacy of peripheral perfusion can be assessed by capillary refill time: normal capillary refill time is less than two seconds. Arterial blood gases are not usually necessary unless airway and breathing assessment thus far have revealed respiratory abnormalities. It is usual for individuals with chest pain to receive a high (60 to 100 per cent) concentration of supplementary oxygen via a non-rebreathe bag to maintain SpO_2 within normal limits. However, unless saturation levels are below 95 per cent there is no evidence to suggest that routine supplementary O_2 provides any real benefit (O'Driscoll et al., 2008). McNulty et al. (2005) concluded that high flow oxygen aimed at maintaining oxygen saturation levels at 100 per cent may increase coronary vascular resistance and reduce coronary blood flow, adversely affecting myocardial oxygen supply. Therefore some

Table 5.4 Normal physiological parameters

- Heart rate: 60–95 beats/min
- Heart rhythm: regular PQRST sinus rhythm
- Systolic BP: 100–140mmHg
- Diastolic BP: 60–90 mmHg
- Respiration: 12–16/min, noiseless and effortless
- Oxygen saturation: >95%

caution with routine administration of supplementary oxygen should be applied and if saturation is above 94 per cent and the mask exacerbates feelings of nausea, sweating and claustrophobia then it is reasonable to remove the mask. However, maintenance of close observation and monitoring of breathing and SpO_2 levels to ensure they remain within normal limits is imperative. Saturation levels below 95 per cent may indicate hypoxaemia and the need for supplementary O_2 therapy to ensure adequate oxygenation of coronary flow to the myocardium. It should be remembered that oxygen dose, method of delivery and target saturation should be based upon accurate assessment and prescribed by a medical practitioner.

Circulation

Circulation assessment via cardiac monitoring (three or five lead) provides a continuous recording of John's heart rate, regularity and rhythm and enables prevention or early detection and treatment of potentially life threatening atrial and ventricular arrhythmias (see Bennett, 2006, for further explanation and ECG interpretation). John's radial pulse should be palpated for 30 seconds to assess pulse volume and skin temperature, which provide a useful indication of perfusion. A regular sinus rhythm between 60 and 95 beats/min is expected. A sinus tachycardia up to approximately 140 beats/min might indicate pain, anxiety or a physiological response to low blood pressure (BP) to maintain an adequate cardiac output. A heart rate below 60 beats/min may be within John's normal range, particularly if he participates in regular vigorous exercise. Alternatively it may indicate a conduction defect in electrical activity across the heart and a potential fall in cardiac output. John's BP may be within normal limits (Table 5.4) or a high BP may be indicative of pain, anxiety or underlying hypertension. A low BP may be normal for John or indicative of failure of the heart to maintain an adequate cardiac output during the acute event. If John's observations are within normal parameters it is safe to record them and re-assess four hours later, during intervention or in response to other evidence of deterioration. Observations that are outside normal parameters should be observed continuously, recorded and reported to medical staff for intervention and repeated as frequently as every ten minutes until a stable trend is established.

A slight rise in John's four hourly temperature recording between 37 and 38 °C during the first 24 hours might be expected as a sign of the acute inflammatory process. A marked increase in temperature above 38 °C may indicate active infection and should be further investigated. During observation and recording of vital signs a brief verbal history of the presenting signs and symptoms can be ascertained from John.

Signs, Symptoms and Symptom Relief

Patients experiencing ACS most commonly present with severe chest pain, although this can vary significantly from one individual to the next as gender (female), age (> 65) and the presence of diabetes can alter pain perception and symptom presentation. At a cellular level an insufficient supply of oxygen to meet myocardial demand provokes anaerobic respiration as a means of energy production, with the consequent accumulation of the by-product lactic acid and excess unused adenosine within the cell. Adenosine and lactic acid stimulate cardiac nociceptors, which transmit pain signals to the medulla via sympathetic afferent fibres located in the upper thoracic and lower cervical spinal cord, giving rise to the experience of chest and arm pain, and cardiac vagal afferent fibres, which convey a feeling of neck and jaw pain (Foreman, 1999). As a consequence ischaemic pain is typically described as diffuse rather than localised central chest pain with radiation into the arms, jaw and neck. John presented with classic characteristics of ischaemic cardiac pain, which include common descriptors such as 'crushing', 'heavy', 'band-like' and 'squeezing'. Ischaemic pain is not 'stabbing' in nature, though occasionally some individuals may describe it as 'sharp' (referring to the intensity rather than knife-like quality) or 'burning'. A localised left or right sided 'sharp' or 'stabbing' chest pain is more likely to be associated with a respiratory cause (Table 5.5). Stable angina may be precipitated by a number of factors, such as exercise, emotional states, a heavy meal, cold weather or an autonomic sympathetically mediated tachycardia. However, severe unstable angina or an acute MI can occur at rest. Although some individuals experience maximal pain from the onset, many describe an increase in intensity over minutes or hours that becomes constant and eventually recedes with intervention. Often the history of the preceding weeks reveals increasing

Table 5.5 Common causes of chest pain

Cardiac	*Non-cardiac*
• Ischaemia: stable angina; unstable angina • Non ST elevation MI (NSTEMI) • ST elevation MI (STEMI) • Dissecting aortic aneurysm • Pericarditis • Myocarditis	• Respiratory: infection, pulmonary embolus, pneumothorax, pleuritis • Gastro-intestinal: oesophagitis, gastritis, spasm, gastric/duodenal ulcer, acute cholecystitis, pancreatitis • Muscular-skeletal • Herpes zoster (shingles) • Anxiety • Referred pain

episodes of similar though less severe pain. Ischaemic pain is not aggravated or relieved by hunger or food (gastric origin) movement or respiration (pericarditic, pleuritic or musculo-skeletal) or non-steroidal anti-inflammatory agents such as Ibuprofen (Table 5.5). Ischaemia is usually relieved by the coronary vasodilating properties of nitrate drugs, though unstable episodes may require successive treatment to secure complete pain relief. Some patients may complain of a consequent headache with continued nitrate therapy due to the associated cerebral vasodilation. If pain persists beyond 30 minutes despite nitrate therapy then MI should be suspected. Pain from myocardial injury and infarction will only respond to opiate therapy such as intravenous (IV) diamorphine (2.5 to 5 mg) or morphine sulphate (10 mg) and for this reason suscard buccal® was removed and John was given intravenous (IV) diamorphine 5 mg. A verbal measure, usually on a 0 to 10 verbal rating scale with 0 being 'no pain' and 10 being 'the worst pain ever', enables John to provide a subjective assessment of his pain and may inform the need for repeated IV diamorphine until complete pain relief is achieved. Continuous assessment of respiratory effort can alert practitioners to the potential depressive effects upon the respiratory centre, in which case IV naloxone® may be required to reverse the opiate effects.

A full assessment, including a range of questions pertaining to chest pain symptoms (Table 5.6), should be performed in the first instance, followed by a re-assessment of John's perception of pain on a 0 to 10 scale until it has completely subsided or with recurrence. Questions related to the locality and characteristics of the pain established during history taking, assessment and clinical examination may reveal the differential diagnosis. However, not all patients experience chest pain, those who do may not always describe the classic descriptive features discussed and caution with over-reliance upon patient history is advised, as a degree of overlap in location and symptom description between patients with cardiac pain and those with non-cardiac chest pain has been suggested (Eslick, 2005). Moreover, for some, chest pain may be over-shadowed by other associated symptoms such as nausea, vomit-

Table 5.6   Assessment of descriptive features of chest pain

- Site
- Radiation
- Character
- Speed of onset and cessation
- Duration
- Precipitating, aggravating & relieving factors
- Severity: 0 to 10 scale
- Associated signs: nausea, sweating, pallor

Table 5.7   Strategies that might help to reduce anxiety during the acute phase

---

1. Adequate, timely pain assessment and relief.
2. Constant reassurance through simple, repetitive, clear, here and now information regarding current treatment and care. Provide careful explanation in answer to questions posed by John.
3. Visibility, approachability and presence enabling John to attract attention easily.
4. Promotion of a professional but compassionate competent manner.
5. Close monitoring may provide a sense of safety for some, though once the intensity of observation is relaxed stress levels may increase

---

ing, breathlessness and syncope. Nausea and vomiting is a common response to pain, hypotension and opiate therapy. It has been specifically associated with infarction of the inferior aspect of the left ventricular myocardium (Culi et al., 2001), though it has also been suggested that infarct size rather than location may be the key factor (Herlihy et al., 2004). The mechanism remains unclear, though stimulus of autonomic receptors in close proximity to the ischaemic zone may trigger the vomiting centre within the medulla. It is therefore customary to administer an anti-emetic such as IV metoclopramide 10 mg in conjunction with opiate therapy and ensure that vomit bowls, tissues and mouthwash are readily available to John. Dyspnoea or shortness of breath may be indicative of left ventricular failure, respiratory disease such as chronic obstructive pulmonary disease or anxiety, and should be thoroughly evaluated as part of the initial ABC assessment. Although they are not definitive physical signs of MI, most patients experience evidence of autonomic sympathetic nervous activation and peripheral vasoconstriction such as profuse diaphoresis (sweating) and pallor mediated by pain and anxiety, which may excite an associated tachycardia and a consequent undesirable increase in cardiac workload. A number of strategies may be employed to help to alleviate some of John's anxiety and tension associated with the gravity of the situation from his perspective (Table 5.7).

Other accompanying signs, such as palpitations, syncope (transient loss of consciousness), dizziness or light headedness, are less common, though they may reflect altered cardiac output, excess vagal stimulation, bradycardia or arrhythmia and should be further observed and investigated. Myocardial ischaemia (insufficient oxygen) and infarction (oxygen deprivation) alter the electrical activity of the affected cells and may be visualised by the ECG.

Specific Investigations

The ECG provides a pictorial image of the electrical activity of the heart. Electrodes (red upper right, yellow upper left, green lower left, black lower

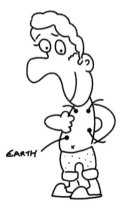

Figure 5.5 Limb lead electrode positions.

right) strategically positioned on the upper and lower limbs or chest sense
and transmit cardiac electrical activity via leads to a monitor (Figure 5.5).
Cardiac monitoring is commonly set to rely upon the green lower left electrode (lead II) to record the heart rate and rhythm. The cardiac monitor
interprets, augments and converts the signal into a wave form on the screen.
A flat isoelectric line corresponds with absent electrical activity within the
heart. An electrical impulse travelling across the heart towards an electrode
is transformed into an upright deflection above the baseline and conversely
an electrical impulse travelling away from an electrode is transcribed as a
downward deflection below the baseline.

Figure 5.6 depicts the normal PqRST complex in lead II of the ECG. The
small, upright, rounded P wave represents the electrical impulse as it travels
across the atria (atrial depolarisation) (Figure 5.7). The PR interval, measured
from the beginning of the P wave to the beginning of the R wave, represents
the time it takes for the electrical impulse to cross the atria and conduct
down through the AV node. As conduction through the AV node is slow and
the electrode at the skin surface is not sufficiently sensitive to sense it the PR
interval is represented as a short flat line after the P wave. The q point or
small negative physiological q wave that follows the PR interval represents
the impulse as it travels across the upper ventricular septum in a left to right
direction. The qRS represents the electrical impulse as it conducts rapidly
down the right and left ventricles (ventricular depolarisation) towards the
electrode (R wave). Once the electrical impulse has conducted across the
entire ventricular muscle mass, ventricular depolarisation is complete and
electrical activity momentarily suspended to allow the ventricles time to
fully contract in response to the electrical impulse. As the electrode can no
longer detect electrical activity the wave returns to the baseline (S wave) to

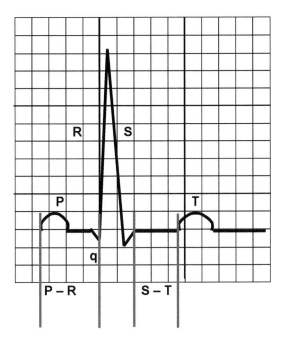

Figure 5.6 The normal PqRST complex.

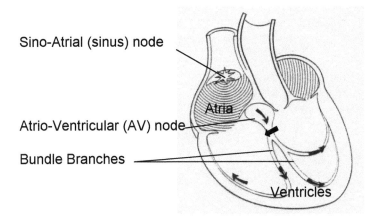

Figure 5.7 Electrical conduction across the heart.

form the flat isoelectric ST segment. In order that the cardiac cells may respond to another electrical impulse they must return to their original electrical state (repolarisation). Atrial repolarisation is not sensed by the surface ECG; however, ventricular repolarisation gives rise to a small, upright, rounded T wave. The 12 lead ECG utilises 10 electrodes placed across the

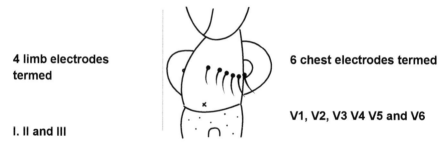

4 limb electrodes termed

6 chest electrodes termed

V1, V2, V3 V4 V5 and V6

I. II and III

Figure 5.8   The 12 lead ECG electrode positions.

chest (Figure 5.8) to provide a PqRST image of the electrical impulse from 12 different viewpoints.

As the muscle mass of the left ventricle (LV) is the greater and tends to sit uppermost in the chest and the majority of electrodes are positioned around the left chest wall, the qRS complexes largely reflect LV depolarisation in most leads (Figure 5.9).

The 12 lead ECG offers visual images of electrical depolarisation and repolarisation of difference aspects of the LV (Table 5.8).

The ECG provides a non-invasive, widely accessible, inexpensive test for the evaluation of chest pain. Ischaemia (insufficient oxygen) and injury (oxygen starvation) initially delay repolarisation of affected cardiac cells, which may translate into an altered ST segment and/or T wave changes on ECG. Depression of the ST segment more than 2 mm below the baseline in

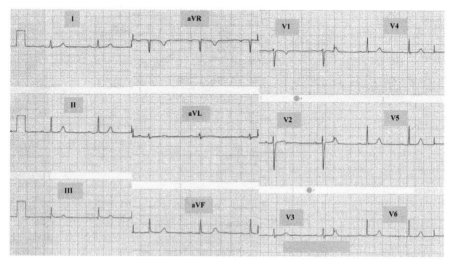

Figure 5.9   Normal 12 lead ECG.

Table 5.8 Twelve ECG leads, corresponding coronary artery and affected area of myocardium

II, III, AVF	Right coronary artery (RCA)	Inferior wall: usually left ventricle (LV). 25% affect the right ventricle inferior wall visualised in V4R, V5R and V6R
I, AVL, V1 to V6	Proximal left anterior descending (LAD)	Left ventricle: extensive anterior region
V1, V2, V3	Left anterior descending (LAD)	Left ventricle: antero septal region
I, AVL, V4, V5, V6	Distal left anterior descending (LAD) or circumflex (Cx)	Left ventricle: antero lateral region
AVR	Right coronary artery (RCA)	Overlooks the right atrium and may be largely ignored

more than two associated (anterior or inferior) leads may be indicative of severe ischaemia and unstable angina (Figure 5.10).

Inversion of the T wave in the opposite direction to the qRS is also an indication, though less reliable, of ischaemia (Figure 5.11). ST segment depression and T wave inversion are relatively non-specific ECG changes that may evolve into a partial thickness non-Q wave MI in approximately 15 per cent of cases or represent unstable or stable angina, though in some instances they may be associated with non-cardiac chest pain.

Elevation of the ST segment more than 2 mm above baseline in more than two associated (anterior or inferior) leads indicates acute myocardial injury and is often the first witnessed ECG sign of acute MI, occurring within minutes of injury and lasting for up to 48 hours (Figure 5.12). The T wave may be superimposed within the elevated ST segment. ST segment changes are transient and will return to the base line as either sufficient

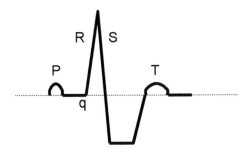

Figure 5.10 ST segment depression.

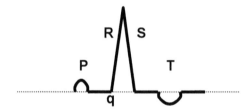

Figure 5.11　T wave inversion.

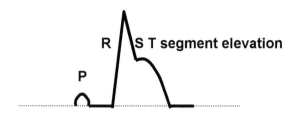

Figure 5.12　ST segment elevation.

oxygen is restored to the cells or cells necrose and become permanently damaged and electrically inert due to cessation of oxygen supply.

As injured cells infarct during the following 24 hours infarct tissue, which extends throughout the full thickness of the left ventricle, may create a pathological Q wave that deflects downwards immediately after the PR interval and whose depth is usually at least one-third the height of the following R wave to reach significance (Figure 5.13). Q waves usually develop as the ST segment begins to return to the baseline at 12 to 24 hours post symptom onset and are permanent indicators of myocardial infarction. T wave inversion in the same leads often occurs at approximately 48 hours post symptom onset as the ST segment returns to the baseline (± Q waves) and may remain on the ECG for up to one year (permanently in some cases). Changes to the qRST complex will occur in the ECG leads that overlook the affected area of the heart. Thus the area of ischaemia or infarction of myocardial muscle and the offending coronary artery can be identified through changes to the qRST complex in the corresponding ECG (Table 5.8). John's 12 lead ECG taken on admission confirmed ST segment elevation in leads I, AVL and V2, V3, V4, V5 and V6 (Figure 5.14), with no Q waves and upright T waves suggesting acute myocardial injury in the anterior region of the left ventricle caused by left anterior descending occlusion. Reciprocal ST segment depression can also be seen in the opposite leads II, III and AVF, which represents an electrical mirror image of the ST elevation. Coronary angiography is, however, necessary to definitively establish the affected coronary artery.

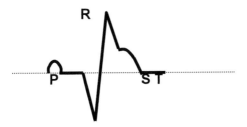

Figure 5.13 Q wave formation.

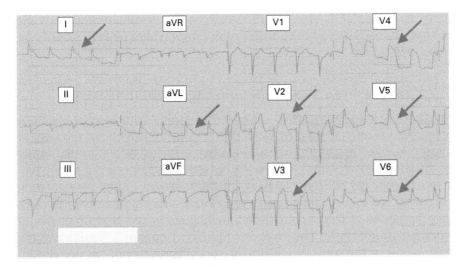

Figure 5.14 John's 12 lead ECG.

A Diagnosis of ST Elevation Myocardial Infarction

John's signs, symptoms and clinical presentation suggest that he has experienced an acute anterior STEMI. At this stage, a decision regarding John's immediate management and care should be reached, which will determine his transfer either to a coronary care unit or to the cardiac catheter laboratories if available on site. Enforced bed rest is initially instigated for John to promote rest and a reduction in cardiac workload, optimise the balance between myocardial oxygen demand and supply, and enable continuous cardiac monitoring and further investigation to confirm the diagnosis and treatment. John is unlikely to have experienced continuous cardiac ECG monitoring and regular 12 lead ECG recording before. The lack of knowledge and experience and the associated enforced restriction in independence may provoke or exacerbate feelings of uncertainty and loss of control and self-esteem, and further raise anxiety and stress. This may promote further sympathetic nervous activity with the undesirable physiological consequence of increased heart rate, BP and thus cardiac workload. Bed rest should therefore be limited to the initial assessment and treatment period and be relaxed as soon as John is pain free, has no evidence of rhythm or heart failure complications and has had any invasive arterial devices removed. Once John is pain free, he should be encouraged to attend to his toilet and hygiene needs as independently as possible and full mobility should be gradually restored. It is equally imperative that an explanation in clear and simple terms of the equipment, monitor tracings and his mobility limits is offered and reinforced if necessary. A full understanding of the method and necessity of close observation can provide a sense of security for some individuals.

Diagnosing a Non-ST Elevation Myocardial Infarction

Although oxygen deprivation is likely to interfere with normal electrical repolarisation of the affected cells, the ECG lacks sensitivity and cannot always be relied upon to provide conclusive evidence of myocardial injury or infarction. ST elevation or new left bundle branch block is a highly reliable indicator (95 per cent) of acute STEMI; however, not all patients present with classic ECG changes and therefore a more substantive diagnosis may be obtained from serum troponin measurement. Three subtypes of troponin (troponin C, TnC; troponin T, TnT; troponin I, TnI), a protein component of the contractile filaments, are present in smooth muscle and cardiac muscle. Oxygen deprivation causes the immediate release of troponin, which is serum detectable from small amounts of myocardial necrosis. As the composition of cardiac TnT and TnI is different to smooth muscle they both provide a sensitive and specific biochemical marker of myocardial damage. The sensitivity of troponin has resulted in a substantial increase in the annual number of diagnosed MIs.

In the UK an estimated 275,000 people have an MI per year, of whom approximately 12 per cent will die, and 1.4 million suffer with angina (DH, 2004). A diagnosis of acute MI with symptoms of ischaemic chest pain unrelieved by nitrate can be made if the serum troponin level is raised, irrespective of whether there is ST segment elevation (STEMI) or not (NSTEMI) on the 12 lead ECG (Fox et al., 2004). TnT or TnI measurement has become the gold standard for diagnosis of MI and different laboratory assays will produce local trust parameters for negative, borderline and positive results (Table 5.9). Negligible myocyte necrosis may release borderline levels of troponin and NSTEMI and STEMI are associated with a positive rise; however, troponin measurement is not without limitations (Table 5.10).

Table 5.9   ACS categories based upon TnI : TnT levels

ACS with UA	= TnI < 0.06 µg/L : TnT < 0.1 µg/L
ACS with myocardial necrosis	= TnI > 0.06–0.5 µg/L : TnT 0.18–1.5 µg/L
ACS with clinical MI	= TnI > 0.5 µg/L : TnT > 1.5 µg/L
	(or CK twice upper limit: 160 U/L on normal reference range)

Note: Normal values differ between men and women and local laboratory test procedures.
Source: British Cardiac Society (Fox et al. 2004).

Table 5.10   Limitations of troponin measurement

1. Biochemical markers are not detectable early after onset of necrosis and therefore a negative sample at admission cannot exclude MI
2. Peak troponin elevation can be up to twelve hours post symptom onset
3. Troponin may remain elevated for two to three weeks, prohibiting use for detecting repeated episodes of myocardial injury
4. Troponin cannot be used to diagnose ischaemia
5. A negative troponin may identify the patient as lower risk but not low or no risk for MI

Table 5.11   Routine venous blood sampling

1. Full blood count (FBC): low Hb (anaemia), raised WBC (infection)
2. Clotting screen: if indicated by current medication, e.g. warfarin
3. Urea and electrolytes (U&E): electrolyte balance and renal function
4. Cholesterol: > 5.0 mmol/L will be treated with statin therapy
5. Random serum blood glucose: > 11 mmol/L may be treated with IV dextrose and insulin (Digami 1 & 2 trials: Malmberg et al. 1999, 2005; Weston et al. 2007)
6. Capillary blood glucose if high or low glucose is suspected, e.g. diabetic patient
7. Liver function tests (LFT): baseline prior to statin therapy, which may alter liver function
8. Creatinine phosphokinase (CK): raised levels indicate the extent of myocardial damage

Venous blood sampling for a range of tests (Table 5.11) should be undertaken, though results may not be readily available for several hours. Elevated levels of serum creatine phosphokinase myocardial band (CK-MB) released during cell necrosis can also diagnose MI; however, the peak elevation time of six to twelve hours post symptom onset limits its use for early definitive diagnosis and necessitates serial sampling at eight to twelve hour intervals. As it is relatively more expensive to test and considered to be slightly less sensitive

Table 5.12 Secondary assessment

- Past medical history (PMH): cardiac and systemic
- Family history (FH)
- Social history (SH)
- Systemic enquiry: general, gastric, urinary, central nervous systems
- Risk factor evaluation (RF)
- Drug history: prescribed, over the counter and recreational
- Full clinical examination: peripheral pulses, jugular venous pressure (JVP), heart and lung sounds, systemic examination
- Chest X-ray and echocardiography

---

than troponin for myocardial necrosis it has largely fallen out of use as an early diagnostic tool. Once the patient is stabilised and early intervention and management have been initiated a more detailed secondary assessment may be elicited (Table 5.12). A definitive diagnosis of STEMI is based upon:

1. History of severe chest pain lasting more than twenty minutes and not relieved by nitrate.
2. ST elevation (or new left bundle branch block pattern) on ECG.
3. Elevated serum cardiac troponin (though treatment should not be delayed awaiting results) means that appropriate treatment and care can be safely initiated for John.

Medical Management Strategies

Accurate and effective assessment and management of acute MI is a multi-professional responsibility. In the UK a range of pre-hospital assessment and treatment initiatives exist across different geographical locations, including specially trained paramedic crews, rapid response and telemetry systems enabling transfer of ECGs to local accident and emergency or coronary care departments for interpretation to facilitate optimal 'call to treatment time'. Paramedic crews are increasingly expected to record and interpret the 12 lead ECG in order that the patient can be transferred to the most appropriate hospital site for immediate management. John's timely arrival in A&E within two hours of onset of ischaemic sounding chest pain and ST elevation on 12 lead ECG make him an ideal candidate for reperfusion therapy. Individuals presenting with a good clinical history and new bundle branch block masking ST segment elevation on ECG are also considered suitable for reperfusion therapy (FTT, 1994). However, not all individuals experience chest pain or have ECG changes and some must await confirmation from

The Case Scenario: Medical Management and Care Issues

At 09.30 hours and within ten minutes of receiving opiate analgesia John reported complete relief from his chest pain. His vital signs were observed and recorded as follows:

> Continuous cardiac rhythm monitoring 86 to 92 beats/min regular sinus rhythm
> BP systolic 90 to 100 mmHg; diastolic 55 to 60 mmHg
> Four-hourly respirations 12 to 16/min
> Continuous O_2 saturation 96 to 98 per cent (24 per cent oxygen via mask commenced by the paramedic crew was discontinued)
> 12 Lead ECG shows ST elevation in leads I, AVL, V2 to V6

A definitive diagnosis of anterior STEMI approximately two hours from onset of symptoms is reached. Medical treatment should be instigated immediately and the continuous monitoring, recording and reporting of vital signs during the acute phase of illness remains an essential aspect of nursing care (NICE, 2007a). Symptom relief, effective communication with John, his close friends and relatives and provision of simple comfort measures are equally important care issues.

Immediate Medical Management
1. What are the current treatment options for an acute STEMI?
2. What factors might inform the choice of immediate management?
3. Explore your local policy regarding immediate treatment for STEMI.
4. What are John's main care issues?

troponin results at twelve hours post symptom onset, taking them out of the reperfusion treatment zone. Moreover, many with chest pain delay seeking help and fail to present for treatment early enough. A number of factors, including gender, age, culture, socio-economic status, experience and misinterpretation of symptoms, transport issues or failing to contact the emergency services, may explain this (Horne et al., 2000; Bird et al., 2009). National campaigns and local initiatives to educate and encourage individuals to report chest pain as soon as possible by contacting 999 aim to improve this situation. The overall aim of immediate reperfusion strategies is to dissolve fibrin rich clot, restore coronary artery patency to limit infarct size and so improve mortality and long-term morbidity.

Primary Percutaneous Coronary Intervention

John may receive an invasive catheter based reperfusion commonly referred to as primary percutaneous coronary intervention or primary angioplasty. PCI requires the immediate transfer of John to the cardiac catheter labs where it can be performed under local anaesthesia with radiographic control. John will receive an oral loading dose of either 600 mg clopidogrel® or 60 mg prasugrel® for their anti-platelet properties (Montalescot et al., 2009). PCI involves passing a small balloon at the tip of a catheter introduced via an artery (usually femoral or brachial) into the occluded coronary artery. The balloon is inflated to re-open the coronary artery and then removed leaving a bare metal or drug eluting stent in place to maintain a rigid support within the artery wall and so resume vessel patency and blood flow (Figure 5.15). During PCI reperfusion a weight-adjusted IV bolus dose

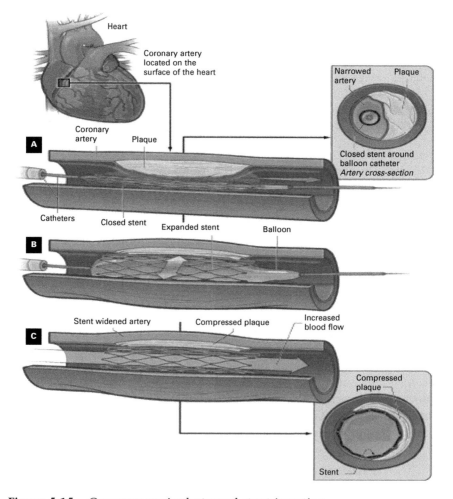

Figure 5.15　Coronary angioplasty and stent insertion.

Source: National Institutes of Health and the US Department of Health and Human Services/National Heart, Lung and Blood Institute. Reproduced with permission.

and infusion of a glycoprotein IIb/IIIa inhibitor such as abciximab® or in John's case bivalirudin® is usually administered (DeLuca et al., 2005). Large randomised controlled trials have revealed that PCI confers a reinfarction, stroke and 2 per cent short term mortality benefit over thrombolytic therapy (Keeley et al., 2003). This benefit was further emphasised with the advent of stent implantation into the offending coronary artery following balloon angioplasty (Nordmann et al., 2004). Consequently primary PCI is the current treatment of choice for patients presenting with STEMI to a hospital with on-site PCI facilities (cardiac catheter lab and cardiac surgical backup), 24 hour interventionalist cover and technical expertise (Antman et al., 2007).

The mortality benefit is, however, time dependent and a delay beyond the recommended 'call-to-balloon' time of 120 to 150 minutes may negatively affect survival benefit (Betriu and Masotti, 2005). Not all UK hospital sites have the facility or expertise to offer primary PCI, which has prompted debate and national enquiry to ascertain whether patients should receive IV thrombolysis on-site or be transferred to the nearest centre for PCI, accepting the risk of a time to reperfusion delay. The DANAMI–2 trial demonstrated a notable reduction in mortality, reinfarction and stroke with primary PCI for patients admitted directly to invasive treatment centres and patients transferred to referral hospitals (Anderson et al., 2003). To date, regional UK policy differs, with some centres providing on-site primary PCI, and some areas routinely transferring patients to an intervention centre, and in the absence of a local PCI service in some districts, pharmacological thrombolytic reperfusion remains the mainstay treatment for STEMI. A national roll-out programme of PCI services across England is feasible, cost effective and now under way, although some geographical challenges are anticipated (DH, 2009). Transfer for primary PCI should always be considered for all high risk patients thought to have large infarctions, those in cardiogenic shock, those with failed thrombolysis and those with a prolonged time from symptom onset to presentation.

Pharmacological Reperfusion Therapy

Alternatively, John may receive thrombolysis therapy if immediate PCI within the 120 to 150 minute time frame from onset of symptoms is not locally available. A decline in 30-day mortality post STEMI from 25–30 per cent in the 1960s and 18 per cent in the mid 1980s to 8–9 per cent in 2002 was largely attributed to the widespread use of thrombolytic therapy, aspirin and coronary interventions (Van de Werf et al., 2003). A wealth of randomised controlled trials has firmly established the use of fibrinolytic therapy (thrombolysis) to treat STEMI since the early 1980s; however, the mortality benefit is also time dependent, with no convincing evidence of benefit beyond twelve hours (GUSTO Investigators, 1993; Boersma et al., 1996). Patients treated within the first hour, frequently referred to as the 'golden hour', have the highest absolute and relative mortality benefit. This well established time dependent factor for thrombolysis supports the 60 minute 'call-to-needle time' and 30 minute 'door-to-needle time' set by the CHD NSF thrombolysis standards (DH, 2000). Several large studies (GISSI 2, 1990; ISIS 3, 1992; GUSTO, 1993) have compared different thrombolytic agents (Table 5.13).

In John's case the ease and speed of administration of IV TNK® with adjunct IV Heparin® or weight adjusted doses of subcutaneous low molecular weight heparin (LMWH) such as clexane® or enoxaparin® would be administered. LMWH, a sub-fraction of standard heparin that has demonstrated a number of clinical benefits, not least removing the need for close aPTT monitoring, has largely superseded IV heparin therapy (ASSENT 3, 2001; Antman et al., 2006). Alternatively in some centres John may receive a single bolus subcutaneous injection of 2.5 mg of fondaparinux®, which selectively inactivates clotting factor Xa and thus reduces the opportunity for further red clot formation (Figure 5.4).

Table 5.13   Thrombolytic agents for STEMI

Agent	Routine use	Administration	Adjunct therapy
Streptokinase® (SK): relatively cheap. Once only use as streptococcal derivative induces antibody response	Acute inferior STEMI and/or > 75 years old unless absolutely contraindicated (Table 5.14)	15,000,000 units in 100 ml of 5% dextrose or 0.9% saline infused over 60 minutes	None (though subcutaneous s/c enoxaparin® is often prescribed until mobility restored)
Alteplase® (tPA) tissue plasminogen activator – approximately 4 times the cost of SK	Acute anterior STEMI, ≤75 years old and all those previously treated with streptokinase unless contraindicated (Table 5.14)	Accelerated regime: 15 mg IV bolus; 50 mg infused over 30 minutes; 35 mg infused over 60 minutes	IV heparin®, s/c enoxaparin® weight adjusted 48 to 72 hours or fondaparinux®
Tenecteplase® (TNK-tPA) – similar cost to tPA	As tPA	Single weight adjusted IV bolus	S/c enoxaparin® weight adjusted 48 to 72 hours or fondaparinux®

Table 5.14   Contraindications to thrombolysis

Absolute contraindications	Relative contraindications
• Haemorrhagic stroke or stroke of unknown origin • Ischaemic stroke within previous 6 months • Central nervous system damage or neoplasm • Recent (within 3 weeks) major surgery/head injury • Gastrointestinal bleed within 1 month • Known bleeding disorder • Aortic dissection	• Transient ischaemic attack within 6 months • Oral anticoagulant therapy (check clotting) • Pregnancy or within 1 week post-partum • Non compressible vascular punctures • Traumatic or prolonged resuscitation • Refractory hypertension (systolic > 180 mmHg) • Advanced liver disease • Infective endocarditis • Active peptic ulcer

Thrombolysis is not without risk and hypotension, usually relieved by temporary cessation of the infusion and elevation of the feet, and rarely requiring IV atropine® or volume expansion, and severe allergic reactions are occasionally associated with IV streptokinase®. Bleeding post thrombolysis with all agents is a major potential complication and observation and early detection is of paramount importance in reducing long-term associated morbidity. The worst outcome is intracerebral haemorrhage, which occurs in 0.5 per cent and may be detected by headache, acute confusional state, visual disturbance, seizure or other new neurological signs. Unfortunately, despite early recognition, diagnosis and possible surgical intervention there is approximately 75 per cent risk of mortality or a permanent neurological deficit, particularly in older adults > 70 years receiving tPA or TNK. There is a 3–13 per cent risk of major non-cerebral bleeding associated with all three agents. Gastrointestinal, retroperitoneal or trauma site bleeding affects less than 5 per cent, though it may be life threatening if undetected, whereas the commonest site around intravenous access is usually self-limiting. Continuous monitoring of John's heart rate and rhythm, BP recording and general observation, particularly of venous puncture sites, should be reported every thirty minutes for the first two to three hours. Superficial bleeding is the most common problem encountered in practice and with vigilance and care is usually limited to localised bruising.

The Case Scenario: Ongoing Care Issues

A brief past medical history and clinical examination revealed that John was previously fit and well and had no apparent contraindications to treatment. John was transferred immediately to the cardiac catheter labs for primary PCI with IV bivalirudin® (an aggressive anti-platelet agent). The procedure revealed occlusion of the proximal left anterior descending artery, which was dilated and implanted with a bare metal stent. The circumflex and right coronary arteries were normal. He had a pre-procedure stat dose of oral prasugrel® 60 mg followed by a daily 10 mg maintenance dose and weight adjusted subcutaneous enoxaparin® was commenced. The medical plan was to commence a daily maintenance dose of aspirin 75 mg, metoprolol® on day one post MI, a loading dose of oral enalapril® on day one post MI if BP stable and simvastatin® 40 mg at night. Bed rest and continuous cardiac monitoring for arrhythmia detection were maintained and a detailed social, family and risk factor assessment was completed.

Nursing Care Issues
1. Consider the appropriate ongoing assessment, monitoring and care required for John, particularly during initial intervention.
2. Explore the potential psychological and social needs for John and his family.
3. Consider what secondary prevention, educational information and advice John will require during the cardiac rehabilitation phase.
4. What complications may arise in the following hours post STEMI?

Ongoing Care Issues and the Role of the Nurse

Immediate Nursing Issues

Following PCI, John's arterial puncture site may be sutured or sealed at the end of the procedure using devices such as the collagen plus angioseal, consisting of an anchor inserted into the artery, a collagen plug that seals the outside and a suture that unites both elements. The angioseal would allow John to sit up immediately post procedure and mobilise within an hour; however, it is relatively expensive and sometimes difficult to deploy. Alternatively, the arterial catheter sheath may remain inserted in the femoral (or brachial) artery post PCI to be removed approximately four to six hours post procedure, with prolonged manual or mechanical pressure applied to the puncture site to ensure adequate stasis. Manual pressure that relies upon direct 'digit to groin' pressure for approximately 10 minutes can be physically arduous and time consuming; therefore mechanical devices such as a 'fem-stop', involving application of an inflatable dome secured over the puncture site with a belt, are often employed. John's arterial sheath and puncture site post removal must be closely observed every 30 minutes for signs of bleeding and the presence of pedal (or radial) pulses on the affected side noted. Removal of the sheath may induce a vasovagal response, leading to a transient bradycardia, sudden hypotension and feeling faint, though this is not common and can be overcome with IV Atropine®. Nevertheless, observation and continuous monitoring of heart rate, rhythm, BP and signs of chest pain or discomfort should continue at least every 30 minutes for the first two hours post procedure and removal of arterial sheath. John must be reminded to inform the nurse if he experiences any chest pain or discomfort during his stay in order that re-assessment and appropriate management can be promptly initiated.

The majority of patients remain haemodynamically stable post reperfusion; however, on occasion some individuals experience a profound hypotension immediately post PCI and may require additional temporary cardiac support from an intra-aortic balloon pump inserted via the arterial catheter sheath, with the same close monitoring for the duration of the therapy. Skin colour and warmth provides a useful visual guide of systemic perfusion and as the kidneys are particularly sensitive to decreased perfusion pressure, urinary output measurement provides a valuable clinical indicator of cardiac output and BP. A 70 kg individual would normally produce at least 0.5 ml/kg/hour and so if John produces less than 35 ml/hour, low cardiac output and BP or in a minority of cases urinary retention due to a reaction to the dye used during PCI, requiring bladder catheterisation, should be suspected.

Aside from immediate coronary angiography a definitive clinical measure of reperfusion success is not currently available. Chest pain relief is affected by a variety of factors, not least opiate therapy and fluctuation in coronary blood flow post infarction, and is therefore not a helpful guide. A repeat ECG at 60 to 90 minutes post reperfusion therapy to assess ST segment resolution may provide some indication of tissue level reperfusion and prognosis, as patients who have $\geq$ 70 per cent ST resolution are thought to have a better prognosis. Following PCI, approximately 20 to 30 per cent of patients do not demonstrate ST resolution despite TIMI flow grade three at the end of the procedure and are more likely to have an unfavourable prognosis (Claeys et al., 1999); however, isolated reliance upon ST segment resolution as an indicator is not recommended. There is some correlation between accelerated idioventricular rhythm and restoration of vessel patency. Therefore a combination of sudden or near complete relief from chest pain, ST segment resolution and accelerated idioventricular rhythm is highly specific for successful reperfusion, though this tends to be evident in only approximately 10 per cent of individuals (see Bennett, 2006, for further explanation of idioventricular rhythm). Further venous blood sampling for troponin or creatinine phosphokinase (CK) is not routinely necessary following a history and ECG diagnosis of STEMI. However, local policies differ and some hospitals may measure one or both biochemical markers at 12 hours post admission as an indication of infarct size. The frequency of observation of vital signs will be determined by the current trend but may be reduced to four-hourly once John is pain free, thrombolysis is successfully infused or four hours post removal of the PCI arterial sheath and there are no obvious signs of complication (Table 5.15).

Table 5.15   Potential complications post-STEMI

---

1. Tachyarrhythmia, bradyarrhythmia or conduction defects (See Bennett 2006).
2. Post infarction ischaemia/angina.
3. Reinfarction: incidence ranges from less than 5% post reperfusion therapy to16% of non-reperfused patients.
4. Acute left ventricular failure: acute pulmonary oedema with or without decreased stroke volume and cardiac output.
5. Congestive cardiac failure: raised pulmonary and systemic venous pressure leading to pulmonary and systemic congestion and decreased cardiac output.
6. Mitral regurgitation: frequency of a new murmur is between 20 and 55%.
7. Pericarditis: sterile inflammation of the pericardium, usually associated with Q wave anterior myocardial infarction causing sharp chest pain, a pericardial rub and effusion and concave ST segment elevation across multiple ECG leads. Incidence has fallen dramatically with reperfusion therapy.
8. Cardiogenic shock: usually signifies severe coronary artery disease and occurs when more than 40% of the left ventricular mass is infarcted and ischaemic.
9. Cardiac rupture: rupture of left ventricular free wall, ventricular septum leading to a ventricular septal defect, the papillary muscle or chordae tendinae.
10. Left ventricular aneurysm: severe persistent infarct expansion and scar tissue development lead to a discrete bulge of the left ventricle.
11. Left ventricular thrombus: usually associated with anterior region infarction and occurs at the site of infarct expansion or apical aneurysm.
12. Left ventricular remodelling: structural and functional changes of the left ventricle, which commence during the acute myocardial infarction and may continue to evolve over months or years and follow a sequence of events. Infarct expansion: thinning and dilation of the infarct zone, which may lead to left ventricular remodelling; dilation of the uninfarcted myocardium leading to hypertrophy; fibrosis and contractile impairment; global change of shape of left ventricle from elongated to spherical.

Adjunct Pharmacological Treatment

NICE (2007b) guidance 48 recommends prescription of a range of cardiac drugs, physical activity, lifestyle modification of diet, smoking habit and alcohol consumption, and invitation onto cardiac rehabilitation programmes for all patients following MI to minimise the risk of further acute events. ISIS 2 confirmed an additional mortality benefit associated with adjunct aspirin therapy with all reperfusion therapies, and it is now standard therapy given to virtually all patients with acute coronary syndrome (ISIS 2, 1988). This explains why John received a stat oral dose of 300 mg of dispersible aspirin for its anti-platelet properties in an effort to disperse the offending platelet-rich 'white clot' rather than for its more traditional analgesic effect. A daily maintenance dose of 75 mg of oral aspirin should be continued indefinitely. The CLARITY trial found that in addition to aspirin, concomitant early oral clopidogrel® therapy for patients with STEMI appeared to confer further benefits in terms of mortality, patency and reinfarction over aspirin alone (Sabatine et al., 2005). Clopidogrel® also provides an effective alternative for individuals who are unable to tolerate the potential gastric irritation sometimes caused by aspirin. A 75 mg daily maintenance dose of clopidogrel® for at least four weeks post STEMI (NICE 2007b) or, in John's case, 10 mg daily of an alternative thioendopyridine called prasugrel® will be prescribed. On day one post acute presentation John is likely to be prescribed a low dose beta blocker such as Metoprolol®; Atenolol® or Carvedilol® might be considered for patients with poor LV function assessed on echocardiography. A significant survival benefit is afforded by angiotensin-converting enzyme inhibitors (ACEI) such as Ramipril®, Enalapril® or Captopril® for post MI patients with evidence of left ventricular dysfunction (Cleland et al., 1993; GISSI 3, 1994; ISIS 4, 1995). Assuming blood pressure was within normal parameters John would commence a graded dose on day one post MI, with 30-minute blood pressure recording for approximately two hours after the first dose to observe for signs of hypotension. Angiotensin receptor 2 antagonists such as Losartan® or Valsartan® may be substituted for patients unable to tolerate the side effects of ACE inhibitors, a tickly cough being a common complaint. Statins (3-hydroxy-3-methylglutaryl coenzyme A (HMG-CoA) reductase inhibitors) such as Pravastatin®, Simvastatin® and Atorvastatin® profoundly reduce plasma cholesterol levels and are instrumental in reducing the incidence of recurring coronary events and improving outcomes post MI (LaRosa et al., 1999). The current national threshold for statin intervention is 5.2 mmol/L but in practice if John's admission serum cholesterol level was found to be more than 4 mmol/L he is most likely to commence a large nightly dose (at least 40 mg) of a statin in view of his evident coronary artery disease. As statins may adversely affect liver function a baseline liver function test is advisable prior to initiation of therapy. Both GISSI 3 (1994) and ISIS 4 (1995) trials failed to establish any benefit from intravenous nitrates or long acting oral nitrates during the acute MI phase. However, intravenous nitroglycerin preparations are used in the treatment of post MI heart failure and recurrent ischaemic pain. Similarly, calcium channel blockers have not demonstrated benefit and are not routinely prescribed post MI. Nifedipine® is generally contraindicated post MI and diltiazem® and verapamil® are reserved for specific treatment of post infarction angina or supraventricular arrhythmias. Opie and Gersh (2004) focus upon the pharmacological action of cardiac drugs in detail.

Psychosocial Concerns

The psychological consequence of the acute and continuing phases of care post STEMI have been well documented and should not be underestimated. A lack of knowledge can lead to misunderstanding and misinterpretation of the situation, and worries and uncertainty related to the implications of having had a 'heart attack', now and in the future, exacerbating fears of the unknown, are common concerns that John may experience. The very speed of symptom onset, diagnosis and intervention during the acute episode exacerbated profound feelings of emotional shock for a group of PCI patients interviewed by Astin et al. (2009). This was further compounded by an apparent mismatch between expectations and reality, which appeared to affect the ability of these patients to make sense of their condition in a coherent manner. This led to a degree of misconception that the condition was 'acute' and treatment 'curative', evading the necessity for longer-term self-management for a chronic condition (Astin et al., 2009). Sudden loss of close communication and contact with family and significant others contributes to feelings of fear, isolation and hopelessness, which may further intensify anxiety. Elevated levels of fear and anxiety during the acute phase may not only prompt the undesirable physiological cardiac effects already mentioned but if overlooked lead to depression and adversely affect long-term rehabilitation and survival (Jowett and Thompson, 2003). Major depression has been reported in up to 20 per cent of patients hospitalised with MI, a further 10 to 17 per cent display significant symptoms of depression and the majority of these patients remain depressed one to four months later (Bush et al., 2005). It is therefore imperative that assessment and management of John's emotional response and adjustment to the immediate phase remain a central aspect of his acute care. Reassurance and appropriate information giving are imperative at all stages of care. Clear, concise, timely and reinforced communication and explanation regarding immediate treatment can help to restore some sense of control over the situation, promote informed decision making, reduce anxiety and enhance compliance with care. Visibility, approachability, empathy and an air of professional competence by health professionals involved in John's care can further endorse this.

Once John has recovered from the acute event, the first of four phases of structured cardiac rehabilitation should be commenced (Table 5.16). Chapter 7 of the NSF for CHD (DH, 2000) recommends that all heart patients be invited to participate in multidisciplinary secondary prevention and cardiac rehabilitation programmes, which offer comprehensive individualised support to change their lifestyle, involving education and psychological input, as well as exercise training. Phase 1 aims to teach, advise, support and promote John's understanding of the MI and treatment received, his return to full independence and behavioural changes he may wish to adopt aimed to restore a full, healthy and happy lifestyle that minimises the risk of further acute cardiac events. However, John's average length of hospital stay following PCI is three to four days (slightly longer post thrombolysis). This and frequent transfers between and within hospitals restrict the available time for healthcare practitioners to offer sufficient, relevant explanation, information and advice on healthy lifestyles, potential behaviour modification and structured exercise programmes to return John to full physical activity, or to discuss his psychosocial and spiritual needs. Further to this the emotional shock of having had a 'heart attack' may influence John's ability to absorb, retain and recall information given. Astin et al. (2008) recommend that information giving be 'staged' to better reflect patient priorities and specific needs and be offered and reinforced prior to and immediately post hospital discharge in the home by specialist nurses to enhance continuity of care and address further information needs. Prior to discharge John specifically needs to:

- be fully informed of all medications prescribed and to receive a clopido-grel®/prasugrel® card;
- know how to deal with future episodes of chest pain and how to use his GTN spray effectively, and be advised to seek professional help if the chest pain is not resolved within 15 minutes;
- know what constitutes a 'healthy heart' diet and exercise regime and be introduced to opportunities to stop smoking in an effort to help him make healthy life choices in the future.

Social support is an essential aspect of physical and psychosocial recovery and so John's home circumstances must also be considered. Although driving a car is permitted one month after a STEMI, John will require a

Table 5.16 Four phases of cardiac rehabilitation

Phase 1 initiates information and advice giving by a cardiac rehabilitation nurse with patient and family prior to discharge and includes:

1. Emotional assessment, reassurance and stress management
2. Risk factor assessment and modification planning
3. Assessment of patient knowledge and understanding of heart disease
4. Accurate, consistent, relevant educational advice about:
   - Coronary heart disease
   - Individual risk factors
   - Drug therapy and chest pain management
   - Healthy diet
   - Smoking cessation
   - Return to usual activities of daily living
   - Return to work
   - Return to sexual activity and issues related to erectile dysfunction
   - Return to driving
   - Holidays, flying and travel abroad
5. Verbal discussion may be supplemented by written leaflets, videos and the Heart Manual (6 week programme)

Phase 2: home visits facilitated by the specialist community cardiac rehabilitation team immediately post discharge for approximately 3 months and including:

1. Pulse and blood pressure monitoring
2. Reinforce lifestyle risk factors and modification
3. Monitor anxiety and depression levels
4. Support patient and family with individual needs

Phase 3: structured exercise programme facilitated by cardiac rehabilitation nurses and trained fitness instructor or physiotherapist 6 to 8 weeks post discharge, including:

1. Educational and psychological support
2. Advice on risk factors

Phase 4: long-term maintenance by primary care practitioners

---

negative exercise stress test before he may be able to resume employment as an HGV driver. This will usually be arranged as an outpatient visit once John has been discharged into the care of the GP and community-based cardiac rehabilitation team. All stages of John's care rely upon a multidisciplinary approach including doctors, nurses, pharmacists, physiotherapists, dieticians, smoking cessation teams, social workers and clinical psychologists in some instances. Comprehensive cardiac rehabilitation programmes are a clinical and cost effective intervention as important as drug therapy in secondary prevention after MI and should be offered to all patients post MI regardless of age, gender, ethnicity, co-morbidity or cardiac function (NICE, 2007b). Evidence suggests that it can reduce mortality by as much as 20 to 25 per cent over three years and can improve health outcomes and quality of life for people with CHD (DH, 2000), yet less than half of eligible patients in the UK access cardiac rehabilitation (Beswick et al., 2004). Cardiac rehabilitation begins before discharge from hospital, though it is largely provided as either home- or community-based programmes where there is an increasing emphasis upon employing strategies to enhance access, participation and retention on programmes.

Summary

Early, accurate assessment, timely intervention and care during the acute phase and entry into a comprehensive cardiac rehabilitation programme should enable John to return to a happy, healthy and active work, social and personal life.

Further Reading

Bennett, D. H. *Cardiac Arrhythmias*, 7th edn (London: Hodder Education, 2006).
Epstein, O., G. D. Perkin, J. Cookson, I. S. Watt, R. Rakhit, A. W. Robbins and G. A. W. Hornett. *Clinical Examination*, 4th edn (London: Mosby International Ltd, 2008).
Gamon, R., T. Quinn and B. Parr. *Emergency Care of the Patient with a Heart Attack* (Edinburgh: Churchill Livingstone, 2006).
Lilly, L. S. (ed.). *Pathophysiology of Heart Disease: A Collaborative Project of Medical Students and Faculty*, 4th edn (Baltimore, MD: Lippincott, Williams & Wilkins, 2007).
Opie, L. H. and B. J. Gersh. *Drugs for the Heart*, 6th edn (Philadelphia: Elsevier Saunders, 2004).
Van de Werf, F., D. Ardissino, A. Betriu et al. 'Management of Acute Myocardial Infarction in Patients Presenting with ST Segment Elevation: The Task Force on the Management of Acute Myocardial Infarction of the European Society of Cardiology', *European Heart Journal*, **24** (2003), 28–66.

References

Anderson, H. R., T. T. Nielson, K. Rasmussen et al. 'For the DANAMI-2 Investigators. A Comparison of Coronary Angioplasty with Fibrinolytic Therapy in Acute Myocardial Infarction', *New England Journal of Medicine*, **349** (2003), 733–42.

Antman, E. M., M. Hand, P. W. Armstrong et al. 'Focused Update of the ACC/AHA 2004 Guidelines for the Management of Patients with ST Elevation Myocardial Infarction: A Report of the American College of Cardiology/American Heart Association Task Force on Practice Guidelines', *Journal of the American College of Cardiology*, **51** (2007), 210–47.

Antman, E. M., D. A. Morrow, C. H. McCabe et al. 'Enoxaparin versus Unfractionated Heparin with Fibrinolysis for ST Elevation Myocardial Infarction', *New England Journal of Medicine*, **354** (2006), 1477–88.

Assessment of the Safety and Efficacy of a New Thrombolytic Regimen (ASSENT) 3 Investigators. 'Efficacy and Safety of Tenecteplase in Combination with Enoxaparin, Abciximab or Unfractionated Heparin: The ASSENT-3 Randomised Trial in Acute Myocardial Infarction', *Lancet*, **358** (2001), 605–13.

Astin, F., S. J. Closs, J. McLenachan, S. Hunter and C. Priestley. 'The Information Needs of Patients Treated with Primary Angioplasty for Heart Attack: An Exploratory Study', *Patient Education and Counselling*, doi:10 1016/j.pec.2008.06.013 (2008).

Astin, F., S. J. Closs, J. McLenachan, S. Hunter and C. Priestley. 'Primary Angioplasty for Heart Attack: Mismatch between Expectations and Reality?', *Journal of Advanced Nursing*, **65**(1) (2009), 72–83.

Barth, J., M. Schumacher and C. Herrmann-Lingen. 'Depression as a Risk Factor for Mortality in Patients with Coronary Heart Disease: A Meta-analysis', *Psychosomatic Medicine*, **66** (2004), 802–13.

Beswick, A. D., K. Rees, I. Griebsch, F. C. Taylor, M. Burke, R. R. West, J. Victory, J. Brown, R. S. Taylor and S. Ebrahim. 'Provision, Uptake and Cost of Cardiac Rehabilitation Programmes: Improving Services to Under Represented Groups', *Health Technology Assessment*, **8**(41) (2004).

Betriu, A. and M. Masotti. 'Comparison of Mortality Rates in Acute Myocardial Infarction Treated by Percutaneous Coronary Intervention versus Fibrinolysis', *American Journal of Cardiology*, **95** (2005), 100–1.

Bird, M. W., A. G. Woods and N. A. Warren. 'Factors Influencing Treatment Delays for Acute Myocardial Infarction', *Critical Care Nursing Quarterly*, **32**(1) (2009), 19–23.

Boersma, E., A. Mass, J. Deckers and M. Simoons. 'Early Thrombolytic Treatment in Acute Myocardial Infarction: Reappraisal of the Golden Hour', *Lancet*, **348** (1996), 771–5.

Bush, D. E., R. C. Ziegelstein, U. V. Patel, B. D. Thombs, D. E. Ford, J. A. Fauerbach, U. D. McCann, K. J. Stewart, K. K. Tsilidis, A. L. Patel, C. J. Feuerstein and E. B. Bass. *Post-Myocardial Infarction Depression* (Rockville: Agency for Healthcare Research and Quality (AHRQ) 310, 2005).

Claeys, M. J., J. Bosmans, L. Veenstra et al. 'Determinants and Prognostic Implications of Persistent ST Segment Elevation after Primary Angioplasty for Acute Myocardial Infarction: Importance of Microvascular Reperfusion Injury on Clinical Outcome', *Circulation*, **99** (1999), 1972–7.

Cleland, J. G., L. Erhardt, G. Murray, A. S. Hall and S. G. Ball. 'Effect of Ramipril on Mortality and Morbidity of Survivors of Acute Myocardial Infarction with Clinical

Evidence of Heart Failure. The Acute Infarction Ramipril Efficacy (AIRE) Study Investigators', *Lancet*, **342** (1993), 821–8.

Culi, V., D. Miri and D. Eterovi. 'Correlation between Symptomatology and Site of Acute Myocardial Infarction', *International Journal of Cardiology*, **77**(2/3) (2001), 163–8.

DeLuca, G., H. Suryapranata, G. W. Stonw et al. 'Abciximab as Adjunctive Therapy to Reperfusion in Acute ST Segment Elevation Myocardial Infarction: A Meta Analysis of Randomised Trials', *JAMA*, **293** (2005), 1759–65.

Denollet, J., S. S. Pederson, C. J. Vrints and V. M. Conraads. 'Usefulness of Type D Personality in Predicting Five Year Cardiac Events Above and Beyond Concurrent Symptoms of Stress in Patients with Coronary Heart Disease', *American Journal Cardiology*, **97** (2006), 970–3.

Department of Health. *National Service Framework for Coronary Heart Disease* (London: HMSO, 2000).

Department of Health. *National Service Framework for Coronary Heart Disease: Winning the War on Heart Disease* (London: HMSO, 2004).

Department of Health. *National Infarct Angioplasty Project (NIAP): Interim Report* (London: HMSO, 2008).

Department of Health. *Coronary Heart Disease National Service Framework: Building on Excellence, Maintaining Progress* (London: HMSO, 2009).

Dubois, C., J. Smeets and C. Demoulin. 'Incidence, Clinical Significance and Prognosis of Ventricular Fibrillation in the Early Phase of Myocardial Infarction', *European Heart Journal*, **7**(11) (1986), 945–51.

Eslick, G. D. 'Usefulness of Chest Pain Character and Location as Diagnostic Indicators of an Acute Coronary Syndrome', *American Journal of Cardiology*, **95**(10) (2005), 1228–31.

Fibrinolytic Therapy Trialists (FTT) Collaborative Group. 'Indications for Fibrinolytic Therapy in Suspected Acute Myocardial Infarction: Collaborative Overview of Early Mortality and Major Morbidity Results from All Randomised Trials of More than 1000 Patients', *Lancet*, **343** (1994), 311–22.

Foreman, R. D. 'Mechanisms of cardiac pain', *Annual Review of Physiology*, **61** (1999), 143–67.

Fox, K. A. A., J. Birkhead, R. Wilcox, C. Knight and J. Barth. 'British Cardiac Society Working Group on the Definition of Myocardial Infarction', *Heart*, **90** (2004) 603–9.

GISSI 2 International Study Group. 'In Hospital Mortality and Clinical Course of 20,891 Patients with Suspected Acute Myocardial Infarction Randomised between Alteplase and Streptokinase with or without Heparin', *Lancet*, **336** (1990), 71–5.

GISSI 3. 'Effects of Lisinopril and Transdermal Glyceryl Trinitrate Singly and Together on Six Week Mortality and Ventricular Function after Acute Myocardial Infarction', *Lancet*, **343** (1994), 1115–22.

GUSTO Investigators. 'An International Randomised Trial Comparing Four Thrombolytic Strategies for Acute Myocardial Infarction', *New England Journal of Medicine*, **329** (1993) 1615–22.

Henkel, D. M., B. J. Witt, B. J. Gersh, S. J. Jacobsen, S. A. Weston, R. A. Meverden and V. L. Roger. 'Ventricular Arrhythmias after Acute Myocardial Infarction: A 20 Year Community Study', *American Heart Journal*, **151**(4) (2006), 806–12.

Herlihy, T., M. E. McIvor, C. C. Cummings, C. O. Siu and M. Alikahn. 'Nausea and Vomiting during Acute Myocardial Infarction and Its Relation to Infarct Size and Location', *American Journal of Cardiology*, **60**(1) (2004), 20–2.

Horne, R., D. James, K. Petrie, J. Weinman and R. Vincent. 'Patients' Interpretation of Symptoms as a Cause of Delay in Reaching Hospital during Acute Myocardial Infarction', *Heart*, **83** (2000), 388–93.

ISIS 2 (Second International Study of Infarct Survival) Collaborative Group. 'Randomised Trial of Intravenous Streptokinase, Oral Aspirin, Both, or Neither among 17,187 Cases of Suspected Acute Myocardial Infarction', *Lancet*, **ii** (1988), 349–60.

ISIS 3 (Third International Study of Infarct Survival) Collaborative Group. 'A Randomised Comparison of Streptokinase versus Tissue Plasminogen Activator versus Anistreplase and of Aspirin plus Heparin versus Aspirin Alone among 41,299 Cases of Suspected Acute Myocardial Infarction', *Lancet*, **339** (1992), 753–70.

ISIS 4 (Fourth International Study of Infarct Survival) Collaborative Group. 'A Randomised Factorial Trial Assessing Early Captopril, Oral Mononitrate and Intravenous Magnesium Sulphate in 58,050 Patients with Suspected Acute Myocardial Infarction', *Lancet*, **345** (1995), 669–85.

Joint European Society of Cardiology (ESC)/American College of Cardiology (ACC) Committee. 'Myocardial Infarction Redefined: A Consensus Document of the Joint ESC/ACC Committee for the Redefinition of Myocardial Infarction', *European Heart Journal*, **21** (2000), 1502–13.

Jowett, N. I. and D. R. Thompson. *Comprehensive Coronary Care*, 3rd edn (London: Bailliere Tindall, 2003).

Keeley, E. C., J. A. Boura and C. L. Grines. 'Primary Angioplasty versus Intravenous Thrombolytic Therapy for Acute Myocardial Infarction: A Quantitative Review of 23 Randomised Trials', *Lancet*, **361**(9351) (2003), 13–20.

LaRosa, J. C., J. He and S. Vupputuri. 'Effect of Statins on Risk of Coronary Disease: A Meta Analysis of Randomised Controlled Trials', *JAMA*, **282** (1999), 2340–6.

Lilly, L. S. (ed.). *Pathophysiology of Heart Disease: A Collaborative Project of Medical Students and Faculty*, 4th edn (Baltimore: Lippincott, Williams & Wilkins, 2007).

McNulty, P. H., N. King, S. Scott, G. Harlman, J. McCann, M. Kozak, C. E. Chambers, L. M. Demers and L. I. Sinoway. 'Effects of Supplemental Oxygen Administration on Coronary Blood Flow in Patients Undergoing Cardiac Catheterisation', *American Journal of Physiology – Heart and Circulatory Physiology*, **288**(3) (2005), H1057.

Malmberg, K., A. Norhammar, H. Wedal et al. 'Glycometabolic State at Admission: Important Risk Marker of Mortality in Conventionally Treated Patients with Diabetes Mellitus and Acute Myocardial Infarction: Long Term Results from the Diabetes and Insulin-Glucose Infusion in Acute Myocardial Infarction (DIGAMI) Trial', *Circulation*, **99** (1999), 2626–32.

Malmberg, K., L. Ryden, H. Wedel et al. 'Intense Metabolic Control by Means of Insulin in Patients with Diabetes Mellitus and Acute Myocardial Infarction (DIGAMI 2). Effects on Mortality and Morbidity', *European Heart Journal*, **26** (2005), 650–61.

Montalescot, G., S. D. Wiviott, E. Braunwald, S. A. Murphy, C. M. Gibson, C. H. McCabe, E. M. Antman and the TRITON-TIMI 38 investigators. 'Prasugrel Compared with Clopidogrel in Patients Undergoing Percutaneous Coronary Intervention for ST-elevation Myocardial Infarction (TRITON-TIMI 38): Double-blind, Randomised Controlled Trial', *Lancet*, **373** (2009), 723–31.

National Heart, Lung and Blood Institute (Part of the National Health Institutes of Health and the US Department of Health and Human Services). *Coronary Heart Disease* (2010). Available from http://www.nhlbi.nih.gov/health/dci (accessed 14 February 2010).

National Institute for Health and Clinical Excellence (NICE). *Acutely Ill Patients in Hospital: Recognition of and Response to Acute Illness in Adults in Hospital* (London: HMSO, 2007a).

National Institute for Health and Clinical Excellence (NICE). *Clinical Guidance 48: Secondary Prevention in Primary and Secondary Care for Patients Following a Myocardial Infarction* (London: HMSO, 2007b).

National Statistics. *Health Statistics Quarterly 34. Death Registration in England and Wales: 2006 Causes* (2007). Available from http://www.statistics.gov.uk (accessed 6 November 2007).

Nordmann, A. J. P. Hengstler, T. Harr et al. 'Clinical Outcomes of Primary Stenting versus Balloon Angioplasty in Patients with Myocardial Infarction: A Meta Analysis of Randomised Controlled Trials', *American Journal of Medicine*, **116** (2004), 253–62.

O'Driscoll, B. R., L. S. Howard and A. G. Davison. 'British Thoracic Society Guideline for Emergency Oxygen Use in Adults', *Thorax*, **63**(suppl. 6) (2008), 1–68.

Ross, R. 'Atherosclerosis – an Inflammatory Disease', *New England Journal Medicine*, **340** (1999), 115–26.

Sabatine, M. S., C. P. Cannon, C. M. Gibson et al. 'Addition of Clopidogrel to Aspirin and Fibrinolytic Therapy for Myocardial Infarction with ST Segment Elevation', *New England Journal of Medicine*, **352** (2005), 1179–89.

Thompson, C. A., J. Yarzebski, R. Goldberg, D. Lessard, J. Gore and J. Dalen. 'Changes over Time in the Incidence and Case Fatality Rates of Primary Ventricular Fibrillation Complicating Myocardial Infarction: Perspectives from the Worcester Heart Attack Study', *American Heart Journal*, **139**(6) (2000), 1014–21.

Van de Werf, F., D. Ardissino, A. Betriu, D. V. Cokkinos et al. 'Management of Acute Myocardial Infarction in Patients Presenting with ST Segment Elevation: The Task Force on the Management of Acute Myocardial Infarction of the European Society of Cardiology', *European Heart Journal*, **24** (2003), 28–66.

Weston, C., L. Walker and J. Birkhead. 'Early Impact of Insulin Treatment on Mortality for Hyperglycaemic Patients without Known Diabetes who Present with an Acute Coronary Syndrome', *British Medical Journal*, **93** (2007), 1542–6.

Yusuf, S., S. Reddy, S. Ounpuu and S. Anand. 'Global Burden of Cardiovascular Diseases. Part 1: General Considerations, the Epidemiologic Transition, Risk Factors and Impact of Urbanisation', *Circulation*, **104** (2001a), 2746–53.

Yusuf, S., S. Reddy, S. Ounpuu and S. Anand. 'Global Burden of Cardiovascular Diseases. Part 2: Variations in Cardiovascular Disease by Specific Ethnic Groups and Geographic Regions and Prevention Strategies', *Circulation*, **104** (2001b), 2855–64.

6

Chronic Obstructive Pulmonary Disease

Liz Cleave

Introduction: Chronic Obstructive Pulmonary Disease in Context (UK Focus)

Chronic obstructive pulmonary disease (COPD) is the global term given to a group of respiratory diseases that are characterised by irreversible airflow obstruction (NCCCC, 2004). COPD encompasses three different diseases: emphysema, chronic bronchitis and chronic asthma. COPD is a preventable and treatable disease (Global Initiative for COPD: GOLD, 2008) relying upon an early diagnosis so that appropriate curative and preventative management can be commenced in an attempt to delay the disease process. A diagnosis should be considered in anyone over the age of 35 presenting with symptoms of dyspnoea, cough and excessive mucus production (BTS, 2006). Preventative measures such as smoking cessation once diagnosis has been confirmed can reduce progression and relieve symptoms (Tashkin and Murray, 2009). Pharmacological medication is an integral aspect of management and aims to delay airflow obstruction. COPD is a complex disease and each person diagnosed with COPD experiences the symptoms and disease course in a unique way, especially the impact the disease has on activities of daily living. Management strategies must reflect the individual experience. Unlike many other common chronic diseases the prevalence of COPD has not declined in recent years and according to data is on the increase (Polkey, 2008). It is a common disease but it is difficult to be certain of the true mortality rate. Some patients die with the disease rather than because of it (Table 6.1) and the causes of death cited in mortality statistics have recently changed, making it difficult to ascertain accurate rates of death caused by COPD. However, COPD produces significant morbidity within the UK and

Table 6.1 COPD statistics

- Prevalence of COPD (estimates) = 1–4% of the population (3 million people).
- Standardised mortality = 35 per 100,000 population for women and 50 per 100,000 population for men.
- Cost to the NHS = £800 million per annum.
- Over 1 in 3 patients admitted with COPD will be readmitted within 30 days.

Source: Department of Health (2010).
Reproduced under the Open Government Licence v1.0.

has a huge resource implication for the National Health Service (in terms of healthcare cost). In late 2009 and early 2010 two important draft consultation documents relating to the strategy and management of COPD were made available for comment.

1. *Chronic Obstructive Pulmonary Disease: Management of Chronic Obstructive Pulmonary Disease in Adults in Primary and Secondary Care (Partial Update)* (NICE, 2009).
2. *Consultation on a Strategy for Services for Chronic Obstructive Pulmonary Disease (COPD) in England* (Department of Health, 2010).

COPD when severe is a complex condition. Therefore, the importance of a full clinical assessment and management of the patient when experiencing an acute exacerbation of COPD sets the scene for the following chapter.

Aim and Learning Outcomes

The Aim

The aim of this chapter is to explore the priorities for accurate assessment and management of an individual presenting with an acute exacerbation of COPD. It briefly identifies and recognises the assessment and management of a patient with stable COPD and then critically explores the management of a patient with an acute exacerbation of COPD (aeCOPD). The case scenario provides the basis for the application of evidence-based theory to support management decisions.

Learning Outcomes

At the end of this chapter the student will be able to:

1. Define what is meant by the term chronic obstructive pulmonary disease (COPD) and recognise the key elements of assessment and management of a patient with stable COPD.
2. Explore and link the pathophysiology to the presenting symptoms associated with aeCOPD.
3. Appreciate the immediate assessment of a patient who experiences aeCOPD.
4. Consider the management of aeCOPD and appreciate the factors indicating a deterioration in the patient's condition.
5. Explore the role of non-invasive ventilation (NIV) in the management of aeCOPD.
6. Consider how acute exacerbation may be prevented.

The Case Scenario: Stable Chronic Obstructive Pulmonary Disease

Arthur is a 55-year-old gentleman who retired early from his job as a welder 18 months ago. He was diagnosed with moderate COPD two years ago. During the last six months of work he reduced his hours to part time because his exercise tolerance rapidly declined. This was mainly due to exertional dyspnoea and a chronic cough that did not allow him to achieve the fine precision required for welding. He had smoked since the age of 16 but gave up smoking 12 months ago following a smoking cessation course suggested by the GP. During the past year his COPD has been relatively stable and he has actively participated in a self-management plan. Six weeks ago Arthur visited the GP practice for his annual influenza vaccination.

Arthur's current medication is:

Short acting B_2-agonists: Salbutamol inhaled two puffs (200 µg) QDS
Short acting anti-cholinergic: Ipratropium bromide inhaled two puffs (400 µg) QDS

Consider the following:

1. Define what is meant by the term COPD.
2. Identify the distinctive features of chronic bronchitis, emphysema and chronic asthma.
3. Explore the pathological changes associated with COPD.
4. Discuss the assessment and management of a person diagnosed with COPD.

The Respiratory System

Respiratory Anatomy and Physiology

An understanding of the underlying normal anatomy, physiology, patho-physiology, clinical features and maintenance therapy of stable COPD is helpful in understanding the assessment and management of an acute exacerbation of COPD (aeCOPD). The purpose of the respiratory system is to enable movement of oxygen from atmospheric air into the bloodstream for delivery to the cells for aerobic energy production and the elimination of the waste product of aerobic respiration, carbon dioxide, from the body. The outer aspect of the respiratory system, composed of the nose, pharynx, larynx and trachea, represents the first point of air entry into the system. The trachea then divides at the carina, forming the right and left main bronchi of each lung, which provide a reservoir for inspired oxygen-saturated air (Figure 6.1). The right lung is separated by invaginations of the

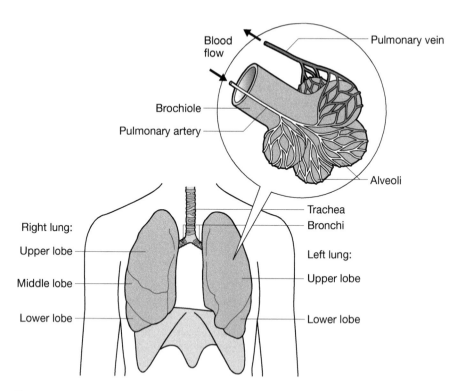

Figure 6.1 The respiratory system.

outer pleural lining into three lobes and the left has two lobes. Each bronchus further subdivides to smaller airways called bronchioles, which finally terminate at the single epithelial-walled alveolar sacs (Figure 6.1). There are approximately 300 million alveoli in the human lung, providing a massive surface area for oxygen to diffuse from an area of high concentration across the semi-permeable alveolar membrane and capillary walls into the pulmonary circulation, where there is a lower concentration of oxygen. Respiration can be subdivided into external and internal respiration.

External Respiration

External respiration is the mechanical process of enabling inspiration of oxygen-saturated atmospheric air (into the lungs) and expiration of carbon dioxide, a waste product of cellular metabolism, from the lungs.

Inspiration is actively controlled by:

1. The movement of ribs upwards and outwards under the influence of the intercostal muscles, leading to an overall increase in lung volume.
2. The contraction and descent of the diaphragm, which is responsible for most of inspiration in healthy adults.

Expiration results from a passive relaxation of intercostal muscles and diaphragm, allowing the lungs to collapse under the influence of their elastic fibres.

External respiration is controlled by the respiratory centre housed within the medulla oblongata of the brain stem. Autonomic nervous impulses arising from the respiratory centre are transmitted via the intercostal and phrenic nerves to respiratory muscles to stimulate a coordinated respiratory movement. Airway tone is also controlled by the autonomic nervous system. Noradrenaline release from sympathetic nerve endings stimulates adrenoreceptors within the bronchial muscular lining, causing bronchodilation. Beta-adrenoreceptor agonists such as salbutamol® mimic this bronchodilatory effect. Alternatively, inhaled stimuli such as smoke, dust or cold

Table 6.2 Glossary of terms

Bronchoconstriction: narrowing of the airway diameter resulting in less airflow available at the alveoli.

Bronchodilation: widening of the airway diameter enabling an increase in airflow.

---

air can activate cough receptors, which trigger reflex bronchoconstriction via vagus parasympathetic nervous activity.

Movement of air in and out of the lungs results from a difference in the pressure in the alveoli and atmospheric pressure. During inspiration atmospheric pressure is greater than alveolar pressure, whereas the reverse is true during expiration. Inspired alveolar oxygen then diffuses across the alveolar membrane into the pulmonary capillary and carbon dioxide moves from the pulmonary capillary back into the alveoli for expiration. Red cell haemoglobin has a high affinity for oxygen, which is transported within the arterial circulation as oxyhaemoglobin to the tissues and cells of the body.

Internal Respiration

Internal respiration describes the process of gaseous exchange at the cells. At a cellular level oxygen is extracted from the capillary blood and utilised by the cell for aerobic energy production. The deoxygenated venous circulation transports the waste product of aerobic respiration, carbon dioxide, back to the lungs for expiration into the atmosphere. Effective respiration must therefore maintain the partial pressure of oxygen (PaO_2) and partial pressure of carbon dioxide ($PaCO_2$) in arterial blood within normal limits (Table 6.3).

Nervous impulses that control respiration are highly influenced by neurogenic and chemical factors. Normal neurogenic influences include:

- a conscious change in respiratory rate and depth;
- impulses from limb receptors in response to exercise and rest;
- impulses from pulmonary receptors sensitive to stretch and irritation;
- impulses from receptors within the respiratory muscles and joints of the chest wall.

Chemical influences occur in response to changes in PaO_2 and $PaCO_2$ detected by peripheral chemoreceptors situated in arterial walls. Chemical influences upon breathing are the following:

Table 6.3 Normal arterial blood gas values

- PaO_2 (partial oxygen) = 11.0–13.0 kPa
- $PaCO_2$ (partial carbon dioxide) = 4.8–6.0 kPa
- pH = 7.35–7.45
- HCO_3 (bicarbonate) = 21–28 mmol/L
- BE (base excess) = –2 to +2
- SaO_2 (saturated arterial oxygen) = 95–100%

1. A rise in $PaCO_2$ is the strongest respiratory stimulant.
2. An increase in hydrogen (H^+) ions in the arterial blood caused by metabolic acidosis will increase ventilation in an effort to remove more CO_2 and therefore reduce arterial pH.
3. Peripheral chemoreceptors in the carotid and aortic bodies respond to a fall in PaO_2 and stimulate the rate of respiration. However, the stimulus is not strong until the PaO_2 falls below 8 kPa. These receptors also respond to an increase in H^+ ions.

Normal Gaseous Exchange

Efficient gaseous exchange also relies upon adequate ventilation of the alveoli and capillary perfusion. When there is inadequate ventilation or perfusion at the alveoli–capillary interface a ventilation/perfusion mismatch leads to ineffective gas exchange, either by the transport of oxygen to or the removal of carbon dioxide from the tissues. Adequate ventilation is dependent on several complex interactions and a failure in one or more of these can lead to a reduced amount of oxygen being available at the interface and a reduction in the removal of carbon dioxide from the blood.

These complex interactions include:

1. Airway resistance, i.e. the diameter of the airways, which determines the ease of airflow within them.
2. Lung compliance, i.e. the ease of lung expansion.
3. Elasticity, i.e. the stretch and recoil of the lung.

Any disruption in the flow of air within the airways can result in respiratory failure. Respiratory failure is when there is insufficient oxygen available at the alveoli–capillary interface and results in a decrease in the arterial level of oxygen (hypoxaemia), also known as type 1 respiratory failure (Table 6.4).

Table 6.4 Definition of respiratory failure

Type 1 respiratory failure
PaO_2 < 8 kPa = reduced arterial blood oxygen, due to a reduction or lack of inspired oxygen. This is termed hypoxaemia.
$PaCO_2$ = normal (or reduced)

Type 2 respiratory failure
PaO_2 < 8kPa
$PaCO_2$ > 6kPa = increased arterial carbon dioxide, due to increased airways resistance and reduced lung compliance. This is termed hypercapnia.

Carbon dioxide levels may be normal. A raised level of carbon dioxide within the blood (hypercapnia) associated with low PaO_2 is known as type 2 respiratory failure (Table 6.4). The effectiveness of gaseous exchange can be measured by examining the arterial blood gas, which measures the arterial level of oxygen (PaO_2) and of carbon dioxide ($PaCO_2$). Blood taken from an artery (normally radial artery) is machine tested to identify the PaO_2 and the $PaCO_2$.

Stable Chronic Obstructive Pulmonary Disease

Chronic Obstructive Pulmonary Disease

COPD is defined as a slowly progressive disorder characterised by irreversible airflow obstruction that does not change markedly over several months. The airway obstruction may be as a result of one or more different disease processes, but results in a loss of normal airway functioning and ineffective gas exchange at the alveoli–capillary interface. The three main diseases that contribute to loss of airflow are chronic bronchitis, emphysema and chronic asthma.

Chronic Bronchitis

Chronic bronchitis is characterised by inflammation and swelling of the lining of the airways, leading to airway narrowing and obstruction, airflow reduction and a consequent fall in alveolar ventilation. Pathological changes include hypertrophy of the mucus secreting glands of the bronchi and an increase in the number of mucus secreting goblet cells. Inflammation and excess mucus secretion can both lead to airway obstruction and to increased likelihood of bacterial infections. Smoking, particularly the number of cigarettes smoked per day, is a major factor in the development of chronic bronchitis. Climate, air pollution, socioeconomic status and employment have also been implicated. Chronic bronchitis, as in Arthur's case, is defined clinically as a daily chronic cough with the production of mucus for at least three months of the year and for two years in a row. Chronic bronchitis and emphysema coexist in many individuals.

Emphysema

Emphysema is defined pathologically as dilatation, permanent enlargement and destruction of the alveoli. The destruction of the alveolar walls reduces the elasticity of the lung, leading to expiratory airflow limitation, and therefore air becomes trapped during expiration. This is due to the loss of elastic recoil within the alveoli, and the trapped air leads to reduced alveolar space and therefore less oxygen availability. Furthermore, as a result of the destruction of the alveoli walls less surface area is available for gas transfer. Alpha1-antitrypsin deficiency has been associated with the development of emphysema at a young adult age; however, not all individuals born with the deficiency develop the disease. Cigarette smoking is largely implicated in disease development and progression.

Chronic Asthma

Asthma is a disease of the airways due to inflammation of the airways and a constriction of the muscles surrounding the airways (bronchospasm). Asthma is largely associated with atopy and allergy to common allergens, such as cats, dogs, house mites, dust, or pollens. Airway bronchospasm is reversible by the use of inhaled bronchodilators such as salbutamol®. In patients with long-standing, poorly controlled asthma, inflammation can lead to chronic scarring and a reduction in airway diameter, lack of airway reversibility and increasing airway resistance. Asthma is generally considered to be a distinct diagnosis, whereas chronic bronchitis and emphysema often coexist and are therefore more often labelled as COPD.

Clinical Signs

Although the above disease processes are distinct from each other, COPD is an amalgamation of different characteristics and shows variation in disease presentation. Table 6.5 offers a summary of the possible various presenting signs of COPD.

Table 6.5 Presenting clinical signs of COPD

Mucus hypersecretion	Airway cell changes resulting in an increased number of goblet cells of the bronchial submucosal glands, as a direct result of an irritation.
Ciliary dysfunction	Airway cell changes resulting in an increase in the size and abnormal functioning of the mucociliary escalator – results in difficulty in expectorating sputum.
Airflow limitation	Loss of bronchial wall and lung elasticity leads to an increase in airway resistance, leading to a reduction in the force of expiration.
Hyperinflation	Loss of lung elastic recoil: air becomes trapped within the lungs.

Source: adapted from Albert et al. (2008).

As a direct result of the physiological changes and effort to achieve alveolar ventilation, the respiratory muscles become weakened by over-inflation and increased airway resistance. Patients experiencing symptoms (dyspnoea) of COPD use their rib cage muscles and accessory muscles (sternocleidomastoids) even during quiet respiration. During exercise or for some patients who struggle for breath with limited movement the use of accessory muscles to assist breathing becomes even more exaggerated.

Common Clinical Features of COPD

Initially people like Arthur with COPD may present with no or minimal symptoms. As the disease progresses, changes in pulmonary function will become more evident and an increasing awareness of dyspnoea and sputum production compels individuals to seek consultation with a medical practitioner as in Arthur's case. A diagnosis of COPD should be considered in patients over the age of 35 years, who have a risk factor (generally smoking but occupation could be noted) and who present with exertional dyspnoea, chronic cough and regular sputum production.

Breathlessness is a subjective experience for the person and an objective scale can be invaluable in providing an objective assessment of the subjective experience. The MRC dyspnoea scale (Fletcher et al., 1959) may be used to determine the severity of dyspnoea experienced (Table 6.6).

It is important that, when reaching a diagnosis of COPD, other respiratory disorders including asthma have been considered and excluded (Table 6.7). The most common similar presentation (airway resistance resulting in reduced airflow) is with patients who have asthma. However, appropriate (inhaled) medication to dilate the airways can reduce the obstruction. Therefore, in asthma airway constriction is reversible,

Table 6.6   The MRC dyspnoea scale

Grade degree of breathlessness related to activities

---

1.   Not troubled by breathlessness except on strenuous exercise.
2.   Short of breath when hurrying or walking up a slight hill.
3.   Walks more slowly than contemporaries on level ground because of breathlessness, or has to stop for breath when walking at own pace.
4.   Stops for breath after walking about 100 m or after a few minutes on level ground.
5.   Too breathless to leave the house, or breathless when dressing or undressing.

Source: adapted from Fletcher et al. (1959).

Table 6.7 Distinguishing clinical features of COPD and asthma

	COPD	*Asthma*
Current or ex-smoker	Nearly all	Possibly
Symptoms under 35 years of age	Uncommon	Common
Chronic productive cough	Common	Uncommon (except in exacerbations)
Breathlessness	Persistent and progressive	Variable
Response to therapy	Partial and incomplete	Good
Nocturnal waking	Uncommon	Common

whereas in COPD there is no such reversibility as the airways are fixed and the airway diameter does not respond to inhaled bronchodilator medication in the same way.

Specific Assessment and Diagnosis of COPD

The importance of a correct and early diagnosis of COPD cannot be emphasised enough, as this will lead to appropriate management (GOLD, 2007). Although some debate has emerged about under- or over-diagnosis of COPD, one key measurement supports the diagnosis of COPD. Spirometry provides an objective measure of the force and volume of expiration. A full respiratory assessment to accompany the spirometry results includes:

1. Assessment of respiratory symptoms: shortness of breath, wheeze, cough and sputum production (consistency, frequency, MC&S, cytology).
2. Detailed history of family respiratory problems, smoking patterns, allergies and occupation.
3. Physical assessment of the chest: palpation, percussion and auscultation and noting finger clubbing and cyanosis.
4. Assessment of chest X-ray, biochemistry, haematology results.

Spirometry investigation is the most useful in determining the severity of airway obstruction, as it measures the volume of air expelled from the lungs after a maximal inspiration breath. Measurements of forced expiratory volume in one second (FEV1) and forced vital capacity (FVC) (Table 6.8) are compared with predicted normal values for the patient's height, age and sex (Russell and Norcliffe, 2008) to give an objective measure of the presence and degree of airway obstruction. FEV1 and FVC are expressed as a percentage of the predicted normal value to give an indication of severity. A normal

Table 6.8   Spirometry definitions

FEV1 (forced expired volume in one second). The amount of breath expired in 1 second following maximal inspiration.

FVC (forced vital capacity) The amount of forceful breath expired following maximal inspiration.

Table 6.9   Severity of airflow obstruction

Severity	*FEV1 as a percentage of predicted FEV1*
Mild	50–80
Moderate	30–40
Severe	< 30

Source: National Collaborating Centre for Chronic Conditions (2004).

reading should be greater than 80 per cent; therefore a result of 66 per cent of predicted FEV1 indicates mild airflow obstruction (Table 6.9).

NICE (2004) recommends annual assessment with spirometry for patients with mild and moderate airflow obstruction and bi-annual for severe airflow obstruction to determine, monitor and manage disease progression (see Booker, 2004, for a detailed description of spirometry).

Management and Maintenance of Stable COPD

Airflow obstruction is irreversible in COPD, though bronchodilators have been used as the principle aspect of management. Arthur was prescribed a short-acting inhaled B2-agonist called Salbutamol (Ventolin®) via a metered dose inhaler (MDI). Bronchodilators stimulate beta receptors within the smooth muscle lining of the bronchioles, causing dilatation. Extensive research has revealed that bronchodilators do not reverse airflow obstruction or produce significant improvements in FEV1, but appear to work by reducing airway smooth muscle tone, increasing airway calibre, and so they help to reduce airway trapping, improve the efficiency of respiratory movements, reduce dynamic hyperinflation and relieve dyspnoea. Salbutamol is the most common bronchodilator drug used in patients with COPD at 2 to 4 µg every six hours or more frequently if symptoms dictate. Once the drug is inhaled it works quickly and the effects last up to six hours (Hennefer and Lawson, 2009). Arthur also had a short acting inhaled anti-cholinergic called Ipratropiun bromide (Atrovent®) which is normally prescribed at 250 to 500 µg four- to six-hourly when alveoli have become enlarged and inflexible.

The mode of action of Atrovent® differs from salbutamol but it results in the same bronchodilator effect, although it takes longer to achieve the same effect. It causes smooth muscle relaxation by blocking nerve impulses that cause bronchoconstriction as a direct result of the disease process. It is effective within 30 to 60 minutes following inhalation and lasts for four to six hours. To obtain maximum control over symptoms inhaled medications are essential, though patient concordance with inhaler therapy must be assessed (Barnett, 2007).

If symptoms persist following use of short-acting drugs in stable COPD, long-acting bronchodilators may be used, though this had not yet been so in Arthur's case. These should be discontinued after four weeks if the patient has not experienced benefit from them. Anwar (2008) provides detailed information regarding bronchodilator use. In stable COPD, the management focus for the health professional is to encourage the patient to stop smoking. There is strong evidence that COPD is aggravated by air pollution and by dusty occupations (Bourke, 2007) but the dominant cause of COPD is cigarette smoking. The sequence of events in respiratory dysfunction is markedly associated with the duration of smoking, depth of inhalation and number of cigarettes smoked. Arthur stopped smoking 12 months ago and by doing so may slow his rate of airway obstruction. He actively participated in a self-management plan that advises individuals how to recognise early signs of deterioration and provides parameters within which Arthur may temporarily increase his bronchodilator therapy and commence a short course of inhaled or oral steroids if symptoms persist. However, the speed of onset from triggers such as respiratory infection sometimes prevents optimal self-management and may necessitate acute admission to hospital.

The Case Scenario: Acute Exacerbation COPD

Arthur had been relatively well until two days ago when he noticed increasing dyspnoea on climbing the stairs. Although he normally had a cough he was aware that he was coughing more often and producing larger amounts of sputum. This morning on waking his sputum colour had changed to a yellow/green thick consistency and he was finding it difficult to expectorate. He contacted his GP, who during a home visit found Arthur's condition to have deteriorated since he had seen him previously, and Arthur was mildly disorientated in time and place. The GP recorded a set of observations below and on the basis of the initial home assessment admitted Arthur to hospital for further assessment and acute management.

The Case Scenario   *continued*

Observations	At home by GP	On admission to A&E
Temperature (°C)	38.4	39
Pulse (beats/min)	102	100
Respiration	22	24
SpO_2 (per cent)	87 on air	89 on air
Arterial blood gases		
PaO_2 (normal 11.0–13.0 kPa)	8.2	
$PaCO_2$ (normal 4.8–6.0 kPA)	6.4	
pH (normal 7.35–7.45)	7.37	

Consider the following:

1. Describe the common signs of a patient presenting with aeCOPD.
2. Explore the possible causes of the exacerbation.
3. Describe Arthur's immediate assessment priorities and initial investigations in an acute exacerbation.

Assessment and Reaching a Diagnosis

Most patients with a mild exacerbation of COPD have unchanged airway limitation or a slight increase and can be managed at home; however, a sudden deterioration in condition or rapid onset of symptoms may need hospital treatment. Arthur's condition is of concern because excessive dyspnoea has confined him to bed; symptom onset was rapid and he shows signs of mild confusion. As Arthur has not experienced this level of dyspnoea and sputum production before and is likely to be anxious and frightened the GP refers Arthur to the A&E for detailed assessment using the ABC approach.

For the purpose of clarity in the written word, the observations are discussed separately here. However, in the clinical setting observations would be taken together, and trends and differences would be noted and reported. Severe exacerbations are associated with a worsening of pulmonary gas exchange because of the inequality between ventilation and perfusion, which can be exacerbated by respiratory muscle fatigue. These symptoms should be assessed with other aspects of the disease process, such as disease frequency and previous other aeCOPD (Rodriguez-Roisin, 2006).

Pathological Changes from COPD to aeCOPD

An exacerbation of COPD can be defined as a worsening of symptoms from their usual stable state (BTS, 2004). In Arthur's case there was evidence of increasing breathlessness and sputum production associated with greater airway inflammation, airflow limitation, mucus hypersecretion, hyperinfla-tions and ciliary clearance. This means that there is a further increase in airway resistance resulting in reduced gaseous exchange at the alveoli–capillary interface. An inflammatory response may be triggered by a range of factors, such as bacterial or viral infection or environmental pollu-tants. The increased inflammatory response seen with aeCOPD is associated with increased white blood cell activity and the release of neutrophils and eosinophils. Airway inflammation, oedema, mucus hypersecretion and bronchial vasoconstriction cause a decrease in ventilation and hypoxic vaso-constriction of the pulmonary arterioles, which impairs perfusion and leads to an increased ventilation/perfusion mismatch.

The Importance of Reassessment

There is no specific method of assessment of exacerbation severity. Prompt re-assessment of reported symptoms is vital for early diagnosis and more intensive treatment of the exacerbation.

Airway

Arthur is currently fully conscious and able to maintain his own airway. However, the risk of respiratory arrest must be considered and therefore close continual observation of airway patency should be employed and basic life support measures must be instigated if airway maintenance deteriorates further (see Chapter 2).

Breathing

Breathing is often the first vital sign to alter in a patient with a deteriorating condition and the potential for respiratory failure. Respiratory failure occurs when there is a decrease in available oxygen (PO_2) for gaseous exchange and may take place with or without changes in the ability to expel carbon diox-ide during expiration.

Arthur is described as dyspnoeic, which means 'difficulty breathing' and is a sign that should prompt a more detailed assessment of breathing. Respiratory rate, regularity, depth, noise and effort should be observed for one minute and should be repeated every 30 minutes to assess for deterioration and to indicate trend. Normal breathing should be 10 to 18 breaths per minute, noiseless and effortless. Arthur's respiratory rate was initially 22, which can be described as tachypnoea (respiratory rate greater than 18). Tachypnoea is an early sign of respiratory distress and a deteriorating clinical condition that can be used as an objective measure of trend. Decreased arte-rial oxygen levels and increased carbon dioxide are detected by arterial sensory chemoreceptors that stimulate the respiratory centre housed within the medulla oblongata to increase stimulation of the intercostal and diaphragmatic muscles, leading to an increase in respiratory rate. Rapid breathing may be shallow and an audible wheeze may be heard on auscultation. Wheezing occurs when air is forced through constricted airways. Immediate observation of Arthur is likely to reveal the use of accessory (sternomastoid and abdominal) muscles to aid breathing. An increased resistance against inspiration caused by obstruction or excess bronchoconstriction may require the use of accessory muscles such as the sternomastoid and scalene muscles for ventilation. Moreover, forced expiration against increased resistance may require the additional force of accessory muscles of the abdominal wall to help push the diaphragm upwards to collapse the lungs. The use of accessory muscles signals an acute exacerbation of COPD. Visible use of accessory muscles in the shoulders, neck and abdomen will make breathing appear difficult (dyspnoea), hard work and laboured, as this type of breathing requires great effort on behalf of the patient. Patients who experience difficulty breathing will appear restless and have difficulty finding a comfortable position, and may show signs of increasing fatigue due to the effort of breathing (BTS, 2004). Posture is therefore very important and while the optimum position to allow air entry would be upright, Arthur may find stability in leaning forward supported by an appropriately positioned table at chest height. Reassurance is essential in gaining the patient's cooperation at a time of respiratory distress. The feeling of dyspnoea and not being able to gain enough breath makes patients panic and feel very anxious. A quiet controlled environment where patients receive reassurance and informed information about immediate management plans and care delivery is essential.

Changes in skin colour may indicate respiratory problems. The consequent fall in available oxygen and rise in carbon dioxide levels may cause skin cyanosis. Initially peripheral cyanosis may be evident as a bluish tinge of the nail beds. Central cyanosis is a sign of worsening respiratory distress and may be visualised as a bluish tinge of the lips, oral mucosa and ears. This is normally detected when the SpO_2 falls below 85 per cent and is considered a late sign of respiratory problems.

The effectiveness of oxygen delivery across the alveolar capillary divide can be measured using continuous non-invasive O_2 saturation (SpO_2) monitoring via a pulse oximeter. SpO_2 provides information regarding the oxygen level within the peripheral perfusion. Airflow limitation and mucus hyper-secretion within the larger airways prevents sufficient O_2 delivery at the alveolar–capillary interface, leading to a reduced SpO_2. On admission Arthur's SpO_2 is 89 per cent on air, which is on the low side of the recommended 88 to 92 per cent saturation level (BTS, 2008) and therefore requires intervention with oxygen therapy. An increased concentration of oxygen delivery should result in an improvement in oxygen saturation. Oximetry can reduce the need for invasive arterial blood gas analysis. However it is not the most reliable method of oxygen saturation monitoring, particularly when the patient is severely ill and has poor perfusion. Arterial blood gas (ABG) analysis will provide a more detailed evaluation of alveolar ventilation. The blood sample is usually obtained from the radial artery via a stab procedure. For respiratory patients the important ABG measures to note are the PaO_2, $PaCO_2$ and pH (Table 6.3). The more serious the interruption of gaseous exchange at the alveolar–capillary interface, the further from normal will be the blood gas measurement. Arthur's initial PaO_2 was low at 8.2 kPa and his $PaCO_2$ was slightly raised at 6.4 kPa. PaO_2 falls reciprocally with an increase in $PaCO_2$ when there is alveolar under-ventilation. Arthur is experiencing a trend towards type 2 respiratory failure (Table 6.4) indicated by hypoxaemia (a decrease in arterial oxygen level) and hypercapnia (a rise in arterial carbon dioxide level). pH is a measurement of the hydrogen (H^+) ion concentration in the blood. Cell metabolism relies upon a normal blood pH value of pH 7.4. A pH of < 7.35 indicates acidosis and > 7.45 indicates alkalosis. The pH is affected by many parameters, including the concentration of CO_2 within the blood. An increased $PaCO_2$ can lead to increased blood acidity recognised as a fall in pH below 7.35. Arthur's arterial blood results indicate an altered pH from 7.4 to 7.37 and a drift towards respiratory acidosis. Simpson (2004) provides a detailed guide to arterial blood gas analysis.

Arthur has a productive cough and is expectorating copious amounts of sputum. While it is important to notice any change in colour or consistency, Brusse-Keizer et al. (2009) identified only a weak association between bacterial load and sputum colour. Therefore colour changes in sputum are important to note but do not necessarily indicate the level or degree of infection. A sputum pot, tissues and mouthwash should be provided in order to collect sputum carefully and safely and enable the collection of a specimen for analysis of microscopy, culture and sensitivity (MC&S). MC&S will detect any bacterial presence and assess the sensitivity and resistance to antibiotic therapy. Arthur's raised temperature of 39 °C, above normal (37–37.4 °C), provides further evidence of an active infection and inflammation.

Circulation

A rapid heart rate > 95 beats per minute is described as a tachycardia. Arthur's heart rate of 102 beats per minute may be abnormally raised for a number of reasons, not least as a result of increased sympathetic activity mediated by feelings of panic and anxiety associated with dyspnoea. It may also indicate a compensatory response to a low PaO_2 concentration sensed by chemoreceptors situated within the arterial walls, which stimulate an increased heart rate to circulate oxygenated blood around the body more quickly. Although a useful mechanism, the increased myocardial workload will demand an increase in oxygen delivery, diverting some of the circulating oxygen away from other organs and tissues and further exacerbating signs of peripheral hypoperfusion. Arthur's pulse and BP should be reassessed regularly during the acute phase and, if they are within normal parameters, this should be repeated every four hours. A blood pressure of more than 140 mmHg systolic and 90 mmHg diastolic may be associated with stress and anxiety or may indicate underlying hypertension, which would require further specific investigation and treatment. A low blood pressure below 100 mmHg systolic may indicate underlying cardiac disease, which again should prompt more specific investigation.

Generalised hypoxia and respiratory acidosis leads to insufficient delivery of oxygen to all the organs and tissues. Cerebral hypoxia may be displayed in a range of ways from mild disorientation in time and place as in Arthur's case to confusion or loss of consciousness in severe cases. At this stage, although conversation will be difficult for Arthur, regular assessment of time and place should be sufficient. However, more formal neurological assessment such as the Glasgow Coma Scale (GCS) should be commenced should his consciousness levels begin to deteriorate (see Chapter 4).

Table 6.10 displays a range of routine venous blood sampling tests that Arthur may undergo to provide vital information about the effects of hypoxia on other major organs.

It is important to establish or exclude other potential causes of respiratory distress, such as pulmonary embolus (PE), pulmonary hypertension, pneumonia, pneumothorax, lung cancer, aspiration or tuberculosis (BTS, 2004). Although the FEV1 was instrumental in an accurate diagnosis of COPD, there is no place for such a measure in an acute exacerbation. A chest X-ray, detailed clinical examination of the respiratory system, including palpation, percussion and auscultation with a stethoscope, and full secondary assessment (Table 6.11) are useful in determining other pathologies.

Table 6.10   Routine venous blood sampling

1. Full blood count (FBC): low Hb (anaemia), raised WBC (infection).
2. C-reactive Protein (CRP): raised suggests active infection.
3. Clotting screen: if indicated by current medication, e.g. warfarin.
4. Urea and electrolytes (U&E): electrolyte balance and renal function.
5. Capillary blood glucose if high or low glucose is suspected, e.g. diabetic patient.

Table 6.11 Secondary assessment

---

1. Past medical history (PMH): respiratory and systemic.
2. Family history (FH) and social history (SH).
3. Systemic enquiry: general, gastric, urinary, central nervous systems.
4. Evaluation of triggers and risk factors.
5. Drug history: prescribed, over the counter and recreational.
6. Full clinical examination: peripheral pulses, jugular venous pressure (JVP), heart and lung sounds, systemic examination.

The Case Scenario: Medical Management and Care Issues

Arthur's past medical history and symptom presentation reflect an acute exacerbation of COPD. Arthur is commenced on 24 per cent oxygen therapy via a venturi mask, nebulised bronchodilator therapy at four-hourly intervals, bed rest and regular observation of respiratory status, including hourly ABGs. The hourly trend following admission in the arterial blood gases reveals a deterioration in PaO_2, $PaCO_2$ and pH levels despite 24 per cent oxygen. The pulse and respiratory rate has increased in compensatory response to worsening respiratory acidosis, decreasing oxygen levels and increasing carbon dioxide levels. Despite the initiation of a course of oral steroids and intravenous broad spectrum antibiotics Arthur's condition remains poor and so non invasive-ventilation (NIV) was introduced.

Observations	1 hour following admission	1 hour post commencing NIV
Temperature (°C)	39.2	39.0
Pulse (beats/min)	108	98
Respiration	24	18
SpO_2 (per cent)	86 on 24 per cent oxygen	92 on entrained air via NIV
Arterial blood gases		
PaO_2 (kPa)	8.0	10.2
$PaCO_2$ (kPa)	7.4	6.9
pH	7.34	7.41

Consider the following:

1. What was the rationale for the change in pharmacological medication to treat aeCOPD.
2. Appreciate the role of oxygen therapy in aeCOPD management.
3. Explore the role of non-invasive ventilation (NIV) in Arthur's management.
4. Identify the key methods employed to prevent further exacerbations.

Medical Management Strategies and Care Issues

The aims of management of a patient with aeCOPD are to:

1. Correct hypoxaemia.
2. Relieve airway obstruction.
3. Treat the presenting infection.
4. Manage any co-morbidities (Seemungal and Wedzicha, 2000).

Early and effective management of aeCOPD can prevent worsening of symptoms (Llor et al., 2008).

Oxygen Therapy

Controlled oxygen therapy plays an important role in optimising the delivery of oxygen to the tissues where hypoxaemia (low PaO_2) has been detected to alleviate the symptoms of dyspnoea. Oxygen therapy is the obvious first line treatment for Arthur but the prescribed dosage must be carefully considered to reflect his underlying respiratory disease.

Normally the respiratory stimulus to breathe, i.e. the 'respiratory drive', is a detected rise in arterial carbon dioxide levels ($PaCO_2$) but in a few patients with long-standing respiratory disease such as COPD the respiratory centre becomes desensitised to high CO_2 levels and so a low PaO_2 becomes the 'respiratory drive'. Therefore high levels of administered oxygen therapy to an individual with COPD may switch off their acquired respiratory drive and lead to respiratory failure. These patients are required to carry an 'alert' card, indentifying the need to be prescribed low levels of oxygen.

The aim of oxygen therapy in Arthur's case is to:

1. Increase the level of oxygen at the alveolar–capillary interface.
2. Maintain oxygen saturations at about 90 per cent (rather than aiming for a normal SpO_2 of 95 to 100 per cent).
3. Increase the arterial oxygen level without risking further carbon dioxide retention (increase in $PaCO_2$) and respiratory acidosis.

Oxygen should be administered in a controlled way and reflect the deviation of oxygen saturation and arterial blood gases from the expected norm. Interpretation of the oxygen saturations and arterial blood gas analysis will give the most accurate picture of effectiveness of gaseous exchange and an indication of the percentage of oxygen that should be given. The most effective (and accurate) method of delivery of oxygen is via a venturi mask where controlled low inspired oxygen concentrations of 24 to 28 per cent (BTS,

2008) can be given through a high flow mask. Some patients may prefer to have the oxygen delivered via nasal cannula, though it can be difficult to assess the percentage of oxygen received, especially as many breathe through their mouth. After one hour of receiving 24 per cent oxygen Arthur's oxygen saturations had decreased from 89 to 86 per cent, the blood pH fell to 7.34 (respiratory acidosis) and carbon dioxide levels increased. This demonstrates that sensitivity to increased $PaCO_2$ is lost and therefore hypoxaemia not hypercapnia is the chief respiratory stimulant. In Arthur's case the oxygen therapy appears to be reducing respiratory drive.

In a patient with COPD maintenance of oxygen saturations at 90 per cent is considered appropriate. Failure to correct the oxygen saturations (SpO_2) to greater than 90 per cent with an oxygen flow rate of 40 per cent may suggest the presence of additional pathophysiology that requires investigation. While objective measurements give a good indication of the success of the oxygen therapy, monitoring Arthur's level of confusion and consciousness is also an important indicator of worsening hypoxaemia. Failure to improve saturation levels (oxygen saturations above 90 per cent) despite oxygen therapy, a fall in pH or a increase in the $PaCO_2$ is an indication of deteriorating respiratory failure and may require ventilation support (non-invasive ventilation, NIV, or intermittent positive pressure ventilation, IPPV).

Inhaled Bronchodilators: Nebulisers

Increased dyspnoea is a result of airway responsiveness to the airflow limitation and increased mucus production. The first line of management is to increase the dose frequency and strength of short-acting bronchodilators. One potential side effect of Salbutamol® is tachycardia. Arthur should be made aware of this and the need to report symptoms such as palpitations as soon as possible. Four-hourly recording of heart rate should also detect signs of increasing tachycardia.

Arthur was prescribed Salbutamol® 5 mg via his MDI but as this method did not provide symptom relief his prescription was changed to nebulised bronchodilator therapy. Arthur's excess respiratory effort, often associated with a peripheral shake, may interfere with his ability to hold and use the device effectively. Boe et al. (2001) showed that there is no real benefit of nebuliser over MDI but anecdotally some patients feel relief from getting the bronchodilators this way. The bronchodilator should be delivered on compressed air (BTS, 2004) rather than oxygen due to the potential effect of high alveolar oxygen tensions on ventilation/perfusion and increasing $PaCO_2$. Ipratropium bromide (Atrovent®) can also be nebulised with the Salbutamol®. The role of the nurse during oxygen/nebuliser therapy is to assist Arthur in gaining maximum effect from the oxygen/nebulised drugs by ensuring correct use of the delivery chamber and assisting him to sit in an upright position to maximise lung expansion. Theophylline® may also be used as an adjunct to the management of aeCOPD, by increasing respiratory drive if there is an inadequate response to nebulised bronchodilators (BTS, 2004; NICE, 2004). Prior to Theophylline® use care must be taken to ensure that Arthur is not taking the drug as part of routine management, as it is easy to exceed the therapeutic range and induce side effects such as nausea and cardiac arrhythmias.

Systemic Corticosteroids

Corticosteroids are given to relieve the symptoms of inflammation, reduce the length of the exacerbation and improve symptoms, although the benefit of corticosteroids has remained contentious. The medication is given by the oral route as opposed to the inhaled route. A more rapid improvement has been demonstrated in patients' FEV1 by giving systemic steroids (de Jong et al., 2007), although other aspects such as hospitalisation and oxygenation may add to the benefits of the steroids (Sayiner et al., 2001). Aaron et al. (2003) found patients treated with Prednisolone® during acute exacerbations took longer to reach subsequent exacerbations. Arthur was commenced on a dose of 30 mg of Prednisolone® for 14 days (NICE, 2004), as longer courses have not been found to be beneficial and increase the risk of side effects (NICE, 2004).

Antibiotics

Antibiotics are commonly prescribed for episodes of purulent sputum (NICE, 2004). The bacteria that have been isolated during exacerbations are generally sensitive to most broad-spectrum antibiotics. There has been some controversy whether antibiotics have benefit in an exacerbation but treatment is usually based on patient symptoms and the purulence of the sputum. Little data exists on the optimum duration of the therapy. As Arthur is experiencing increased sensation of breathlessness, increased sputum production and an observed colour change to the sputum, intravenous antibiotics have been prescribed. The antibiotic chosen may be dictated by antibiotic policies and local resistance patterns but it is generally agreed that the drug of choice (Amoxycillin®, Doxycycline®, Erythromycin®) will cover common pathogens such as *Haemophilus influenzae*, *Moraxella catarrhalis* and *Streptococcus pneumoniae*. It is not considered necessary to take sputum samples prior to initiating antibiotics except where patients do not appear to be responding to treatment or to check whether the correct antibiotic has been prescribed. Safety of drug prescribing should be detailed regarding previous administration of antibiotics or to determine any drug allergies or details of drugs that may interact. It should also be noted that aeCOPD is not always caused by infection, as air pollutants and adverse weather conditions may lead to an exacerbation.

Non-invasive Ventilation

Non-invasive ventilation (NIV) has become pivotal in the management of patients with aeCOPD (RCP National Guidelines, 2008), particularly for individuals whose arterial blood gases show no improvement following initial management with bronchodilators, oxygen therapy, corticosteroids and antibiotics (NICE, 2004). An arterial blood gas pH of 7.35 or less is an indication that the patient requires NIV (Seemungal and Wedzicha, 2008). NIV can reduce the intubation rate and mortality in patients presenting with aeCOPD and should be considered as a treatment option within the first 60 minutes of arrival in hospital. NIV augments tidal volume and decreases the work of breathing by initiating a slower, deeper breath reflecting a more normal physiological pattern of breathing, where inspiration and expiration parameters on the NIV machine are independently set to reflect individualised breathing pattern. The inspiratory phase improves alveolar ventilation and as a direct result of this decreases carbon dioxide, decreases dyspnoea and ultimately decreases the use of accessory muscles. In the expiratory phase of breathing, NIV forces an extra breath of air into the lung to splint the alveoli open at the end of respiration, therefore increasing the time of respiration, and this in turn increases gas exchange, decreasing carbon dioxide and increasing oxygen. This ultimately improves the ventilation/perfusion mismatch. Arthur continued to struggle with his breathing despite being compliant with the optimum drug management offered. A repeat arterial blood gas analysis after one hour of management revealed a worsening of respiratory failure and therefore the decision was made to initiate NIV. NIV involves positioning a very tight fitting mask over the mouth and/or nose to aid assisted ventilation (Figure 6.2). However, in addition to the underlying dyspnoea, the forced ventilation during expiration and the tight fitting mask can cause feelings of claustrophobia, sweating, facial sores and anxiety, and may limit patient compliance with the device. Sensitive management is essential to promote compliance at this critical time. Initially allowing the patient to hold the mask without strap fixing may decrease the anxiety and the patient may tolerate the air delivery from the machine more readily. The selection of low initial inspiratory and expiratory pressures allows the patient to become used to the forced inspiration and expiration prior to being increased to achieve maximum NIV therapy. Simple explanation, reassurance, visibility, approachability and easy methods of communication with nurses and family

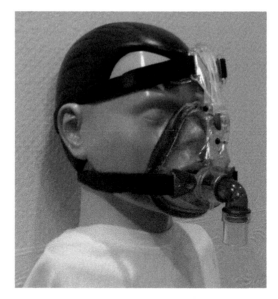

Figure 6.2   Non-invasive ventilation mask.

Table 6.12   NIV observations

Initial NIV observations include:
- Respiratory rate
- Heart rate
- Level of consciousness
- Chest wall movement
- Ventilator synchrony

may help Arthur to cope and tolerate his treatment. During NIV therapy observations should be monitored every 30 minutes during the first four hours (Table 6.12) and adequate fluid management, nutrition and communication should be planned, implemented and evaluated within Arthur's care delivery plans.

Bed rest also necessitates careful planning of toilet and hygiene needs, especially mouth and eye care, pressure area care, including facial points beneath the NIV mask, and passive limb exercises to avoid deep vein thrombosis. Regular arterial blood gas analysis via several arterial stab wounds will require localised manual pressure to achieve stasis, and regular observation of the sites for bleeding, oozing or signs of infection such as redness and soreness. Arterial blood gas analysis provides evidence of improvement of alveolar ventilation and assessment of Arthur's ABG after one hour of NIV reveals an improved pH from 7.34 to 7.41, indicating less respiratory acidosis; the PaO_2 has increased from 8.0 to 10.2 kPa and the $PaCO_2$ has decreased from 7.4 to 6.9 kPa, indicating a positive response to prescribed treatment. Jarvis (2006) provides a useful overview of the research evidence for NIV. For some patients NIV is not successful in correcting the arterial oxygen and carbon dioxide levels and the decision to proceed to full intubation must be considered. This can be a difficult decision and the thoughts, beliefs and opinion of the patient and family must be carefully considered to ensure the patient is fully informed of the possible treatment options available.

Preventing Exacerbations

A positive partnership between the patient and the GP will enable the patient to recognise the symptoms of deterioration (Decramer et al., 2008). Early treatment can be initiated and prevent further deterioration of the patient's lung function. Arthur and his GP had worked together to develop a self-management plan and this was used successfully when he began to experience a change in symptoms. Self-management plans reduce hospital admissions and patients report an improved quality of life following their introduction to them (Bourbeau et al., 2006).

Other strategies that may prevent hospital admission include:

1. Annual influenza vaccinations and pneumonococcal vaccinations.
2. Education and health promotion related to smoking.

If patients with diagnosed COPD continue to experience exacerbations then the GP may consider the following:

1. Inhaled steroids with patients who are experiencing more than two acute exacerbations of COPD in a 12-month period and if the FEV1 is < 50 per cent predicted.
2. Long-acting bronchodilator therapy such as salmeterol®.
3. Using combined therapy of long-acting bronchodilator and inhaled steroids.

Summary

COPD is a complex disease and annual review is suggested for patients experiencing mild symptoms in stable COPD and biannual for more severe disease. Acute exacerbations of COPD (aeCOPD) can be successfully managed within primary care, but due to the severity of symptoms experienced the patient may require hospital admission. Acute exacerbations of COPD present a burden both to the patient in terms of quality of life and to the health service in cost (Haughney et al., 2005), but successful treatment of acute exacerbations can prevent further deterioration in the patient's lung function. Thorough assessment of a patient experiencing an acute exacerbation will inform the management to optimise treatment availability. A critical aspect of the management of the patient is to recognise the physical and psychological impact the 'stable' disease can have on the activities of daily living and the anxiety and fear that often accompanies an acute exacerbation. Guidelines (BTS, NICE, NCCCC and GOLD, USA) inform practitioners of the researched evidence base for care delivery.

Further Reading

Anwar, A. 'Bronchodilators: Uses and Prescribing Rationale', *Nurse Prescribing*, **6**(5) (2008).

Barnett, M. 'Chronic Obstructive Pulmonary Disease: A Phenomenological Study of Patients' Experiences', *Journal of Clinical Nursing*, **14** (2005), 805–12.

Booker, R. 'Chronic Obstructive Pulmonary Disease: Importance of Diagnosis', *British Journal of Nursing*, **13**(4) (2004).

Harris, S. 'COPD and Coping with Breathlessness at Home: A Review of the Literature', *British Journal of Community Nursing*, **12**(9) (2007).

Jarvis, H. 'Exploring the Evidence Base of the Use of Non-invasive Ventilation', *British Journal of Nursing*, **15**(14) (2006).

NICE, National Collaborating Centre for Chronic Conditions. *Chronic Obstructive Pulmonary Disease: Management of Chronic Obstructive Pulmonary Disease in Adults in Primary and Secondary Care* (2004). www.nice.org.uk/pdf/CG012_niceguidelines.pdf

Simpson, H. 'Interpretation of Arterial Blood Gases: A Clinical Guide for Nurses', *British Journal of Nursing*, **13**(9) (2004).

References

Aaron S. D., K. L. Vandemheen and P. Herbert. 'Outpatient Oral Prednisolone after Emergency Treatment of Chronic Obstructive Pulmonary Disease', *New England Journal of Medicine*, **348** (2003), 2618–25.

Albert R. K., S. G. Spiro and J. R. Jett. *Clinical Respiratory Medicine* (Philadelphia: Mosby Elsevier, 2008).

Barnett, M. 'Improving Drug Concordance in Patients with COPD', *Nursing Prescribing*, **5**(5) (2007).

Boe J., J. H. Dennis, B. R. O'Driscoll, T. T. Bauer, M. Carone and B. Dautzenberg. 'European Guidelines on the Use of Nebulisers', *European Respiratory Journal*, **18** (2001), 228–42.

Bourbeau J., J. P. Collet, K. Schwartzman, T. Ducruet and D. Nault. 'Economic Benefits of Self Management Education in COPD', *Chest*, **130**(6) (2006).

Bourke, S. J. *Respiratory Medicine*, 7th edn (Oxford: Blackwell Publishing, 2007).

Brusse-Keizer, M. G. J., A. J. Grotenhuis, H. A. M. Kerstjens, M. C. Telgen, J. van der Palen, M. G. R. Hendrix, P. D. L. P. M. van der Valk. 'Relation of Sputum Colour to Bacterial Load in Acute Exacerbations of COPD', *Respiratory Medicine*, **103** (2009), 601–6.

British Thoracic Society. 'Management of Acute Exacerbations of COPD', *Thorax*, **59**(suppl. 1) (2004), 1–232.

British Thoracic Society. *The Burden of Lung Disease*, 2nd edn (London: British Thoracic Society, 2006).

British Thoracic Society. 'BTS Guidelines for Emergency Oxygen Use in Adult Patients', *Thorax*, **63**(suppl. VI) (2008) iv1–vi68.

Decramer, M., L. Nici, S. Nardini, J. Reardon, C. L. Rochester, C. M. Sanguinetti and T. Troosters. 'Targeting COPD Exacerbation', *Journal of Respiratory Medicine*, **102**(suppl. 1) (2008), S3–S15.

De Jong Y., S. M. Uil, H. P. Grotjohan, D. S. Postma, A. M. Kerstjens and J. W. K. van den Berg. 'Oral or IV Prednisolone in the Treatment of COPD Exacerbations', *Chest*, **132**(6) (2007).

Department of Health. 'Improving Care for Patients with Chronic Obstructive Pulmonary Disease', Press release 2006/0241.

Department of Health. *Facts about COPD* (2010). www.dh.gov.uk/en/Healthcare/Longtermconditions/COPD/DH

Fletcher C. M., P. C. Elmes and M. B. Fairbairn. 'The Significance of Respiratory Symptoms and the Diagnosis of Chronic Bronchitis in a Working Population', *British Medical Journal*, **ii** (1959), 257–66.

GOLD. *Global Initative for Chronic Obstructive Lung Disease. Pocket Guide to COPD Diagnosis, Management and Prevention. A Guide for Healthcare Professionals* (New York: Gold, 2008).

GOLD Executive Summary. 'Global Strategy for the Diagnosis, Management and Prevention of Chronic Pulmonary Obstructive Disease', *American Journal of Respiratory and Critical Care Medicine*, **176**(6) (2007), 532–55.

Haughney, J., M. R. Partridge, C. Vogelmeier, T. Larsson, R. Kessler, E. Stahl, R. Brice and C. G. Lofdahl. 'Exacerbations of COPD: quantifying the patient's perspective using discrete choice modelling', *European Journal of Respiratory Medicine*, **26**(4) (2005), 623–9.

Hennefer, D. and E. Lawson. 'Pharmacology: A Systems Approach: Respiratory System', *British Journal of Healthcare Assistants*, **3**(3) (2009).

Llor, C., J. Molina and K. Naberan. 'Exacerbations Worsen the Quality of Life of Chronic Obstructive Pulmonary Disease Patients in Primary Healthcare', *International Journal of Clinical Practice*, **62** (2008), 585–92.

National Collaborating Centre for Chronic Conditions (NCCCC). 'Chronic Obstructive Pulmonary Disease. National Clinical Guideline on Management of Chronic Obstructive Pulmonary Disease in Adults in Primary and Secondary Care', *Thorax*, **59**(suppl. 1) (2004).

National Institute for Clinical Excellence (NICE). *Chronic Obstructive Pulmonary Disease: Management of Chronic Obstructive Pulmonary Disease in Adults in Primary and Secondary Care* (London: NICE, 2004).

Polkey, M. I. 'Chronic Obstructive Pulmonary Disease', *Medicine*, **36**(4) (2008), 213–17.

Rodriguez-Roisin, R. 'COPD Exacerbations: 5 Management', *Thorax*, **61** (2006), 535–44.

Royal College of Physicians (RCP). *Non-invasive Ventilation in Chronic Obstructive Pulmonary Disease: Management of Acute Type 2 Respiratory Failure. Concise Guidance to Good Practice. National Guidelines. Number 11* (London: RCP, 2008).

Russell, R. and J. Norcliffe. 'Chronic Obstructive Pulmonary Disease: Management of Chronic Disease', *Medicine*, **36**(4) (2008).

Sayiner A., Z. A. Aytemur, M. Cirit and I. Unsal. 'Systemic Glucocorticosteroids in Severe Exacerbation of COPD', *Chest*, **119** (2001), 726–30.

Seemungal, T. and J. A. Wedzicha. 'Acute Exacerbations of Chronic Obstructive Pulmonary Disease: Treatment and Prevention', *Medicine*, **36**(4) (2008).

Tashkin, D. P. and R. P. Murray. 'Smoking Cessation in Chronic Obstructive Pulmonary Disease', *Respiratory Medicine* **103**(7) (2009), 963–74.

7

Acute Kidney Injury

Mark Bevan

Introduction

Acute kidney injury (AKI) replaces the once commonly used term acute renal failure (ARF). This is an international initiative by the Acute Kidney Injury Network (AKIN) to standardise practice and improve patient outcome (Mehta et al., 2007). While both terms may be used interchangeably, AKI implies a spectrum of kidney damage that ranges from mild impairment to outright organ failure and will be used throughout this chapter. AKI is a condition that can affect anyone with an acute illness; it can complicate chronic illness or be the sole disease affecting a person. AKI is not inevitable in acute or critical illness and in many cases is preventable and it is seen in acute care wards but can also be found in the primary care environment (Hegarty et al., 2005). It is estimated that between 25 and 30 per cent of intensive care patients develop AKI, with 5 to 6 per cent of these requiring renal replacement therapy (Clarkson et al., 2007).

It is difficult to estimate the incidence of AKI due to a lack of consistent information. However, there is some emerging evidence. An early community-based study found that 51 patients per million population (pmp) with AKI were being referred to specialists (Feest et al., 1993). This study used a serum creatinine of > 500 μmol/L (normal range 60 to 125 μmol/L: Provan and Krentz, 2002) as a definition of AKI, which is a considerable elevation demonstrating severe renal impairment. These authors found an overall incidence of 140 episodes of AKI pmp per year. A Scottish study examined the incidence of AKI, which was defined as a creatinine level of ≥ 300 μmol/L with severe AKI at ≥ 500 μmol/L. The overall incidence of AKI was 620 pmp, with severe AKI being 102 pmp. They also noted a marked increase in incidence with age: for example, the incidence of AKI in the 0 to 19 age group was 30 pmp but it was an astonishing 4,266 pmp in the over 80 age group (Khan et al., 1997). A similarly high incidence of AKI in older adults

159

has also been observed in England. A more recent study re-examined the incidence of AKI in the Grampian region of Scotland and found the incidence to be 1,811 pmp/year and the median age to be 76 (Ali et al., 2006). The higher incidence in this study reflects the use of lower creatinine levels to indicate AKI ≥ 150 µmol/L for males and ≥ 130 µmol/L for females. This study also found the incidence of AKI in patients who already had chronic kidney disease (CKD) to be 336 pmp/year (median age 80.5 years). What these selected studies demonstrate is that AKI is a common condition and is increasing in incidence, especially within the older age group (Waiker et al., 2006).

Acute kidney injury has proved difficult to define given its broad spectrum and lack of quality evidence (Mehta et al., 2007; Davenport and Stevens, 2008). According to AKIN acute kidney injury occurs when there is 'an abrupt (within 48 hours) reduction in kidney function currently defined as an absolute increase in serum creatinine of ≥ 26 µmol/L, a percentage increase in serum creatinine of ≥ 50 per cent (1.5 fold from base line), or a reduction in urine output (documented oliguria of less than 0.5 ml/kg/h for > 6 hours)' (Mehta et al., 2007, p. 3). These criteria (Table 7.1) require at least two serum creatinine levels within 48 hours for diagnosis and will take into account variables such as body mass index, gender and age. AKI is marked by a rapid but potentially reversible decline of kidney function, which results in a retention of nitrogen-based waste products of metabolism such

Table 7.1   Criteria for diagnosis of acute kidney injury

AKI network stage	*Serum creatinine (SCr) criteria*	*Urine output criteria*
1	SCr ≥ 26.4 µmol/L Or SCr ≥ 150–200% from base line	< 0.5 ml/kg/hr for > 6 hr
2	SCr > 200–300% from base line	< 0.5 ml/kg/hr for > 12 hr
3	SCr > 300% from base line Or SCr ≥ 354 µmol/L with an acute rise of ≥ 44 µmol/L in ≤ 24 hr Or Initiated on RRT (irrespective of stage at time of initiation)	< 0.3 ml/kg/hr for 24 hr Or Anuria for 12 hr

Source: Adapted from Mehta et al. (2007).

as urea and creatinine and in most cases a reduction in urine output (Clarkson et al., 2008). Understanding this information enables nurses to play an important role in the assessment, continuous monitoring, prevention and management of AKI in the patient.

Aim and Learning Outcomes

Aim

The aim of this chapter is to explore the priorities of early accurate assessment, prevention and nursing and medical management of the individual presenting with acute kidney injury

Learning Outcomes

At the end of this chapter the reader will be able to:

1. Define acute kidney injury and distinguish between the differing manifestations of AKI.
2. Identify and explain the pathophysiological basis of the presenting signs and symptoms of AKI.
3. Identify and explain the immediate nursing and medical assessment, specific monitoring and key investigations required to enable an accurate and timely diagnosis.
4. Explore the evidence basis for immediate priorities of medical and nursing management, with a particular focus upon pharmacological and invasive interventions.
5. Appreciate the role of different health professionals in acute assessment and management of AKI.
6. Recognise the common complications associated with AKI.

The Case Scenario: The Presenting Complaint

Ralph is an 80-year-old man who lives in an elderly care home. He is usually mobile and self-caring. The staff, in the home, report that over the past four days Ralph has become increasingly lethargic and drowsy following treatment for a chest infection (treated with oral Amoxicillin® 500 mg three times daily for seven days). He was found on the floor of his room by morning staff; they are unsure of how long he had been lying there. He has been taking no food and very little fluids and has had several episodes of vomiting over the past two days. On examination Ralph is

The Case Scenario   *continued*

drowsy but responsive to questioning, though a little disorientated. He is also irritable and has a headache. His skin is dry, he has a minor petechial rash on his upper chest and lower neck and has an unproductive cough. He complains of anorexia, nausea and has vomited once (100 ml bile-stained fluid). His bladder is not palpable.

His vital signs were recorded as:

Pulse: 110 beats/minute sinus tachycardia
BP: lying = 90/40 mmHg; standing = 80/40 mmHg
Jugular venous pressure (JVP): unrecordable
Oxygen saturations (SpO$_2$): 92 per cent on room air
Temperature: 37.7 °C
Glasgow Coma Scale: 14 (E4, V4, M6)
Weight: 75 kg

Ralph's past medical history reveals:

Type II diabetes mellitus since age 65
Osteoarthritis of left hip
Hypertension since age 60
Urinary hesitancy awaiting urological investigation

Ralph's current medication is:

Metformin® 2 g divided with meals
Bendrofluazide® 5 mg daily
Ibuprofen 400 mg eight-hourly

A provisional diagnosis of acute kidney injury is made.

Consider the following:

1. With reference to the underlying pathophysiology describe what is meant by acute kidney injury.
2. What are the common signs and symptoms associated with AKI?
3. What further investigations need to be carried out to identify a definitive diagnosis?

Acute Kidney Injury

The medical review of Ralph's clinical features suggests that he has AKI. However, unless one knows how to interpret these clinical features it will not be clear how this conclusion was made. One way in which to make sense of these clinical features is to start with some indication of the causes of AKI. Initial assessment should be comprehensive to help determine the cause of AKI and to ensure appropriate treatment (Stevens et al., 2008), and should include physical assessment and investigations (Table 7.2).

Table 7.2   Summary of assessment of AKI patients

Assessment	*Content*
History	Presenting condition, symptoms, past medical history, drug history, family history, social history
Clinical examination	Vital signs (BP, P, resps)
	Level of consciousness
	Intravascular volume (skin turgor, mucous membranes, BP lying and standing, orthostatic pulse change)
	JVP
	Pulse oximetry
	CVP, pulmonary artery catheter
	Peripheral capillary return
	Weight
	Systems: cardiovascular, respiratory, gastrointestinal, neurological, dermatological eyes, nails, oedema
Urine	Output, volume
	Appearance and content (cells, crystals, blood, protein, glucose, pH, ketones, SG)
	Culture
	Biochemistry: sodium, protein, creatinine clearance
Blood	Estimated GFR: creatinine
	Biochemistry: sodium, potassium, chloride, bicarbonate, calcium, phosphate, pH, magnesium, urea
	Blood gases
	LFTs: CK, amylase, albumin
	Cholesterol
	Immunology
	Culture
ECG	LVF, dysrhythmia, MI
Imaging	Ultrasound, X-ray, CT scan, MRI, urography, nuclear medicine, angiography, cystoscopy
Biopsy	Kidney diseases
Nutritional status	Malnutrition
Medication	Nephrotoxins, inappropriate drugs

Acute kidney injury has many causes but is generally classified into three groups, known as pre-renal, intrinsic and post-renal. While each group is discrete in its content it is worth noting that there may be considerable overlap, especially with pre-renal and intrinsic causes. The causes of AKI are summarised in Figure 7.1.

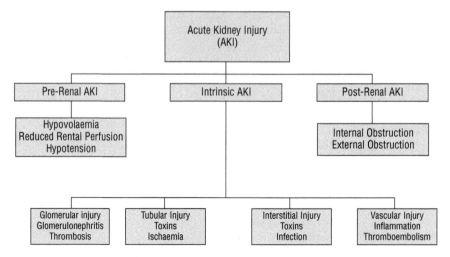

Figure 7.1 Causes of acute kidney injury.

Pre-renal Acute Kidney Injury

The causes of pre-renal AKI can be identified from the term 'pre-renal', occurring before the kidney, whereby AKI is a secondary event, with the primary event occurring elsewhere in the body. In order to understand how an illness or disease elsewhere in the body can affect the kidney some knowledge of renal physiology is required. The kidneys produce urine, which is made up of water, waste products of metabolism, hormones and drugs. The production of urine occurs within 1.2 million (approximately) functional units called nephrons housed within each kidney (Figure 7.2).

The cellular activity of the kidney requires a huge amount of oxygen. In fact, while the kidney only occupies 1 per cent of total body weight it uses 10 per cent of the body's oxygen requirements (Cohen, 1986). The kidney's high oxygen consumption is proportionate to the amount of sodium reabsorption, which is a vitally important function for maintaining fluid balance. However, the cells in the nephrons function at very low oxygen saturation levels of 1.3–2.9 kPa (normal is 12–15 kPa) and therefore are very sensitive to change. The kidney requires 1200 mL of blood per minute, which is one-fifth of cardiac output, in order to produce 1 mL of urine per minute (Koeppen and Stanton, 2001). Kidney blood flow causes a filtration pressure within the glomerulus of about 60 mmHg, which in turn produces a glomerular filtration rate (GFR) of approximately 125 mL/min/1.73 m^2 (Koeppen and Stanton, 2001). The key point here is that given all these factors the kidney is susceptible to alterations in its blood supply and oxygenation and this is where pre-renal causes affect kidney function.

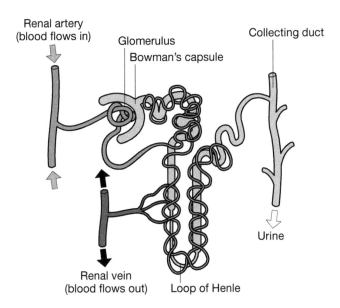

Figure 7.2 The nephron.

In order to provide 1200 mL/min of blood to the kidney certain factors need to be in place. These factors are the need for an effective pump (the heart), an effective circulating volume (the blood), appropriate volume pressure (blood pressure) and a patent vasculature (blood vessels). Any change to one or more of these factors may cause a reduction of kidney perfusion significant enough to cause injury. Major causes of pre-renal AKI cause a rapid loss of GFR and a reduction in urine output (oliguria). Typical causes of pre-renal AKI are hypotension of any cause, congestive cardiac failure, diuretic use and haemorrhage (Table 7.3).

Loss of significant volumes of fluid will lead to a low blood pressure and reduced kidney perfusion. Volume depletion is by far the major cause of

Table 7.3 Examples of causes of pre-renal AKI

Cause	*Examples of common problems*
Cardiac	Congestive cardiac failure, cardiac surgery, arrhythmia
Volume	Burns, bleeding, vomiting, diarrhoea, diuresis
Vascular resistance	Shock, antihypertensive treatment, NSAIDs, ACE inhibitors, hepatorenal syndrome
Vascular patency	Renal artery thrombosis, abdominal aortic aneurysm (AAA), bilateral renal artery stenosis

Table 7.4   Causes of volume depletion

Total intravascular depletion	Effective volume depletion
• Haemorrhage	• Reduced cardiac output: congestive cardiac failure, pulmonary embolism, cardiogenic shock
• Renal fluid loss: diuretics, osmotic diuresis (such as glycosuria)	
• Gastrointestinal loss: vomiting, diarrhoea and nasogastric aspiration	• Peripheral vasodilation: sepsis, anaphylaxis, cirrhosis, antihypertension medication
• Skin fluid loss: burns, sweating	
• Third space syndrome: pancreatitis, peritonitis	

Source: Adapted from Faubel et al. (2005).

pre-renal AKI and can be divided into two groups. One is total intravascular depletion, where intravascular volume is reduced, and the other is effective volume depletion due to arterial under-filling, where there is adequate volume (Faubel et al., 2005) (Table 7.4).

However, additional factors, including commonly used drugs such as non-steroidal anti-inflammatory drugs (NSAIDs), are known to cause vasoconstriction of the arterioles of the kidney, thus reducing GFR. Therefore it is important that a range of possible causes are considered. In Ralph's case, his clinical history reveals a number of clues that may point to pre-renal AKI as a possible cause. The clinical information indicates Ralph is hypotensive, his fluid intake has been low, he has vomited, though the frequency is not known, and he is taking medication (Bendrofluazide® and ibuprofen), which all carry the risk of reducing renal perfusion.

Intrinsic Acute Kidney Injury

In contrast to pre-renal AKI, where a physiological insult occurs elsewhere in the body, intrinsic AKI points to the kidney as the source of the problem. Intrinsic simply means something specific to the kidney, whereas pre-renal AKI is extrinsic or from without the kidney. Other words used synonymously with intrinsic are intrarenal, renal or parenchymal, and each points to problems with the functional parts (nephrons) of the kidney. The structures of the kidney that are affected are the microcapillaries (glomeruli, afferent and efferent arterioles), the tubular cells and the interstitium, which is the tissue that surrounds the nephrons (Figure 7.3). It is also important to note that if pre-renal AKI occurs this will have an impact upon the nephron and cause tubular cell death, also known as acute tubular necrosis (ATN). Examples of intrinsic AKI can be found in Table 7.5.

Table 7.5 Examples of causes of intrinsic acute kidney injury

Vascular	Glomerular	Tubular	Interstitial
• Renal artery thrombosis • Surgical cross clamping • Polyarteritis nodosa • Haemolytic uraemic syndrome • Malignant hypertension	• Goodpasture's syndrome • Henoch-Schoenlein purpura • Infective endocarditis • Wegener's granulomatosis	• Ischaemia • Haemorrhage • Nephrotoxins, e.g. vancomycin • Myoglobin (muscle damage) • Haemoglobin (haemolysis)	• Drug-induced: antibiotics, NSAIDs, diuretics • Infection: bacterial, viral, tuberculosis

The glomerulus is where filtering of the blood occurs (Figure 7.3). Filtration is driven by blood pressure and so a fall in blood pressure will cause a decline in the GFR. The filtration barrier is made up of three structures: the endothelial cells of the blood vessel, the basement membrane and the epithelial cells of the Bowman's capsule. This glomerulus has a size restriction (anything over 42 angstroms is retained) and is also negatively charged to prevent substances such as proteins from escaping into the urine (Koeppen and Stanton, 2001). Any pathological process that damages this structure alters its function by inhibiting filtration or essentially making it more permeable to larger substances, such as in protein (albumin) leakage (seen in diabetes mellitus) or red blood cell leakage (as found in glomerulonephritis). As already noted, the nephron is made up

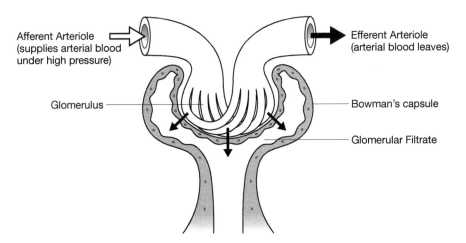

Afferent Arteriole
(supplies arterial blood under high pressure)

Efferent Arteriole
(arterial blood leaves)

Glomerulus

Bowman's capsule

Glomerular Filtrate

Figure 7.3 The glomerulus.

of highly active cells and it is here where wholesale and fine tuning reabsorption of essential substances such as water, sodium and potassium as well as the secretion of excess and toxic substances occurs. These cells are responsible for maintaining the chemical balance of extracellular fluid by manipulating substances such as sodium and potassium. Damage to these cells will alter the ability to maintain chemical homeostasis and the removal of toxins.

Intrinsic diseases that affect the kidney can be primary to the kidney or as part of a systemic disease. Where the disease is part of a systemic disease such as systemic lupus erythematosis (SLE) kidney function cannot be affected by manipulating external factors such as maintaining circulating volume. Diseases that affect the microcapillaries involve the blood vessels or the capillary bundle known as the glomerulus. There are inflammatory conditions of blood vessels such as polyarteritis nodosa and Wegener's granulomatosis, large vascular disease such as renal artery thrombosis, renal vein thrombosis and surgical cross-clamping as found in abdominal aortic aneurysm repair. Conditions that affect small vessels include thrombocytopaenic conditions such as pre-eclampsia, scleroderma, malignant hypertension and haemolytic uraemic syndrome (HUS), which is often caused by *E. coli* H0157:H7 contamination of food. In these conditions there is damage to the endothelial cells of the blood vessels and stimulation of the clotting cascade (Salama, 2002).

Intrinsic AKI: Glomerular Disease

There are diseases of the glomerulus that alter the structure of the glomerular filtration barrier, causing haematuria and proteinuria. They are usually immunologically mediated and cause the condition known as glomerulonephritis. Proteinuria can be very severe and in some cases in excess of 3 grams in 24 hours can be lost, which is known as nephrotic, whereas less than 2 grams in 24 hours is called nephritic. Such conditions include Henoch–Schönlein purpura, Goodpasture's syndrome, infective carditis and post-infectious glomerulonephritis (often streptococcal infection). Patients with these diseases are usually very ill, with skin lesions and often a rash (Holley, 2001). Ralph has a petechial rash, which may indicate an intrinsic cause to his AKI. Alternatively his rash could have been caused by local capillary trauma due to coughing during his chest infection. The blood cells found in the urine of patients with glomerulonephritis are often misshapen and lumped together in 'casts' as they progress through the tubules. Haematuria can be non-visible and only found by urine dipstick testing, or visible. This simple test aids diagnosis of intrinsic disease of the kidney.

Intrinsic AKI: Tubular Disease

Damage to the renal tubules (acute tubular necrosis: ATN) is caused in 50 per cent of cases by a reduction in blood flow (ischaemia) to the kidney and in 35 per cent of cases by a nephrotoxic substance (Faubel et al., 2005). Ischaemic causes of ATN have already been identified in pre-renal AKI; however, nephrotoxins are multiple and in theory any substance is potentially toxic to the kidney. Due to the rich blood supply to the kidney and the ability to concentrate toxins in high levels the kidney is particularly vulnerable to toxic substances (Clarkson et al., 2008). Nephrotoxins can be drugs such as aminoglycoside antibiotics, including Gentamicin® and Vancomycin®; cancer drugs such as Cisplatin®; anaesthetic drugs such as Enflurane®; antiviral drugs such as Acyclovir® and immunosuppressive drugs such as Ciclosporin®. Nephrotoxins can also come from within the body, such as haemoglobin (from haemolysis), myoglobin (from muscle damage) and uric acid. Each of these nephrotoxins will damage the tubular cells to varying degrees, which may be sufficient to prevent function or lead to cell death. Subsequent tubule blockage leads to cellular casts or debris in the urine.

Intrinsic AKI: Interstitial Disease

Interstitial disease of the kidney occurs when an inflammatory process is initiated in the cells between nephrons. Commonly inflammation occurs as a consequence of hypersensitivity to drugs but it can also be caused by infection or systemic disease such as SLE (Baker, 2002). Infectious causes can be direct, as found in upper urinary tract infection leading to pyelonephritis, or they can be systemic, such as streptococcal, staphylococcal, HIV and hepatitis A. Drugs that induce acute interstitial nephritis (AIN), include many perceived safe drugs such as antibiotics (ampicillin, erythromycin), non-steroidal anti-inflammatory drugs, Ranitidine®, diuretics (Furosemide®, thiazides), paracetamol and aspirin (Baker, 2002). It is likely that any drug has the potential for initiating hypersensitivity in a person and causing kidney injury. Patients with AIN frequently present with pyrexia, rash, joint pain, hypertension, fluid retention and possible signs of systemic disease. It can occur at any time after exposure to the drug and is not dose dependent.

There are a number of possible causes in Ralph's case. He may have ATN due to low blood pressure but he has also had an infection and was treated with an antibiotic. Further to this Ralph has been taking ibuprofen (a NSAID) and bendrofluazide® (a diuretic), which may indicate interstitial nephritis. Ralph has a rash on his chest, which is a possible sign of a vasculitic disease, and protein in his urine could indicate glomerular damage. This information adds to the complexity of assessment of someone with AKI and by no means can it be assumed that the cause is pre-renal or intrinsic at this point.

Post-renal Acute Kidney Injury

Post-renal AKI relates to conditions that interfere with the flow of urine from the tip of the papillae (renal pyramids) to the tip of the urethra. Obstruction is the usual cause, with elderly men being most at risk due to prostatic hypertrophy and/or cancer (Table 7.6).

In these conditions patients usually present with reduced (oliguria) or loss of urine output (anuria), urinary retention, loin pain and possibly fever. Anuria usually suggests urinary tract obstruction; otherwise it is unusual in AKI (Hilton, 2006). Urinary retention and bilateral kidney obstruction will eventually cause back pressure into the kidney tubules, which counteracts the pressure across the filtration barrier of the glomerulus, thus reducing glomerular filtration rate and renal blood flow. This in turn would eventually cause an intrinsic AKI due to ischaemia of the tubular cells. This additional information adds more possibilities to the cause of Ralph's AKI. Ralph has a reduced urine output, which may be symptomatic of obstruction, especially as he has a history of urinary hesitancy, not uncommon for a man of his age. Ralph also has diabetes mellitus, which is known to cause papillary necrosis, which obstructs the ureters with necrotic tissue. Each of these potential causes requires investigation to differentiate cause and initiate appropriate management.

Table 7.6   Examples of causes of post-renal acute kidney injury

Intraureteral obstruction	Bladder and urethral obstruction	Obstruction by external pressure
• Stones • Papillary debris caused by drugs, diabetes, stricture • Blood clots • Myeloma	• Urethral stricture • Prostatic hypertrophy/cancer • Tuberculosis • Spinal cord injury • Multiple sclerosis • Diabetes mellitus	• Malignancy: rectal, ovarian, uterine, cervical • Fibroids • Crohn's disease • Haemorrhage • Aortic aneurysm

Risk Factors for Acute Kidney Injury

It is important to note what factors increase the risk of AKI (Table 7.7). In relation to Ralph increased age is a risk factor for AKI. The reason for this is multi-factorial, including multiple co-morbidities, but one major reason is that kidney function of older people lacks renal reserve. This means that the kidney has an age-related reduced GFR which, when put under stress, such as dehydration, cannot compensate effectively (Bevan, 2001, 2005). The elderly kidney is also sensitive to the effects of drugs, especially NSAIDs, which cause vasoconstriction and may be implicated in Ralph's AKI (Pannu and Halloran, 2002). Underlying chronic kidney disease, often identified by proteinuria or cardiovascular disease (especially hypertension and renovascular disease), is also a risk factor in that it will affect the kidney's ability to respond to injury. In addition, diabetes mellitus causes long-term vascular damage to the kidneys (see Chapter 9). These three factors immediately place Ralph at high risk for AKI. Surgery, especially cardiac surgery, predisposes individuals to AKI and accounts for 25 per cent of hospital-acquired AKI (Lamiere et al., 2005) and hypotension is a major risk factor that is increased with the use of diuretics. The increase in organ transplantation is contributing to more cases of AKI due to the use of immunosuppressive therapy (Lamiere et al., 2005).

In summary, an understanding of the underlying causes of AKI can inform the assessment strategy employed in Ralph's case. It is apparent that Ralph has a number of potential causes for his condition. His history of potential hypovolaemia and hypotension may suggest pre-renal AKI, whereas possible intrinsic causes such as his medication may have caused acute tubular necrosis. Finally, Ralph may also have a urinary system obstruction that may have contributed to his kidney injury.

Table 7.7   Risk factors for AKI

- Increased age
- Diabetes mellitus
- Underlying kidney disease
- Cardiac disease
- Proteinuria
- Diuretic use
- Volume depletion
- Multiple myeloma
- Cardiac surgery
- Smoking in the elderly

The Case Scenario: The Immediate Assessment Priorities

Samples of blood and urine taken for analysis from Ralph revealed the following results:

Capillary blood glucose: 8.5 mmol/L
Venous blood biochemistry – urea and electrolytes (U&Es)
  Urea: 40 mmol/L
  Creatinine: 330 μmol/L
  Na^+: 133 mmol/L
  K^+: 6.9 mmol/L
  Cl^-: 107 mmol/L
  HCO_3: 19 mmol/L
  Cholesterol: 7.5 mmol/L
  CK: 180 iu/L
  Calcium: 2.2 mmol/L
  Pi: 1.2 mmol/L
  Glucose: 10 mmol/L
Venous blood liver function tests (LFTs)
  Albumin: 35 g/L
  Bilirubin: 10 μmol/L
  ALT: 15 iu/L
  Alkaline phosphate: 123 u/L
  Lactate: 2.0 iu/L
  CRP: 72
Venous blood haematology
  Hb: 13.2 g/dL
  HCT: 0.45 L/L
  WCC: 22×10^9/L
  Platelets: 10×10^9/L
Immunology
  ANA, ANCA, complement, protein electrophoresis, Anti-GBM all tested normal
Virology
  No HIV, hepatitis A or B
Urinalysis
  Protein +
  pH 6
  No other abnormality
  Urine output: 150 mL in 8 hours
  Sodium: 10 mmol/L
  Fractional excretion Na: < 1 per cent
  Urine osmolarity: 1250 mOm/kgH$_2$O

The Case Scenario *continued*

Immediate Assessment
1. How does the information gleaned so far help with the next step of assessment?
2. Devise a comprehensive acute assessment plan for Ralph and explain the rationale for each measure.
3. How is AKI differentiated from chronic kidney disease?
4. How is Ralph's level of kidney function calculated?
5. Re-examine Ralph's biochemistry results then calculate his eGFR at http://www.renal.org/eGFRcalc/GFR.pl and consider what it means with respect to the amount of kidney function he has.

Assessment and Reaching a Diagnosis

Notwithstanding other aspects of assessment, namely ABCDE identified in Chapter 2, assessment will focus upon specific issues related to Ralph and AKI. However, it is important to note that assessment of airway, breathing and circulation is essential especially because AKI is potentially a life threatening condition. There must be appropriate prioritisation in the assessment of Ralph because focusing upon the wrong issues may prove fatal for someone with AKI.

Airway and Breathing

While conscious, Ralph will be maintaining his own airway; however, his SpO_2 at 92 per cent suggests a degree of hypoxaemia. It is therefore important to observe and document his respiratory rate, depth and rhythm and sounds regularly and to monitor oxygen saturations using pulse oximetry continuously. Oxygen therapy should be commenced at 40 per cent via face mask in an effort to increase the SpO_2 above 95 per cent.

Circulation

Retention of electrolytes, in particular potassium, due to renal failure can lead to serious cardiac arrhythmias. Therefore Ralph requires continuous cardiac monitoring to assess his heart rate, regularity and rhythm. He is documented as having a sinus tachycardia, which may be a compensatory response to his low blood pressure (BP). Ralph's BP should be recorded at least every four hours as an indication of improvement or deterioration. Central venous pressure (CVP) measurement may also be useful in assessing Ralph's circulatory fluid status but will require insertion of a wide bore catheter into the jugular vein attached to a litre infusion of 0.9 per cent sodium chloride to enable regular measurement (see Chapter 3).

Disability

Assessment of Ralph's altered consciousness must be undertaken. Altered consciousness is a trigger factor for initiating urgent treatment in an attempt to prevent deterioration (NICE, 2007). Ralph's conscious level should prompt a bedside capillary blood glucose measurement, particularly as he has a history of type 2 diabetes and hasn't eaten well recently. His capillary and venous blood glucose are on the upper side of normal but not sufficiently abnormal to account for his drowsiness. Drowsiness is a common clinical feature in AKI. If other potential factors such as hyper- or hypoglycaemia, hypoxia and hypotension are excluded, altered consciousness occurs in AKI due to the accumulation of uraemic toxins. Vanholder et al. (2003) identified 90 potential uraemic toxins, including urea, creatinine, parathyroid hormone, guanidines, ammonia and peptides. These substances are poorly understood: for example, urea only has a very minor effect and is believed not to be the cause of uraemic symptoms, requiring accumulation with other substances to have an effect (Meyer and Hostetter, 2007). It is worth noting that uraemia does not mean high urea levels in the blood but literally means 'urine in the blood': that is to say, the products normally seen in the urine are retained in the blood but at abnormal levels.

Uraemia causes altered neurosensory function, presenting with cognitive impairment such as defects in memory, attention and concentration. Unrelieved uraemia will lead to coma and death. Clinical signs and symptoms of uraemia can be found in Table 7.8. Ralph's consciousness level must be monitored using the Glasgow Coma Scale (or equivalent) for deterioration (see Chapter 4) and the frequency of assessment will be determined by his condition, level of consciousness and potential for deterioration. Ralph currently has a GCS of 14 so every 15 to 30 minutes may initially be sufficient; however, there must be a nursing initiative to increase the frequency of testing should his condition deteriorate. Drowsiness in uraemia is a sign of very high accumulation of uraemic toxins. Patients with chronic kidney disease can usually tolerate high levels of uraemic toxins and are not usually drowsy in the way Ralph is; therefore his symptoms appear to point towards AKI, where drowsiness is more likely.

Table 7.8 Signs and symptoms of uraemia (some features may be dependent upon underlying cause)

System	Uraemic signs and symptoms
Neurological	Altered consciousness, irritability, reduced concentration and memory numbness, weakness, tremor, stupor, coma, hearing disturbance
Respiratory	Dysponea, orthopnoea, haemoptysis, nose bleed, sinusitis
Cardiovascular	Palpitations, arrhythmias, pericarditis, cardiac failure, hypotension
Gastrointestinal	Nausea, vomiting, diarrhoea, thirst, abdominal pain, acid reflux, bleeding, hiccup, stomatitis, fetor, gastritis, gastric/enteral ulceration, bleeding
Genitourinary	Haematuria, proteinuria, frequency, dysuria, suprapubic pain, altered urine output, loin pain, colic
Musculoskeletal	Arthralgia, muscular pain, cramp
Skin	Rash, pruritis, bruising, jaundice, hypothermia, dry skin, oedema, uraemic frost
Eyes	Red eyes, oedema
General	Fever, malaise, insomnia, weight loss
Haematological	Anaemia, thrombocytopenia (bleeding), altered white cell function

Specific Investigations

A range of specific investigations are required to reveal the exact cause of Ralph's apparent kidney failure and presenting signs and symptoms. Table 7.9 outlines investigations for a general approach to assessment of causes of acute kidney injury.

Estimating the Level of Kidney Function

Creatinine is a substance that is also thought to be of limited toxicity. Normal kidney function usually excretes all creatinine, unlike urea, of which about 60 per cent is reabsorbed. Creatinine is a by-product of muscle metabolism and reflects total muscle mass. Because of its complete removal by the kidney it is a useful marker for glomerular function. It is used as a means for estimating kidney function. Current recommendations advise the use of the

Table 7.9 Investigations for assessment of AKI

Investigation	Specific test content	Reason for test
Urea and electrolytes	Urea and creatinine	Creatinine to estimate kidney function and hydration (Ur:Cr ratio)
	Sodium	Assess level and hydration
	Potassium	Assess level and cardiac risk
	Calcium	Assess level and differentiate CKD, High levels cause AKI, low in rhabdomyolysis
	Phosphate	Assess level and differentiate CKD
	Chloride	Assess level; acidosis/alkalosis
	Magnesium	Assess level, (may be low)
	Bicarbonate	Acidosis/Alkalosis
	Urate	Assess level pre-eclampsia (high uric acid levels are implicated in pre eclampsia and lead to AKI)
	Lactate	Tissue ischaemia/under perfusion, assess lactic acidosis
eGFR	Estimate glomerular filtration rate	Assess level of kidney function
Liver function test	Albumin	Assess level; may be low in glomerulonephritis
	Creatine kinase	Assess level for muscle damage (myoglobin)
	Amylase	Assess level;Pancreatitis may cause AKI
	Bilirubin, AST, ALT	Haemolysis, liver disease may cause AKI
Arterial blood gases	pO_2	Assess oxygen level for oxygenation
	pCO_2	Assess acidosis, CO_2 retention
Full blood count and coagulation studies	Haemoglobin	Asses for anaemia, need for transfusion
	White cell count	Indicator of infection
	Platelets	Level and coagulopathy (e.g. DIC)
	Group and save	Transfusion
	Haematocrit	Assess anaemia/hydration
	INR	Clotting screen

Inflammation and immunology	ESR	Indicator of inflammation
	CRP	Non-specific marker for inflammation and infection
	ANA, ANCA, Anti-GBM, IgA, IgM, IgG, electrophoresis, complement, antistreptlysin	Specific glomerular disease tests e.g. SLE, vasculitis, myeloma
Infection	Blood Culture	Infection: sepsis may cause or prolong AKI
	Urine culture	Infection: may cause interstitial nephritis, prolong AKI
	Virology	Hepatitis A B, HIV
Urinalysis	Dipstick	Assessing for blood, protein, infection
	Electrophoresis	Specific test for multiple myeloma which causes AKI
	Albumin creatinine ratio	Assess glomerular damage
	Creatinine clearance	To assess kidney function/damage
	Volume	Assesses urine output/kidney function and prescribe volume replacement
Imaging	Chest X-ray	Evidence of pulmonary oedema, LVF
	Renal Ultrasound	Assess kidney structure, size and signs of obstruction
	X-ray Kidney Ureter Bladder	Obstruction, stones, abdominal masses
	CT/MRI	Assess kidney structure
	Isotopes studies	Assess renal perfusion, cortical necrosis, vascular obstruction
	Biopsy	Assess ATN, suspected intrinsic AKI
Cardiac	ECG	Assess cardiac function: LVF, dysrhythmia

estimated glomerular filtration rate method (eGFR), which uses age, race, creatinine and sex to calculate kidney function, rather than the Cockroft–Gault formula (Renal Association, 2008). Some caution is needed in AKI because eGFR is normally used for chronic kidney disease. The eGFR is requested at the same time as obtaining U&Es but there are many eGFR calculators available on the internet. Using the Renal Association (2008) calculator Ralph's GFR is 19 mL/min/1.73m^2 (normal: about 100 mL/min/1.73m^2 without signs of kidney disease), which means he has about 20 per cent of his kidney function remaining.

Differentiating between AKI and CKD

It is important to establish whether Ralph has AKI or CKD to ensure that he gets the appropriate treatment. Not only is Ralph a prime candidate for AKI but his increased age, diabetes and hypertension make him a prime candidate for CKD. Ralph may have underlying kidney disease and be presenting with an acute-on-chronic episode or with end-stage renal disease (ESRD). Drowsiness is a common symptom of AKI but can also manifest in ESRD (National Collaboration for Chronic Conditions, 2008; Hsu et al., 2008). People with

---

The Case Scenario: Medical Management and Care Issues

Ralph is diagnosed with acute kidney injury and he does not appear to be showing any signs of improvement. A radial artery sample is taken for blood gas analysis and the following results received:

Arterial blood gases (ABGs)
PO$_2$: 10.6 kPa
PCO$_2$: 8.1 kPa
Base excess: −1
Anion gap: 18
pH: 7.31

Immediate Medical Management
1. What two urgent priorities of management and care can you identify for Ralph?
2. How would these two priorities be managed?
3. What fluid replacement regime would best suit Ralph's needs?
4. What are Ralph's main care issues?
5. What are Ralph's additional management priorities?
6. Examine the blood gas results carefully and consider what might be done.

CKD usually have an absence of acute illness, and also present with anaemia, nocturia, long duration of symptoms, hyperphosphataemia and hypocalcaemia (Hilton, 2006). Renal ultrasound will identify the size of the kidney, as those with CKD will typically have small kidneys (< 9 cm), though diabetes may preserve kidney size for some time. Ralph's clinical features and history indicate his problem is acute in nature rather than chronic.

Medical Management Strategies

Acute kidney injury is a life threatening condition and it is therefore important that priorities for management are promptly identified. Principles of AKI management can be found in Table 7.10, where some immediate concerns such as hyperkalaemia and fluid resuscitation are noted.

Hyperkalaemia

Ralph demonstrates signs that are potentially life threatening and may override the initial desire to find an underlying cause. The two immediate concerns are his high potassium level (hyperkalaemia), which is 6.9 mmol/L (normal range 3.2–5.0 mmol/L), and hypovolaemia. In the first instance causes of hyperkalaemia should exclude pseudohyperkalaemia caused by test tube haemolysis, prolonged tourniquet tightness, leucocytosis and infusion arm sampling to avoid inappropriate treatment. Additional causes of hyperkalaemia include potassium supplementation, gastrointestinal bleeding and

Table 7.10 Principles of management of AKI

- Identify and correct cause
- Optimise cardiac output and renal perfusion
- Restore urine flow
- Accurate fluid balance, daily body weight
- Review drugs: stop nephrotoxic drugs, adjust doses and monitor blood levels
- Identify, avoid and treat complications, e.g. hyperkalaemia, fluid overload, acidosis, hyper-/hyponatraemia, hyperphosphataemia
- Optimise nutritional support: calories, potassium restriction, minimal nitrogen
- Vigilant monitoring for infection and treat aggressively.
- Minimise the use of indwelling lines and catheters: remove if unnecessary
- Avoid, identify and treat bleeding tendency
- Initiate dialysis before uraemic complications occur
- Expert nursing care

Source: adapted from Lameire et al. (2005) and Hilton (2006).

in Ralph's case potassium retention due to loss of kidney function (GAIN, 2008). Ralph's medication must be considered and any drug that may cause hyperkalaemia – for example, ibuprofen – should be discontinued, if possible, without causing additional medical problems. Alternative medication may be required. The effects of hyperkalaemia are neuromuscular and cardiac but demonstrate few symptoms. Patients may complain of vague abdominal sensations or skeletal muscular weakness but more importantly they may develop cardiac arrest. Cardiac arrest occurs because of decreased membrane excitability, neuromuscular depression and cardiac arrhythmias (Weisberg, 2008). In view of this, Ralph must be closely monitored by continuous ECG for progressive hyperkalaemic changes, which occur in sequence with elevating hyperkalaemia, as seen in Table 7.12. The degree of hyperkalaemia requires immediate attention. Treatment must be instigated urgently, especially if the potassium is over 6.5 mmol/L or ECG changes are present. The aim is to reduce Ralph's potassium and limit his risk by the following principles:

1. Remove any potential high potassium medications or supplements.
2. Cardio protection: medical or advanced nurse practitioner administration of prescribed 10 ml 10 per cent intravenous calcium gluconate, repeat if necessary. This drug does not reduce potassium level but 'protects' the heart from excess potassium excitability.

Table 7.11   Drugs that can cause hyperkalaemia

- Angiotensin converting enzyme inhibitors (ACEI)
- Angiotensin II receptor blockers (ARB)
- Non-steroidal anti-inflammatory drugs (NSAIDs)
- Digoxin
- Spironolactone, especially in those with underlying renal insufficiency

Table 7.12   ECG changes in hyperkalaemia

- Peaking ('tenting) of T waves: $K^+ > 5.5$ mmol/L
- Flattening and disappearance of P waves: $K^+ > 6.5$ mmol/L
- Prolonged PR interval
- Progressive widening of QRS complex: $K^+ > 6.5$ mmol/L
- Deepened S waves and merging with T waves
- Sine wave patterns
- Ventricular fibrillation and asystolic cardiac arrest: $K^+ > 12.0$ mmol/L

Source: Adapted from Steddon et al. (2006)

3. Shift potassium from the blood to the cells:
   - Administration of a prescribed slow intravenous infusion of 50 mL of 50 per cent glucose (over 5 minutes).
   - Effects may last up to 60 minutes.
   - Monitor U&Es for hypokalaemia 30 minutes after each administration.
   - Administer prescribed insulin (15 iu Actrapid®) and dextrose (50 mL of 50 per cent) infusion. Effects are seen within 15 minutes and last between two and four hours.
   - Monitor blood potassium 30 minutes after each administration then hourly.
   - Monitor blood glucose level with a blood glucose monitor 30 minutes after administration then hourly and treat hypoglycaemia with prescribed dose of 10 per cent glucose.
   - The process can be repeated after four hours.
   - Nebulised salbutamol (which drives potassium into the cells) 10–20 mg may be used in conjunction with insulin and glucose providing an additive effect. Effects are seen within 15–30 minutes and last for two hours. Monitor for tachycardia and palpitations.
4. Removal from the body:
   - Oral calcium resonium (which binds with potassium in the gut) 15 g with lactulose®, though this is slow to work ($\geq$ 2 hours).
   - Dialysis only when first line treatments fail to control potassium level or if severe hyperkalaemia ($\geq$ 7 mmol/L) is present (GAIN, 2008).

Insulin and glucose is the most effective means for conservatively keeping the potassium low but may be improved with nebulised salbutamol (Mahoney et al., 2005). Insulin works by increasing cellular uptake of potassium by increasing intracellular sodium. Intravenous access will be necessary for infusions and strict fluid balance monitoring of all intake and output commenced. All fluid volumes, including intravenous fluids, nasogastric feeds and oral fluids, must be entered onto the fluid balance chart. All types of fluid output, including urine, vomit, and wound drainage, should be measured and documented accurately. Urine output may need to be assessed on an hourly basis.

Volume Depletion

The next priority for Ralph is his fluid status. Ralph is displaying evidence of volume depletion, which if not treated may cause permanent damage to the kidney as well as more systemic problems such as hypovolaemic shock, leading to inadequate tissue oxygenation and multiple organ failure (Ragaller, Theilen and Koch, 2001). Volume depletion is evident in Ralph in a number

Table 7.13 Assessing circulating volume

- Pulse
- Blood pressure
- JVP or CVP
- Peripheral perfusion
- Lung crackles
- Dyspnoea

Table 7.14 Volume depletion: test results

Hypovolaemia
- Blood sodium variable dependent upon loss: low/normal/high sodium level
- Raised urea:creatinine ratio
- Increase urine specific gravity
- Increased urine osmolality
- Haematocrit variable dependent upon cause, e.g. low in blood loss

Dehydration
- High blood sodium level (> 145 mmol/L)
- Raised blood osmolality
- Elevated haematocrit
- Urine specific gravity above 1.030

of clinical features (Table 7.13). Most noticeably, Ralph's jugular venous pressure is unrecordable, which means it is low (normal 0 to 3 cm above the sternal angle). Ralph is also tachycardic with a heart rate of 110 beats per minute and his BP is low and falls when standing. This effect is known as a postural drop or orthostatic hypotension and is a classic sign of hypovolaemia. However, in a systematic review of studies of clinical signs of hypovolaemia, hypotension was frequently absent in supine patients. Orthostatic hypotension is also present in 10 per cent of normovolaemic adults under 65 years old and up to 30 per cent of normovolaemic adults over 65 years old (McGee et al., 1999). Tachycardia is a normal response to volume depletion in an attempt to ensure vital organs receive blood. A postural increase of pulse rate by 30 beats/min or more upon standing is an accurate sign of hypovolaemia (McGee et al., 1999).

A reduced fluid intake, vomiting, continued use of diuretic medication and mild pyrexia all indicate uncontrolled fluid loss and fluid imbalance, which may be further substantiated when Ralph's test results are examined. Biochemistry results show Ralph's sodium level to be 133 mmol/L (normal range: 135–145 mmol/L), rendering him hyponatraemic. There are many

Table 7.15 Some causes of hyponatraemia

Low plasma osmolality	*Normal or raised plasma osmolality*	*Syndrome of inappropriate anti-diuretic hormone (SIADH)*
• Vomiting • Diarrhoea • Diuretic use • Excess fluid replacement • Congestive cardiac failure • Cirrhosis and ascites	• Hyperglycaemia • Acute uraemia • Alcohol • Mannitol infusion • Amino acid infusion • Sickle cell syndrome	• Stress • Nausea and vomiting • Pain • Trauma/surgery • Infection • Stroke • Meningitis • NSAIDs

Note: Osmolality is the measure of osmoles of solutes (e.g. sodium, chloride, glucose) per kg of solvent (blood).
Source: adapted from Crook (2006).

causes of hyponatraemia (Table 7.15) that need to be considered when assessing Ralph's condition.

Hyponatraemia is an important sign because it indicates volume depletion rather than dehydration. Dehydration means a loss of intracellular water, which would increase plasma sodium levels. In contrast, volume depletion describes a loss of sodium (and water) from extracellular space caused by bleeding, excessive vomiting or diarrhoea. Ralph's sodium is low and points towards volume depletion, but there are other clues. Ralph's urea and creatinine levels are raised due to retention by the kidney (not urinary retention), but also in comparison to each other the urea is disproportionally high. This is caused by passive re-absorption of urea in the kidney (creatinine is not re-absorbed), which occurs in hypoperfusion of the kidney but also increased catabolism, steroid therapy, gastrointestinal bleeding and the use of tetracyclines. As a result the high urea level must be interpreted with caution (Goldberg, 2002). Analysis of Ralph's urine also reveals a low sodium content, less than 10 mmol/L (normal about 100 mmol/L), and a fractional excretion of sodium (FeNa) of less than 1 per cent (normal 1–2 per cent). This is typical of pre-renal AKI and demonstrates tubular sodium reabsorption in an effort to retain water to expand the circulating blood volume. Conversely, intrinsic AKI has a FeNa of greater than 2 per cent, meaning the tubules are unable to reabsorb sodium, which is lost in what urine there is (MacPhee, 2002). Urine osmolality is also high, indicating concentrated urine, and in Ralph's case it is in excess of 500 mosm/kg H_2O, indicating pre-renal AKI. Ralph's urine output (oliguria) is reduced to 150 mL in eight hours

Table 7.16   Glossary of terms

Oliguria: a urine output of less than 1 ml/kg/hour or less than 400 ml/24hours

Anuria: a urine output of less than 100 ml/24 hours

Non-oliguric AKI: high urine volumes but of poor quality

(Table 7.16). Non-oliguric AKI can also occur where normal amounts of urine are passed but of poor quality, but this type has a better prognosis. Oliguria occurs when the kidney is attempting to retain water in the body, thus concentrating the urine, or when little urine is being made due to kidney damage. Oliguria is often followed by a polyuria (> 3 litres/24 hr) phase due to recovery of kidney function but an initial inability to concentrate effectively, and usually resolves in a few days. All these points direct attention to the fact that Ralph is hypovolaemic, which needs to be addressed. Addressing these problems will require close and frequent monitoring of Ralph's fluid balance, which would include daily weight, hourly urine output, insensitive loss such as sweating and faecal loss (which is estimated a being $\geq$ 500 mL/24 hr) measurements and all fluid input. Central venous pressure monitoring provides for a more accurate assessment of blood volume (see Chapter 3).

Managing Hypovolaemia

Ralph is hypotensive, hypovolaemic and in need of urgent fluid resuscitation. Fluids are required to return normal circulating volume, elevate his blood pressure, increase renal perfusion and reverse pre-renal AKI. The general 'rule of thumb' is to replace lost fluid with its equivalent. Ralph's blood pressure is not low enough to warrant the need for colloid (e.g. human albumin solution) infusion for immediate improvement, and in fact evidence suggests that colloids appear to offer no survival benefit over crystalloids (e.g. 0.9 per cent sodium chloride) in critically ill patients (Perel and Roberts, 2007). Colloids are also thought to cause a hyperoncotic renal failure and should be used sparingly. In view of this Ralph needs a crystalloid infusion and 0.9 per cent sodium chloride is most appropriate. Dextrose or dextrose/sodium chloride saline are inappropriate because they would quickly distribute among total body water with little vascular filling effect. Mannitol also plays no part in fluid management except when a patient has rhabdomyolisis, which causes nephrotoxicity from damaged muscle myoglobin. The amount of 0.9 per cent sodium chloride needed is dependent upon the extent of Ralph's hypovolaemia, his age and what it takes to restore his blood pressure. Given Ralph's advanced age it may be advisable to infuse 200 to 300 mL of 0.9 per cent sodium chloride over 10 minutes. Any improvement in BP, pulse, CVP and oliguria would prompt further infusions until Ralph is normovolaemic. Great care is needed to avoid over-hydration, which would cause cardiac failure, pulmonary oedema, respiratory distress, hypertension, peripheral oedema and elevated JVP. Medical and nursing staff should endeavour to maintain urine output with fluid infusions by matching input with urine output plus 30 ml (for insensible loss) or maintaining a CVP of 8 to 12 cmH$_2$O. Ralph's AKI may move into the polyuric phase, which could increase the risk of further volume depletion as well as potassium depletion. Once again fluid balance becomes an essential monitoring activity for the AKI patient.

In some instances patients with AKI are commenced on diuretic infusions in an attempt to maintain a urine output. Ralph is prescribed a diuretic (Bendrofluazide®) but this kind of drug is ineffective when GFR is below 30 mL/min/1.73m^2 and should be discontinued. The diuretic drug of choice is Furosemide® and may be given as an infusion. This is controversial treatment with no evidence of its clinical benefit to AKI patients; however, it is thought to promote diuresis but should only be used in patients with adequate circulating volume (Lamiere et al., 2005; Ho and Sheridan, 2006). Dopamine infusion at an alleged 'renal dose' has been shown not to improve patient outcome and has additional risks and so is not recommended for AKI patients (Kellum and Decker, 2001; Stevens et al., 2008). In some instances of deterioration such as in septic shock (but not hypovolaemic shock) it may be necessary to provide blood pressure support and thus renal perfusion with the use of inotropic drugs such as Dopexamine® or norepinephrine. However, given Ralph's health history the use of inotropic drugs is not necessary.

Table 7.17   Stages of AKI

Initiation: reduction in renal blood flow by 30–50% = oliguria phase

Extension: continued cell hypoxia, inflammatory response, cell death = oliguria/anuria phase

Maintenance: proximal cortical cell regeneration and proliferation = oliguria/anuria phase

Recovery: tubular cellular regeneration and proliferation = diuresis phase, development of concentration gradient and return to normal output

---

Managing Acidosis

Ralph's arterial blood gases (ABGs) show a low oxygen level of 10.0 kPa (normal > 10.6 kPa), a high carbon dioxide level of 8.1 kPa (normal range 4.7–6 kPa) and a low but not life threatening pH of 7.31 (normal range 7.35–7.45). The anion gap is 18 (normal range 8–16) and base excess is –1 (diagnostic range –3 to +3). These results indicate that Ralph is hypoxic and in need of oxygen. He is also retaining acid, which is demonstrated by high carbon dioxide level, low pH, high anion gap and negative base excess. The kidney is responsible for maintaining long-term acid–base balance by removal of acids from the body and reconstituting bicarbonate into the blood for buffering excess acids. Should the kidney fail then it can no longer remove acids and produce bicarbonate, which leads to metabolic acidosis. Indeed this is the case for Ralph, though his low oxygen level may be caused by his chest infection, resulting in respiratory acidosis. Ralph's acidosis is best dealt with by treating the underlying cause so fluid resuscitation is essential. Treatment with bicarbonate is not recommended unless Ralph's pH falls below 7.1 because it in fact generates more CO_2 when reacting with hydrogen ions and also delivers a large dose of sodium. Providing oxygen therapy would be beneficial in order to keep Ralph's oxygen saturation level at 95 per cent or higher with a non-rebreathe mask at 15 litres per minute until blood gas values stabilise. Then a 24 per cent venturi mask or nasal cannulae at 2 litres per minute can be used. Naturally this may change with frequent monitoring, which is determined by the patient's condition (O'Driscoll et al., 2008).

One additional point to consider is Ralph's diabetes medication. Metformin® is associated with lactic acidosis production in reduced kidney function and so would probably be discontinued. Treatment of Ralph's diabetes in the short term can be with insulin and glucose (as used in the treatment for hyperkalaemia) but will require reappraisal for long-term treatment.

Ongoing Care Issues and the Role of the Nurse

Ralph was found lying on the floor and had been there for an indeterminate period. The reason for this is unclear; however, from an AKI perspective this may be important. Long-term pressure upon muscle tissue (crush injury) leads to tissue hypoxia and tissue death. Muscle tissue breakdown is known as rhabdomyolysis and releases myoglobin, which is nephrotoxic. A common presentation of this condition in AKI is brown urine (in about 50 per cent of cases) that tests positive for blood upon urine dipstick test, limb swelling, myalgia, hypocalcaemia and hyperkalaemia. Elevations in blood

The Case Scenario: Ongoing Care Issues

Ralph is very ill and requires close observation. He has been commenced on an IV dextrose and insulin infusion to control his elevated plasma potassium and his diabetes. He has an intravenous infusion of 0.9 per cent sodium chloride with 10 minute bolus infusions of 200 mL until his blood pressure is within normal limits. He will then require a continuous infusion set according to hydration and urine output. He may have been given additional medication such as calcium resonium, salbutamol nebuliser and Furosemide®. Ralph's fluid balance must be monitored closely to avoid under- or over-hydration. He is also receiving oxygen therapy to treat hypoxia and acidosis. He requires bed rest and continuous cardiac monitoring for arrhythmia detection. A detailed social, family and risk factor assessment was completed.

Nursing Care Issues
1. Consider the appropriate ongoing assessment and monitoring required for Ralph.
2. Discuss in detail Ralph's immediate care issues.
3. What is important about Ralph being found on the floor and acute kidney injury?
4. Why should the nurse be concerned with infection control and the patient with acute kidney injury?
5. What are Ralph's nutritional requirements and how can they best be provided?
6. What are the indications for initiating renal replacement therapy (RRT)?
7. What types of RRT are available to support the treatment of AKI?

levels of amylase and very high levels of creatine phosphokinase (CK) after 12 hours would indicate rhabdomyolysis. Vigilance is required in the assessment and monitoring of patients with AKI who have been involved in this kind of situation.

Infection and Acute Kidney Injury

Ralph has been treated for a chest infection but it would appear that this has not been successful. Ralph is pyrexial and has an elevated white cell count and c-reactive protein (CRP), all indicating infection. Naturally this will require treatment with an appropriate antibiotic and the collection of samples of urine, sputum and blood for culture, bacteriology and virology. Uraemia renders a person at increased risk of infection because white cells develop functional abnormalities that reduce the ability to adhere to and destroy invading organisms (Meyer and Hostetter, 2007). There is also a reduction in the number of circulating white cells and the response to microorganisms. This is an important care issue because infection will account for a mortality rate of 76 per cent in patients with AKI and sepsis (Steddon et al., 2006). Sepsis is also a major risk factor for AKI and may delay recovery. The acutely ill patient is at risk of infection from a number of sources, particularly where invasive procedures are needed. The incidence of acquired hospital infection has been reported as up to 8.8 per cent, with lung infection accounting for 26 per cent, abdominal infection at 23 per cent, vascular access at 16 per cent, urinary tract at 10 per cent and wound infections at 6 per cent (Hoste et al., 2004). Catheterisation to assess urine output is a common procedure in the AKI patient but frequently causes infection. Ralph has known urinary retention, which may make urine output assessment difficult, and so an indwelling catheter may be necessary. This will require increased awareness and caution by the nurse in the prevention of infection. Invasive procedures should be minimised and catheters removed when not needed, such as when there is anuria. Constant vigilance is needed when monitoring the AKI patient, especially around vascular access sites and urinary catheters.

Nutritional Requirements

While Ralph is unwell and may be anorexic and nauseated (common uraemic symptom) he will require nutritional support (Table 7.18). Malnutrition with AKI will independently increase Ralph's risk for morbidity and death (Stevens et al., 2008). Fiaccadori et al. (2009) observed severe malnutrition in approximately 40 per cent of patients with AKI on intensive care units. Ralph is at risk of protein-energy wasting, characterised by the loss of lean-body mass and fat mass (Fiaccadori et al., 2009). He is also at risk of protein catabolism, hyperglycaemia due to insulin resistance and decreases in trace elements, water soluble vitamins (except vitamin C) and vitamins A and E. Malnutrition exacerbates the inflammatory state found in patients with AKI. Nutritional support requires a multidisciplinary approach, including a dietician to calculate Ralph's needs, and should commence within 24 hours of admission. Enteral feeding is preferred in order to avoid complications associated with parenteral feeding. Each person requires individual assessment, which avoids blanket approaches to nutrition. In some instances protein restriction may be necessary to prevent nitrogen build-up but is unlikely in most cases due to the frequency of catabolism. Protein intake, often given as amino acids, can vary between 0.8 and 1.8 g/kg/day. Ralph will also need a high calorific intake to attenuate catabolism and this can vary, depending upon need, from 20 to 35 non-protein kcal/kg/day. In

Table 7.18   Goals of nutritional support

- Prevent protein = energy wasting
- Preserve lean-body mass and nutritional status
- Avoid metabolic derangements
- Avoid complications
- Improve wound healing
- Support immune function
- Minimise inflammation
- Improve antioxidant activity
- Reduce mortality

Source: Fiaccadori et al. (2009).

Ralph's case a minimum of 1,500 kcal/day are necessary and in many instances in excess of 2000 kcal/day may be given (Stevens et al., 2008). Nutritional demand may increase in hypercatabolism or if Ralph needs renal replacement therapy and supplementation of trace elements, vitamins and electrolytes, and fluid restrictions may be necessary and should reflect Ralph's fluid status and urine output.

Renal Replacement Therapy

Many of the conservative measures for managing Ralph's condition may be inadequate to control metabolic imbalances caused by AKI. To prevent further deterioration renal replacement therapy may be initiated (Table 7.19). It is generally believed that early initiation of RRT is beneficial to patient outcome but precise optimal time is unclear and remains a clinical decision (Stevens et al., 2008). Ralph may require RRT if he does not improve soon. There are three options: peritoneal dialysis, intermittent haemodialysis or haemofiltration and continuous haemodialysis or haemofiltration.

Each method of RRT has advantages and disadvantages (Table 7.20). In each instance Ralph would need some form of access, either a peritoneal dialysis catheter or a central venous catheter. RRT brings an additional set of challenges for the AKI patient, such as the additional invasive treatment and anti-coagulation.

Ralph's medication must be discontinued for the immediate situation as the action and metabolism of some drugs may be affected by reduced kidney function (Table 7.21). Most drugs are eliminated from the body by the kidney, which makes it essential to consider this in AKI. In many instances problems of toxicity or accumulation can be overcome by reducing the dose; however, this requires knowledge of GFR. Many drugs will require reduced dosage due to margins of safety from toxicity. Some drugs such as

Table 7.19   Indications for renal replacement therapy

Clinical indications	Biochemical indications
Urine output < 0.3 mL/kg/24hr or absolute anuria for 12 hr	Refractory hyperkalaemia > 6.5 mmol/L
AKI with multiple organ failure	Serum urea > 30 mmol/L
End organ damage: encephalopathy, myopathy, neuropathy, pericarditis, bleeding	Refractory electrolyte abnormalities: hypo/hypernatraemia, hypercalcaemia
Refractory fluid overload	Refractory metabolic acidosis: pH $\leq$ 7.1
Poisoning and drug overdose	Tumour lysis syndrome with hyperuricaemia and hyperphosphataemia
Severe hypo-/hyperthermia	Urea cycle defects and organis acidurias: hyperammonaemia, methymalonic acidaemia
Create intravascular space for infusions: blood, plasma, nutrition	For additional information consult the Renal Association Standards (2008) on AKI

Table 7.20   Advantages and disadvantages of renal replacement therapy

Modality	Patient haemodynamic instability	Solute clearance	Volume control	Anti-coagulation
Peritoneal dialysis (PD)	Yes	Moderate	Moderate	No
Intermittent haemodialysis (HD)	No	High	Moderate	With/without
Hybrid techniques	Possible	High	Good	With/without
CVVH	Yes	Moderate/high	Good	With/without
CVVHD	Yes	Moderate/High	Good	With/without

CVVH: continuous haemofiltration. CVVHDF: continuous haemodialfiltration.

Source: adapted from Stevens (2008).

Vancomycin® and Genatmicin® will require careful monitoring of therapeutic levels with repeated doses altered accordingly. Wherever possible nephrotoxic drugs should be avoided in order to minimise any further injury to the kidney.

Ralph will need expert nursing care to help him through his illness,

Table 7.21   Effects of reduced kidney function upon drugs

- Increased drug sensitivity
- Reduced drug and/or metabolites excretion
- Decreased toleration of side effects
- Some drugs become ineffective

Table 7.22   Essential nursing skills for patients with AKI

Expert nursing focus	Example AKI patient problems
Comfort	Fatigue, fever, myalgia, pain, insomnia
Infection control	Risk of infection in urinary catheters, vascular access, respiratory, gastrointestinal, wounds
Mouth care	Uraemic ulcers, anorexia, vomiting, thirst, infection
Skin care	Uraemic itching, wound care, fever, oedema, pressure care, delayed wound healing, infection, ischaemia
Hydration and fluid balance	Under/over hydration, fluid restrictions, intravenous fluids
Nutrition	Anorexia, nausea, vomiting, gastritis, dietary restrictions, malnutrition, nasogastric feeding
Medications management	Drug dose alteration, side effect surveillance, prevention of nephrotoxins
Symptoms management	Headache, irritability, erractic memory, confusion, pulmonary oedema
Oxygenation	Pulmonary oedema, LVF, infection
Elimination	Urinary catheter, urinary obstruction, infection, diarrhoea, constipation
Health surveillance: safety	Hypotension, bleeding, dyspnoea, hyperkalaemia, fluid overload, infection
Psychological support and education	Anxiety, depression, metabolic cognitive changes

which will include a multidisciplinary approach. Nursing care will include essential aspects of patient comfort and safety, such as skin care, mouth care and hydration, because of the multiple effects of uraemia. Examples of essential nursing skills as applied to AKI patients can be found in Table 7.22.

In addition disease-specific knowledge is needed to minimise risks from potential complications such as infection, and management of additional problems such as nausea, vomiting, pain and itching must be assessed and implemented. Psychological care remains essential, as does accurate and sensitive communication. The prognosis for AKI over the years has remained relatively unchanged at around 50 per cent. Critically ill patients who develop AKI and require RRT generally have a poor prognosis, with mortality rates exceeding 60 per cent, and unsurprisingly mortality is higher in older patients (Bagshaw, 2008). Between 8 and 22 per cent of critically ill patients will not recover renal function and will require RRT on a permanent basis. The risk of mortality does not stabilise until after one year following discharge from hospital (Morgera et al., 2008). In one study only 57 per cent attained complete recovery of kidney function, with the remaining 43 per cent attaining partial recovery (Morgera et al., 2008). If kidney function had not recovered within 6 to 12 months of AKI there was no further recovery of function. Two per cent of AKI survivors proceed to end-stage kidney disease. There is a 76 per cent chance of recovery from a single cause but multiple causes of AKI only have a 30 per cent chance of kidney function recovery (Bagshaw, 2008). Therefore should Ralph recover he will need long-term follow-up to monitor his kidney function along with his diabetes, hypertension and arthritis.

Summary

A patient presenting with AKI requires a comprehensive assessment and management strategy that utilises both general and specific knowledge. Developing knowledge of specific medical conditions can enhance a nurse's ability to care and manage a patient. While it is acknowledged that some conditions appear more complex than others this should not prevent nurses from learning to care for such patients. Integration of nursing care and medical knowledge enables the development of nursing expertise that can only benefit the patient and enhance the nurse's confidence.

References

Ali, T., I. Khan, N. Simpson, G. Prescott, J. Townend, W. Smith and A. McLeod (2007) 'Incidence and Outcomes in Acute Kidney Injury: A Comprehensive Population-based Study', *Journal of the American Society of Nephrology*, **18** (2007), 1292–8.

Bagshaw, S. M. 'Short and Long-term Survival after Acute Kidney Injury', *Nephrology, Dialysis and Transplantation*, **23** (2008), 2126–8.

Baker, R. 'Acute Interstitial Nephritis', in P. Glynne, A. Allen and C. Pusey (eds), *Acute Renal Failure in Practice* (London: Imperial College Press, 2002).

Bevan, M. 'Renal Disease in the Older Person', *Nursing Older People*, 13(6) (2001), 21–5.

Bevan, M. 'Renal Function', in H. heath and R. Watson (eds), *Older People: Assessment for Health and Social Care* (London: Age Concern, 2005).

Clarkson, M. R., J. J. Friedewald, J. A. Eustace and H. Rabb. 'Acute Kidney Injury', in *Brenner and Rector's The Kidney*, 8th edn (Philadelphia: Saunders Elsevier, 2008).

Cohen, J. J. 'Relationships between Energy Requirements and Na^+ Reabsorption and Other Renal Functions', *Kidney International*, **29** (1986), 32–40.

Crook, M. A. *Clinical Chemistry and Metabolic Medicine*, 7th edn (London: HodderArnold, 2006).

Davenport, A. and P. Stevens. 'Module 5: Acute Kidney Injury', *Clinical Practice Guidelines*, 4th edn, www.renal.org/guidelines (London: UK Renal Association, June 2008).

Faubel, S., C. L. Edelstein and R. E. Cronin. 'The Patient with Acute Renal Failure', in R. W. Schrier (ed.), *Manual of Nephrology*, 6th edn (Philadelphia: Lippincott Williams and Wilkins, 2005).

Feest, T. G., A. Round and S. Hamad. 'Incidence of Severe ARF in Adults: Results of a Community Based Study', *British Journal of Medicine*, **306** (1993), 481–3.

Fiaccadori, E., M. Lombardi, S. Leonardi, C. F. Rotelli, G. Tortorella and A. Borghetti. 'Prevalence and Clinical Outcome Associated with Pre-existing Malnutrition in Acute Renal Failure: A Prospective Cohort Study', *Journal of American Society of Nephrology*, **10** (1999), 581–93.

Fiaccadori, E., G. Regolisti and A. Cabassi. 'Specific Nutritional Problems in Acute Kidney Injury, Treated with Non-dialysis and Dialytic Modalities', *Nephrology Dialysis Transplantation Plus*, doi:10.1093/ndtplus/sfp017 (2009), 1–7.

GAIN. *Guidelines for the Treatment for Hyperkalaemia in Adults* (Belfast: GAIN, 2008).

Goldberg, L. 'Biochemical Investigations', in P. Glynne, A. Allen and C. Pusey (eds), *Acute Renal Failure in Practice* (London: Imperial College Press, 2002).

Hegarty, J., R. Middleton, M. Krebs, H. Hussain, C. Cheung, T. Ledson, A. Hutchison, P. A. Kalra, H. Rayner, P. Stevens and D. O'Donoghue. 'Severe Acute Renal Failure in Adults: Place of Care, Incidence and Outcomes', *Quarterly Journal of Medicine*, **98**(8) (2005), 661–6.

Hilton, R. 'Acute Renal Failure', *British Medical Journal*, **333** (2006), 786–90.

Ho, K. M. and D. J. Sheridan. 2006 'Meta-analysis of Frusemide to Prevent or Treat Acute Renal Failure', *British Medical Journal*, **430** (2006), 330, BMJ Online BMJ, doi:10.1136/bmj.38902.605347.7C, available at http://www.bmj.com/cgi/rapid-pdf/bmj.38902.605347.7Cv1

Holley, J. 'Clinical Approach to the Diagnosis of Acute Renal Failure', in A. Greenberg (ed.), *Primer on Kidney Disease*, 3rd edn. (San Diego: Academic Press, 2001).

Hoste, E. A., S. I. Blot, N. H. Lameire, R. C. Vanholder, D. de Bacquer and F. A. Colardyn. 'Effect of Nonsocomial Bloodstream Infection on the Outcome of Critically Ill Patients with Acute Renal Failure Treated with Renal Replacement Therapy', *Journal of American Society of Nephrology*, **15** (2004), 454–62.

Hsu, C. Y., J. D. Ordonez, G. M. Chertow, D. Fan, C. E. McCuloch and A. S. Go. 'The Risk of Acute Renal Failure in Patients with Chronic Kidney Disease', *Kidney International*, **74** (2008), 101–7.

Kellum, J. A. and J. Decker. 'Use of Dopamine in Acute Renal Failure: A Meta-analysis', *Critical Care Medicine*, **29**(8) (2001), 1526–31.

Khan I. H., G. R. Catto, N. Edward, and A. M. MacLeod. 'Acute Renal Failure: Factors Influencing Nephrology Referral and Outcome', *Quarterly Journal of Medicine*, **90** (1997), 781–5.

Koeppen, B. M. and B. A. Stanton. *Renal Physiology*, 3rd edn (St Louis: Mosby, 2001).

Lamiere, N., W. van Biesen and R. Vanholder. 'Acute Renal Failure', *The Lancet*, **365** (2005), 417–30.

McGee, S., W. B. Abernathy and D. L. Simel. 'Is This Patient Hypovolaemic?', *Journal of the American Medical Association*, **281**(11) (1999), 1022–9.

MacPhee, I. 'Urine Output and Urinalysis', in P. Glynne, A. Allen and C. Pusey (eds), *Acute Renal Failure* (London: Imperial College Press, 2002).

MacTier, R. 'Acute Kidney Injury – Best Practice and Staging System', *British Journal of Renal Medicine*, **13**(2) (2008), 19–21.

Mahoney, B. A., W. A. D. Smith, D. S. Lo, K. Tsoi, M. Tonelli and C. M. Clase. 'Emergency Interventions for Hyperkalaemia', *Cochrane Database of Systematic Reviews*, **2** (2005), art. no. CD003235. DOI: 10.1002/14651858.CD003235. pub2.

Mehta, R. L., J. A. Kellum, S. V. Shah, B. A. Molitoris, C. Ronco, D. G. Warnock, A. Levin and the Acute Kidney Injury Network. 'Acute Kidney Injury Network: Report of an Initiatiative to Improve Outcomes in Acute Kidney Injury', *Critical Care*, **11**(2) (2007), http://ccforum.com/content/11/2/R31

Meyer, T. W. and T. H. Hostetter. 'Pathophysiology of Uraemia', in *Brenner and Rector's The Kidney*, 8th edn (Philadelphia: Saunders Elsevier, 2007).

Morgera, S., M. Schneider and H. H. Neumeyer. 'Long-term Outcomes after Acute Kidney Injury', *Critical Care Medicine*, **36** (2008), S193–7.

National Collaboration for Chronic Conditions. *Chronic Kidney Disease: National Clinical Guideline for Early Identification and Management in Adults in Primary and Secondary Care* (London: Royal College of Physicians, 2008).

National Institute for Clinical Excellence. *Acutely Ill Patients in Hospital: Recognition of and Response to Acute Illness in Adults in Hospital* (London: National Institute for Clinical Excellence, 2007).

O'Driscoll, B. R., L. S. Howard and A. G. Davison. 'BTS Guidelines for Emergency Oxygen Use in Adults', Thorax, **63**(suppl. VI) (2008), vi1–vi10

Pannu, N. and P. F. Halloran. 'The Aging Kidney', in A. Greenberg (ed.), *Primer on Kidney Disease*, 3rd edn (San Diego: Academic Press, 2002).

Perel, P. and I. G. Roberts. 'Colloids versus Crystalloids for Fluid Resuscitation in Critically Ill Patients', *Cochrane Database of Systematic Reviews*, **4** (2007), art. no. CD000567. DOI: 10.1002/14651858.CD000567.pub3.

Provan, D. and A. Krentz. *Oxford Handbook of Clinical Laboratory Investigations* (Oxford: Oxford University Press, 2002).

Ragaller, M. J. R., H. Theilen and T. Koch. 'Volume Replacement in Critically Ill Patients with Acute Renal Failure', *Journal of the American Association of Nephrology*, **12** (2001), S33–S39.

Renal Association. *eGFR Calculator* (2008), http://www.renal.org/eGFRcalc/GFR.pl

Salama, A. 'Haemolytic Uraemic Syndrome and Thrombocytopaenic Purpura', in P. Glynne, A. Allen and C. Pusey (eds), *Acute Renal Failure in Practice* (London: Imperial College Press, 2002).

Steddon, S., N. Ashman, A. Chesser and J. Cunningham. 'Acute Renal Failure', in S. Steddon, N. Ashman, A. Chesser and J. Cunningham (eds), *Oxford Handbook of Nephrology and Hypertension* (Oxford: Oxford University Press, 2006).

Stevens, P., A. Davenport, S. Kanagasundaram and A. Lewington. *Acute Renal Failure (Acute Kidney Injury), Clinical Practice Guidelines* (London: The Renal Association, 2008).

Vanholder, R., R. de Smet, G. Glorieux et al., for the European Uremic Toxin Work Group (EUTOX). 'Review on Uremic Toxins: Classification, Concentration, and Interindividual Variability', *Kidney International*, **63** (2003), 1934–43.

Waiker, S. S., G. C. Curhan, R. Wald, E. P. McCarthy and G. Chertow. 'Declining Mortality in Patients with Acute Renal Failure', *Journal of the American Society of Nephrology*, **17** (2006), 1143–50.

Weisberg, L. S. 'Management of Severe Hyperkalaemia', *Critical Care Medicine*, **36**(12) (2008), 3246–51.

8

Small Bowel Obstruction

Beverley Gallacher

Introduction

Small bowel obstruction is a common reason for admission to hospital and surgical consultation (Foster et al., 2006), accounting for between 12 and 16 per cent of surgical admissions annually (Maglinte et al., 2003). It is most common in people who have had previous surgery during which the bowel has been handled, as this predisposes the formation of adhesions. Adhesions are created when the sections of the bowel adhere or 'stick' together, a process that impairs small bowel function and its ability to transport partially digested food. A small bowel obstruction is said to occur when the contents of the small bowel fail to move forward (Urden et al., 1996).

The general consensus is for surgical treatment for large bowel obstruction; however, there is a difference of opinion regarding the need for surgical treatment for small bowel obstruction (Hayanga et al., 2005; Williams et al., 2005; Foster et al., 2006), particularly if the cause of the small bowel obstruction is adhesions. Cox et al. (1993) found that in 123 patients admitted with adhesive small bowel obstruction, the obstruction resolved without surgery in 85 cases (69 per cent); 75 of these resolved within 48 hours and the remaining 10 within 72 hours. Patients who did not require surgery in the study were managed medically and regularly assessed for signs of deterioration as an indication for surgical intervention. Cox et al. (1993) concluded that most adhesive small bowel obstructions resolve with medical treatment within 48 hours; however, they also state that if the patient shows no signs of resolution within 48 hours, surgical intervention should follow. Assessment is therefore the key to management of the patient. The need for surgery is determined by a number of factors (Table 8.1). The degree of obstruction (complete or partial) and the development of strangulation are important, as 'patients with complete obstruction are at substantial risk of strangulation' (Hayanga et al., 2005, p. 11), and this

Table 8.1 Factors that determine medical or surgical intervention

Factor	Treatment
Partial obstruction	Conservative/medical
Complete obstruction	Surgical
Strangulation	Surgical

Source: Adapted from Hayanga et al. (2005).

doubles the mortality associated with small bowel obstruction from 10 to 20 per cent (Hayanga et al., 2005). Strangulation occurs as a result of impaired blood flow to and from the bowel and leads to necrosis of the bowel wall. This necrotic tissue can then become gangrenous and, as a consequence, bleeding into the lumen of the bowel and peritoneal cavity can occur, eventually leading to perforation (Doherty and Way, 2006). The contents of the lumen will thus contain blood, necrotic tissue, bacteria and toxic bacterial products, which can enter the circulation through lymphatic vessels and the peritoneum and cause septic shock and peritonitis (Doherty and Way, 2006). It is therefore important not only to be able to identify small bowel obstruction, but to also distinguish between complete and partial obstruction and to determine whether strangulation has occurred, in order to best manage the patient.

Aim and Learning Outcomes

The Aim

The aim of this chapter is to provide you with the knowledge required to understand the nursing assessment, care and management of a patient suspected of having a small bowel obstruction.

Learning Outcomes

At the end of this chapter the reader will be able to:

1. Identify possible causes of bowel obstruction.
2. Explain the pathophysiological basis of the presenting signs and symptoms of small bowel obstruction.
3. Recognise the immediate assessment, specific monitoring and key investigations required to enable an accurate and timely diagnosis.

4. Describe and explore the ongoing nursing assessment and monitoring required to establish whether the obstruction requires medical or surgical intervention.
5. Appreciate the role of different health professionals in acute assessment and management of small bowel obstruction.

The Case Scenario: The Presenting Complaint

Mrs Brown is an 82-year-old lady with a two-day history of intermittent, colicky, cramping abdominal pain and bloating. Mrs Brown is alert and tells you that she is in some pain, although this has been relieved somewhat by 10 mg IM morphine given in casualty. Mrs Brown has vomited twice this morning and so is now 'nil by mouth'. An intravenous infusion of 1 litre of 0.9 per cent sodium chloride has been commenced to infuse over eight hours. On arrival to the ward Mrs Brown's vital signs are recorded as follows:

Pulse: 84 beats per minute
Blood pressure: 150/80 mmHg
Respiratory rate: 18 breaths per minute
Temperature: 36 °C

Mrs Brown lives alone but is accompanied by her son, who lives locally and is her next of kin. A provisional diagnosis of small bowel obstruction has been made.

Consider the following:

1. Describe the structural anatomy of the gastrointestinal tract.
2. Explain how the gastrointestinal tract functions to enable the digestion and absorption of food and drink.
3. Does Mrs Brown's presentation represent an acute and urgent situation?
4. Describe the pathophysiological basis for Mrs Brown's presenting signs and symptoms.
5. List some of the common causes of bowel obstruction.

Structure and Function of the Gastrointestinal Tract

Mrs Brown has a two-day history of abdominal pain and bloating, she has started to vomit and her pain has increased sufficiently for her to seek medical help, which may indicate an acute presentation of bowel obstruction. A large proportion of small bowel obstructions resolve with medical management alone. Resolution is defined as the absence of abdominal pain, reduced abdominal distension, the passage of flatus and/or faeces, and the successful intake of food and drink without recurrence of symptoms (Cox et al., 1993). However, although many obstructions resolve spontaneously, some will not and symptoms worsen, indicating the need for surgical removal. If a deterioration in symptoms is not acted upon swiftly, Mrs Brown could develop hypovolaemic shock and the bowel could perforate, resulting in peritonitis, which is associated with increased mortality. The situation is not urgent at the moment as Mrs Brown's vital signs are within normal limits and her pain has been relieved by morphine. However, she is seriously ill and will require close monitoring as her symptoms could worsen and her condition deteriorate. In order to appreciate the severity and impact of small bowel obstruction a basic knowledge and understanding of the normal anatomy and physiology of the gastrointestinal tract is necessary.

Brief Overview of the Gastrointestinal Tract

Figure 8.1 illustrates the gastrointestinal tract. The bowel, also known as the intestine, is divided into two sections based upon the diameter of the lumen, and includes the small bowel and large bowel. The diameter of the small bowel varies between 4 cm at the stomach and 2.5 cm at the junction with the large intestine. The large bowel has a diameter of 7.5 cm (Martini, 2009). The purpose of the gastrointestinal tract is to transfer modified nutrients, water and electrolytes from ingested food into the body's internal environment (Sherwood, 1993). Modification of ingested nutrients is necessary as most food eaten is in the form of molecules that are too large to pass from the bowel into the blood or lymph (internal environment). Large molecules are 'modified' or broken down into small ones that can 'pass' or be absorbed by mechanical and chemical processes.

The Small Bowel

The small bowel achieves mechanical digestion through peristalsis and segmentation. Peristalsis is the rhythmical muscular contraction that breaks down and pushes partially digested food through the gastrointestinal tract. The muscular layer responsible for peristalsis is known as the muscularis externa (Figure 8.2). Segmentation is a similar process to peristalsis; however, muscular movement is both forwards, towards the anus, and backwards.

The large and small bowel have the same common structure as the whole of the gastrointestinal tract, which can be divided into four layers (Figure 8.2). The inner mucosal layer is the surface from which intestinal secretions

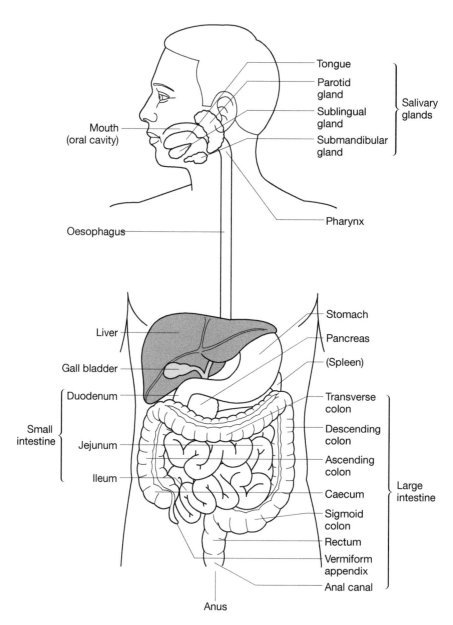

Figure 8.1   The gastrointestinal tract.

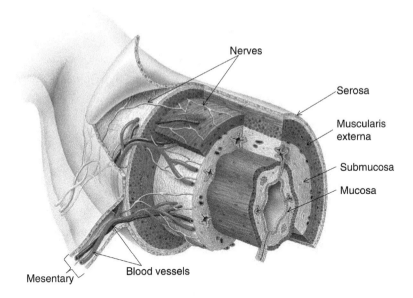

Figure 8.2 The layers of the gastrointestinal tract.
Source: Seeley, R. et al.: *Essentials of Anatomy and Physiology 4th Edition* (2002). © The McGraw-Hill Companies, Inc. Reproduced with kind permission.

are produced and through which absorption of essential water and nutrients into the circulation occurs. Anatomically the mucosal layer is made up of thousands of villi and microvilli, which increase the surface area over which secretion and absorption can take place. The second layer is the sub-mucosa, which contains blood and lymphatic vessels and a nervous network called the Meissner's plexus. These are all vital for transporting the absorbed products of digestion, and for stimulating the secretion of digestive juices from the mucosa, respectively. The third layer is composed of two layers of muscle (the stomach has an additional third layer) arranged in a longitudinal and circular manner. Rhythmical contractions of the muscle layers are responsible for peristalsis and segmentation. The final outer layer is the serosa, which is a serous membrane composed of epithelium and connective tissue. Below the diaphragm the serosa is called the peritoneum. The peritoneum is a double membrane, one of which forms the outer layer of the gastrointestinal tract (visceral peritoneum) and the other of which lines the abdominal cavity (parietal peritoneum). This can best be thought of as similar to the two layers that are formed when a fist is pushed into an inflated balloon. If an inflated balloon was inserted into the abdominal cavity and then the abdominal organs were placed on top of it, the balloon would envelop the organs in the same way as the peritoneum (Figure 8.3).

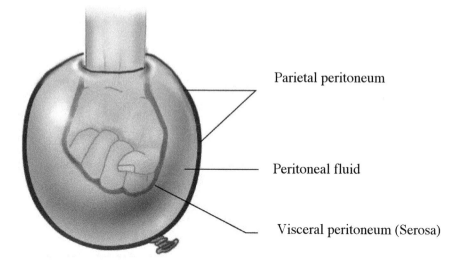

Parietal peritoneum

Peritoneal fluid

Visceral peritoneum (Serosa)

Figure 8.3   Illustration of the double layer peritoneum.

Source: Seeley, R. et al.: *Essentials of Anatomy and Physiology 4th Edition* (2002). © The McGraw-Hill Companies, Inc. Reproduced with kind permission.

Between the two layers of the peritoneum lies a thin layer of serous, 'peritoneal' fluid, which acts as a lubricant enabling the bowel to move within the abdominal cavity with as little friction as possible. Peristalsis moves partially digested food along the gastrointestinal tract while segmentation allows it to thoroughly mix with digestive chemicals such as bile and pancreatic and intestinal enzymes that are secreted into the small bowel (Figure 8.4).

Bile is produced by the liver and secreted via the right and left hepatic ducts (Figure 8.4) for storage in the gall bladder before being released by the relaxation of the hepatopancreatic sphincter, in response to hormonal stimulation. Sphincter relaxation also allows the entry of pancreatic enzymes via the pancreatic duct into the small bowel.

Bile and enzymes thoroughly mix with the food via segmentation. Bile does not contain enzymes, but does contain bile salts, which emulsify lipids (fats). Normally lipid and water do not mix unless an emulsion is created. Bile converts large lipid droplets into many small droplets that are suspended in the watery contents of the intestine, creating an emulsion. This process increases the surface area of the lipid droplets over which the enzyme lipase can act, thus speeding up the chemical digestion of lipid.

Enzymes play a key role in chemical digestion and act as catalysts in the digestive process. Catalysts are compounds that accelerate chemical reactions without being permanently changed or consumed themselves

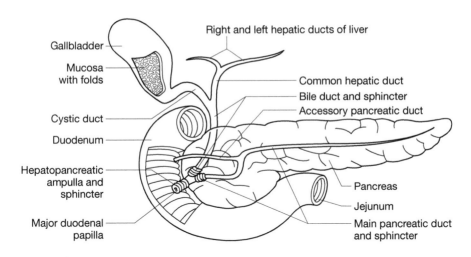

Figure 8.4 The duodenum and related organs.

(Martini, 2009). Digestive enzymes speed up the breakdown of food into absorbable molecules. There are three main classes of enzymes, determined by the food group they act upon (Table 8.2).

The approximate quantity of fluid that is ingested and secreted into the gastrointestinal tract per day is shown in Table 8.3.

In addition to the daily intake of fluids by mouth, approximately 7 litres of fluid are produced by the intestine every day (Martini, 2009). Much of this liquid will be absorbed from the lumen of the gut into the blood, along with the small absorbable nutrient molecules produced from the mechanical and chemical digestion of food, such as monosaccharides and amino acids. Indeed, the prime function of the small bowel is to facilitate the final stages of digestion and to absorb the nutrients generated into the blood and lymph. Ninety per cent of nutrient absorption occurs in the small intestine and the rest occurs in the large intestine (Martini, 2009). This is achieved via large circular folds, 'plicae circulares', villi and microvilli (see for example Martini, 2009). See Martini (2009) for detailed mechanisms of digestion and absorption.

Table 8.2 Enzyme classification

Food group	Enzyme group	Absorbable units	Example
Carbohydrate	Carbohydrase	Monosaccharides	Glucose
Protein	Protease	Amino acids	Tryptophan
Lipid	Lipase	Fatty acids + glycerol	Linoleic acid + glycerol

Table 8.3   Quantity of fluid within the gastrointestinal
tract in 24 hours

Source	Daily quantity (mL)
Food and drink	2,000
Saliva	1,500
Gastric secretions	1,500
Bile	1,000
Pancreatic secretions	1,000
Intestinal secretions	2,000

The close proximity of blood and lymphatic vessels to the absorptive mucosal surface facilitates their transport. Monosaccharides and amino acids are absorbed into the blood, and fatty acids and glycerol are largely absorbed into the lymph via lymphatic vessels (also known as lacteals).

The Large Bowel

The large bowel connects the end of the ileum to the anus. Its four main functions are absorption of water, compaction of intestinal contents into faeces, absorption of vitamins generated by the bacteria that occupy it and storage of faeces prior to defecation.

Bowel Obstruction

Definition and Classification of Bowel Obstruction

Intestinal obstruction 'is defined as partial or complete obstruction of the small or large bowel that impedes the natural progression of digestive processing' (Shelton, 1999). Mrs Brown's presenting symptoms of a two-day history of intermittent, cramping abdominal pain, bloating and vomiting typify the halting of digestive processing associated with small bowel obstruction.

There are two broad types of bowel obstruction: mechanical and paralytic (Table 8.4). Mechanical obstruction is caused by a physical blockage of the intestinal lumen – for example, by a cancerous growth – and paralytic obstruction relates to the halting of peristalsis caused by neuromuscular disorders such as multiple sclerosis, vascular disorders such as a mesenteric thrombosis or temporary problems such as post-operative paralytic ileus.

Table 8.4   Classification of bowel obstruction

	Type of obstruction	*Definition*
Causes	Mechanical	Lumen physically obstructed with mass or narrowed opening
	Paralytic	Halted peristalsis – causes build up of intestinal contents
Type of lesion	Intrinsic	Obstruction involves lumen or bowel wall
	Extrinsic	Obstruction is external to bowel
Onset	Acute	Usually single occurrence and rapid onset of symptoms
	Chronic	Repeated episodes of partial or complete obstruction due to an ongoing risk factor
Extent	Partial	Lumen partly open – some movement of bowel contents, but activity slowed
	Complete	Total occlusion of lumen – build up of intestinal contents proximal to obstruction
Location	High small bowel	Occurring in duodenum and jejunum
	Low small bowel	Occurring in jejunum and ileum
	Large bowel	Occurring in the large intestine

The Causes of Bowel Obstruction

Mechanical obstruction occurs when something physically halts the progression of the contents of the gastrointestinal tract. The intestine may be blocked from the inside by the severe inflammation of inflammatory bowel disease, thickened pancreatic secretions of cystic fibrosis, tumour growth into the lumen or the presence of the parasitic worm ascaris, although this is more common in children living in less developed nations (Gil et al., 2006) (Table 8.5).

Extrinsic causes that originate from outside the intestine can be a tumour and, in women, endometriosis and pregnancy, when the foetus physically presses on the bowel. Obstruction during pregnancy is uncommon, with a reported incidence of 1 in 16,709 deliveries (Hayanga et al., 2005). The bowel can also twist (volvulus), loop back on itself (intussusception) or protrude through a weak spot in the muscular wall of the abdomen (hernia), which can result in obstruction (Figure 8.5). External pressure on the herniated bowel impairs its venous drainage and the resultant swelling and oedema can cause it to become permanently trapped (incarcerated). With

Table 8.5   Causes of bowel obstruction

Congenital	Intussusception; cystic fibrosis; Meckel's diverticulum; Hirschprung's disease
Mesenteric vascular disease	Bowel ischaemia
Neuromuscular diseases	Multiple sclerosis; myasthenia gravis; paralytic ileus
Other intrinsic causes	Crohn's disease; ulcerative colitis; volvulus; foreign body in GI tract; abdominal trauma
Infectious diseases	Cytomegalovirus; ascariosis; tuberculosis
Other extrinsic causes	Adhesions (post-operative or radiation induced); endometriosis; tumours; pregnancy; abdominal hernia

time, this can compromise the blood supply to the gut and the herniated bowel may become strangulated, leading to ischaemia and necrosis.

Lastly, adhesions can cause bowel obstruction, and with an approximate incidence of 60 per cent this is by far the most common cause of small bowel obstruction in developed nations (Hayanga et al., 2005; Doherty and Way, 2006; Foster et al., 2006). Adhesions are bands of scar tissue that cause organs and tissues to stick or bind together and commonly occur following

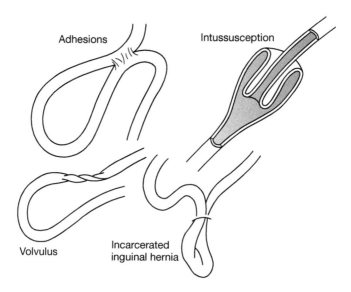

Figure 8.5   Adhesions, volvulus, hernia and intussusception.
Source: Porth, C.: *Pathophysiology 7th Edition* (Lippincott, Williams and Wilkins, 2004). Reproduced with kind permission of Wolters Kluwer Health.

surgical operations. The trauma and inflammation associated with surgical procedures triggers the leakage of plasma and the deposition of fibrin. Fibrin is one of the key factors that cause adhesions. Fibrin is naturally broken down by the enzyme plasmin, which is itself produced in an inactive form called plasminogen. Plasminogen is converted to plasmin in the presence of plasminogen activator, produced by the peritoneum. Adhesions are associated with reduced levels of plasminogen activator, levels that are further lowered by the abrasions and drying that occur during the manual handling of the bowel during an operation (Garden et al., 2007). Ultimately the low levels of plasminogen activator mean that fibrin is not broken down and adhesions are created. Adhesions can also follow irradiation of the bowel: for example, after radiotherapy treatment. Mrs Brown's history may reveal some clues to the potential cause of obstruction in her case.

Pathophysiology Associated with Bowel Obstruction

Once the bowel has become obstructed the contents can not move forward beyond the obstruction. As a result the contents 'build up' and 'back up' as fluid and food are ingested. The excess buildup of intestinal contents characteristically results in vomiting. Typically when the bowel is obstructed there is heightened peristalsis proximal to the obstruction in an attempt to force the contents of the bowel past the obstruction, often causing abdominal pain. Mrs Brown has experienced both vomiting and pain. Beyond or 'distal' to the obstruction peristalsis is reduced. The absence or presence of peristalsis can be assessed by listening for bowel sounds with a stethoscope, normally performed by a doctor or advanced nurse practitioner.

In addition to partially digested food, the bowel becomes distended with gastrointestinal secretions and gas, from swallowed air, which are unable to move beyond the obstruction and which create additional pressure on the gut wall. The intestinal distension stimulates the secretion of fluid, electrolytes and succus entericus (intestinal juice) into the bowel, producing further distension, which stimulates further secretion in a positive feedback manner (Hayanga et al., 2005). As this continues, the increased pressure of fluid in the lumen acts directly on the four tissue layers that make up the bowel wall (Figure 8.2), compressing the mucosal blood and lymphatic vessels of the mucosa. Compression of the blood vessels produces an increase in blood pressure or hydrostatic pressure. As a result normal capillary fluid exchange is compromised and the increase in hydrostatic pressure forces excess leakage of fluid and electrolytes from the capillaries into the surrounding interstitial tissues. At the same time, compression of the lymphatic vessels impairs their ability to drain away excess tissue and interstitial fluid, which naturally accumulates in health back into the blood stream (Hayanga et al., 2005). Therefore fluid accumulates in the interstitial space around the bowel and eventually leaks through the mucosa into the gut lumen. If the pressure continues to build within the bowel, fluid will eventually also move through the visceral peritoneum into the peritoneal cavity. Movement of interstitial fluid into the lumen of the bowel triggers a local inflammatory response that increases mucosal permeability, further exacerbating the movement of fluid into the lumen. The altered permeability of the mucosa also facilitates the movement of electrolytes within the interstitial fluid (which originated from the circulation) into the lumen itself, which will be detected as a loss of serum electrolytes. The large shift of fluid from the circulation to the lumen of the bowel results in further intestinal distension, hypovolaemia and dehydration and may result in hypovolaemic shock.

The pressure created by the accumulation of fluid and gastric contents in an obstructed bowel, exerted upon the four tissue layers of the bowel, may result in the perforation of the visceral peritoneum. This gives rise to the serious complication of peritonitis, which carries a high risk of mortality. Clinical signs and symptoms that suggest peritonitis is imminent or has occurred are rebound tenderness, muscular rigidity and spasm, guarding of the abdomen and often the patient adopting a lying position on their side with hips and knees flexed, which reduces peritoneal irritation (Melander, 2004). In addition there can be a marked increase in abdominal pain, which is not relieved by analgesia accompanied by pyrexia. Though they are not yet evident Mrs Brown requires careful observation for these signs, which should be reported immediately to senior nursing and medical staff, as it is likely that surgical intervention would need to follow as a matter of urgency. Every effort should be made to avoid this by relieving the obstruction before perforation occurs. Lastly, compression of blood vessels can lead to a compromised circulation in the bowel, which could result in necrosis and strangulation.

Assessment and Reaching a Diagnosis

Mrs Brown will be anxious about her condition and will find herself in an unfamiliar environment on the ward. It is therefore important that the nurse endeavours to reduce her anxiety by introducing herself in a friendly confident manner, explaining to her where she is and what is likely to happen to her in the near future. It is now recognised that people fall into one of two groups when it comes to innate coping styles. Some people,

The Case Scenario: The Immediate Assessment Priorities

The initial assessment of signs, symptoms and observations indicates that Mrs Brown is seriously ill and could develop hypovolaemic shock and/or peritonitis and she may require surgery to relieve the obstruction. She is nursed in a bed close to the nurse's station that has piped oxygen and suction. A nurse chaperones and assists the doctor to complete a full clinical examination, making a mental note of the discourse between the doctor and Mrs Brown. During this time, Mrs Brown's past medical history is confirmed as a colectomy for cancer of the colon five years ago and a cholecystectomy 30 years ago. She does not take any regular medication and is allergic to penicillin. Mrs Brown's pain has eased following morphine 10 mg, which was given in casualty two hours ago; however, her abdomen is quite distended. Venous blood samples are collected and a provisional diagnosis of suspected small bowel obstruction is documented. Mrs Brown is nil by mouth and requires insertion of a nasogastric tube.

Consider the following:

1. Given the large volumes of fluid constantly produced within the small bowel, what problem is Mrs Brown likely to experience at this time?
2. What are the immediate assessment priorities in Mrs Brown's case and what is the rationale for each measure?

'vigilant copers', require copious amounts of information as too little makes them more anxious, whereas 'avoidant copers' should receive small amounts of information as too much increases anxiety (Mitchell, 2000). Mrs Brown will know and have her preference considered. Mrs Brown should be reassured that her condition will be closely monitored every 30 minutes for the next 24 hours in an effort to ensure her safety and comfort and to reduce anxiety (Mitchell, 2000). A reduction in pain and abdominal distension and a return of normal bowel sounds would suggest that the obstruction had resolved spontaneously and the need for surgery abated, whereas an increase in the severity of symptoms would indicate the need for surgical laparotomy to resolve the obstruction. The nurse should communicate this information to Mrs Brown and her son, ideally at the same time, as he will be able to reinforce and clarify what his mother has been told, should she require it. Involving relatives in this way is thought to further reduce patient anxiety (Mitchell, 2000).

The Preliminary Assessment

A systematic ABCDE approach to assessment is advocated.

Airway and Breathing

As Mrs Brown is conscious, alert and verbally participating in her assessment on the ward it is obvious that her airway is patent. However, episodes of vomiting are a potential source of airway obstruction and so an ongoing assessment of airway should continue. Mrs Brown's respiratory rate is 18 breaths per minute and the depth is normal. Oxygen saturation is 97 per cent, which is within normal parameters, and therefore she does not need oxygen therapy at this stage. Mrs Brown's respiratory status should be observed and documented every 30 minutes to establish a trend and provide early indication of any deterioration until her abdominal symptoms have been relieved and her condition considered stable.

Circulation

Pulse and blood pressure (BP) will also be assessed initially at 30 minute intervals as they can provide an early indication of hypovolaemic shock (see Chapter 3). Mrs Brown's observations should be carefully compared against her admission results and normal parameters. Circulation can also be assessed indirectly by measuring Mrs Brown's urine output as the first process in urine formation, filtration, is determined by the blood pressure. A fall in blood pressure lowers the glomerular filtration rate (see Chapters 3 and 7), thus reducing urine output. As intestinal obstruction can result in fluid movement from the blood into the intestine and latterly the peritoneal cavity, a fall in blood pressure and subsequent urine output may be observed. Insertion of a urinary catheter to enable accurate hourly monitoring of urine output is a priority and an hourly urine measurement of at least 0.5 to 1 mL/kg/hr is considered satisfactory (Bassett and Makin, 2000). Strict measurement and recording of fluid balance should be maintained. Inspection of the skin and oral mucosa for dryness can also help assessment of the presence of dehydration but a more accurate measure of circulatory volume would be central venous pressure (CVP) monitoring (see Chapter 3).

Disability

Disability or altered state of consciousness should be assessed, although this is often one of the first obvious judgements nurses make when they communicate and interact with the patient. Mrs Brown is alert and communicating freely at this stage and there is no cause for concern. However, if her blood pressure falls sufficiently and she develops hypovolaemic shock her consciousness levels may alter and prompt more specific assessment such as the AVPU (see Chapter 2) or Glasgow Coma Scale (see Chapter 4).

Exposure

Exposure is important to assess in surgical patients as skin integrity can be compromised during bed rest and while in the operating theatre itself. As a result, pressure areas should be observed on admission and an assessment undertaken to determine whether a specific pressure-relieving mattress is required. This assessment should be carried out in accordance with the RCN (2001) recommendations for pressure ulcer risk assessment and prevention. Four-hourly peripheral temperature is also an assessment priority, as pyrexia may indicate perforation of the bowel and acute peritonitis.

Signs, Symptoms and Immediate Nursing Care

Mrs Brown's most obvious problems are nausea, vomiting and pain. A vomit bowl, tissues and plain water mouthwash should be within easy reach as Mrs Brown's mouth is likely to feel extremely dry as a result of the restriction of oral fluids (Whiteing and Hunter, 2008). Lubricant may be applied to her lips if appropriate (Randle et al., 2009). As the small bowel is obstructed, the section distal to or beyond the obstruction will not be active in absorbing fluid and nutrients. This, coupled with the vomiting, will contribute to dehydration, electrolyte imbalances and malnutrition. Therefore assessment of the amount, colour and consistency of vomit is important and should be documented clearly on the fluid balance chart.

A nasogastric tube is passed to remove fluid and accumulated air or gas in the gastrointestinal tract and thus relieve pressure. It should also relieve vomiting and thus prevent aspiration, and limit the effect that further swallowed air would have on the abdominal distension (Doherty and Way, 2006). Once a nasogastric tube has been inserted via the oesophagus, aspirate should be checked for acidity by turning blue litmus paper red to ensure that the tip is situated in the stomach and not the lungs. Nasogastric tubes can be used to administer nutritional feeds; however, in Mrs Brown's case it will only be used to relieve her symptoms. For this to be effective the tube should be aspirated every 30 to 60 minutes initially, depending on the volume of the aspirate. Between aspirations the tube can be left on 'free drainage' and attached to a drainage bag. If single use syringes are used it is important that they are discarded into the clinical waste stream after every aspiration attempt. Aspirate from a high small bowel obstruction is likely to have a yellowish green colour and reflects a high proportion of bile. Aspirate from a patient with a low small bowel obstruction is likely to be a darker colour and is described as faeculent, as it contains faecal-like sediment that has an offensive odour. The removal of fluid and gases from the stomach will also help to relieve some pain, distension and discomfort.

Vomiting can lead to dehydration, and although intravenous fluids have been commenced, the intravenous infusion site should be inspected for patency in case it has dislodged from the vein during transit (infiltration or 'tissued') and the infusion checked against the prescription for accuracy of fluid and rate administration. Intravenous access is vital to replace plasma and fluid secreted into the intestinal lumen. IV 0.9 per cent sodium chloride infused at a litre every four to eight hours dependent upon the degree of dehydration is usually favoured; however, a dextrose/sodium chloride infusion may be indicated if blood glucose levels are below 4 mmol/L.

Pain assessment is an important means of establishing the site, character and intensity of the abdominal pain. Mrs Brown should be able to locate where the pain is and describe its character, which typically would be intermittent, colicky and cramp like as it relates to spasm of the dysfunctional intestine. A verbal rating scale, such as 0 for no pain and 10 for the worst possible pain, allows Mrs Brown to verbalise the pain from her perspective and provides a benchmark against which the effect of pain relief can be measured. IV morphine 5 to 10 mg dependent upon Mrs Brown's body mass should relieve the pain but discomfort from abdominal distension may still be present. Regular pain assessment at 30-minute intervals or if prompted by Mrs Brown should be maintained and documented in the clinical notes. A failure to alleviate the pain at all or worsening pain should be reported to senior nursing and medical staff immediately, as it may signal perforation of the bowel.

As Mrs Brown is likely to be in bed for a prolonged period of time it is vital that she wear thigh length thrombo-embolus deterrent stockings (TEDs), in order to prevent the complication of a deep vein thrombosis (DVT) (NICE, 2007). The graduated compression they provide facilitates the venous return of blood in the legs, preventing stasis, which is the perfect condition for the development of a venous thrombosis. Mrs Brown's legs should be measured to ensure the correct size TEDs are fitted. Prophylactic subcutaneous heparin or a weight-adjusted dose of low molecular heparin such as clexane® would normally be prescribed to prevent deep vein thrombosis (Geerts et al., 2001). Finally, encouraging Mrs Brown to bend and flex her knees and ankles while in bed will improve venous return, reducing blood stasis and hence DVT formation.

Specific Investigations

Abdominal girth measurements are one way of assessing abdominal distension. It is important to measure the abdomen in the same place every time and it should therefore be marked with a pen. A disposable tape measure should be used and can be left in situ to promote patient comfort.

Abdominal inspection by the doctor requires Mrs Brown to lie flat and she will need explanation and assistance from the nurse to achieve this position. The general shape and contours of the abdomen would be noted: a visible swelling, for example, could indicate a hernia, which could relate to the cause of the obstruction. Surgical scars are important to note as they indicate previous surgical procedures, which could suggest adhesions. Visible movement and pulsation of the abdomen is assessed, as marked visible rippling is strongly suggestive of bowel obstruction (Springhouse, 2004).

Bowel sounds are listened for by auscultation with a stethoscope. When the bowel is dilated, stretch receptors are activated, resulting in reflex peristaltic contractions (Garden et al., 2007), the effects of which can be heard with a stethoscope as bowel sounds. Peristalsis is increased proximal to the obstruction and the bowel is described as hyperactive. Hyperactive bowel sounds are 'loud, high-pitched tinkling sounds that occur frequently' (Springhouse, 2004, p. 405) and typically in bowel obstruction the sounds coincide with the patient experiencing abdominal cramps. The bowel distal to the obstruction collapses as fluid and gas no longer enter it and peristalsis is reduced or absent (Garden et al., 2007). The bowel is therefore hypoactive and sounds are heard very infrequently. Generally, people with a high small bowel obstruction have hyperactive bowel sounds in the left upper quadrant of the abdomen, and hypoactive bowel sounds elsewhere. A low small bowel obstruction is associated with hyperactive bowel sounds in the left and right upper quadrants of the abdomen, with hypoactive bowel sounds elsewhere.

Abdominal percussion and palpation, by their very nature, may alter bowel activity and can affect bowel sounds and should therefore be performed after auscultation. Percussion consists of listening to the sounds made by tapping the abdomen with the hand or finger. It can determine the presence of fluid and air in the abdomen which, if present, is heard as a clear, hollow, drum-like sound. Palpation involves first light and then deep touch, to assess the nature and tenderness of the abdominal organs and the presence of fluid. An abdominal mass may be identified on palpation and may signify the cause of the obstruction. Percussion and palpation may, however, be painful for Mrs Brown; therefore painful areas should be assessed last, and the procedures may be postponed as radiological investigations can provide similar information.

Diagnostic Imaging

Diagnostic imaging provides information that often cannot be obtained by patient history and assessment of clinical signs and symptoms alone. There is, however, some debate as to the most reliable type of imaging. An analysis of five studies to determine the accuracy of abdominal plain films in determining bowel obstruction revealed variability between 46 and 80 per cent (Furukawa et al., 2003). A study comparing abdominal plain film with CT scan suggested very little difference between them in identifying a small bowel obstruction (Maglinte et al., 1996), but Suri et al. (1999) found CT (94 per cent accuracy) to be more accurate than plain film (75 per cent accuracy). Although the clinical accuracy of abdominal plain film is debatable, it remains the first imaging procedure in patients with suspected bowel obstruction (Furukawa et al., 2003) and its use is advocated by the EAST Practice Parameter Workgroup for Management of Small Bowel Obstruction (2007). Suri et al. (1999) also found that CT could accurately determine the cause of obstruction more frequently than plain films (87 compared to 7 per cent). It is particularly valuable in identifying ischaemic changes associated with strangulation, and specific types of obstruction such as closed loop obstruction, both of which require urgent surgical intervention (Furukawa et al., 2003). 'A closed loop obstruction is a form of mechanical intestinal obstruction where two points of the intestine along its course are obstructed at a single site' (Furukawa et al., 2003, p. 346). Diagnosis of small bowel obstruction has become faster and easier since the development of multidetector CT scanners (Desser and Gross, 2008). Unlike conventional CT scanners, these are able to generate multiple slices through the abdomen simultaneously, increasing the speed at which images are generated. This, coupled with the high resolution achieved, will make it an increasingly important tool in the future.

Medical Management Strategies

Continuous unrelieved pain of increasing severity and a distended abdominal girth suggest that Mrs Brown's obstruction has not resolved spontaneously and her observations reveal deterioration in her haemodynamic status. Movement of fluid and electrolytes from the circulation into the intestinal lumen will result in a fall in blood pressure, which will initially be compensated for by an increase in heart rate and peripheral vasoconstriction. If the fluid loss is not reversed compensation will fail to maintain the blood pressure and a decrease will be observed. In turn the renal glomerular filtration rate will fall, leading to a decrease in urine output below 0.5 mL/kg/hr. Mrs Brown's increased pulse, low BP and poor urine output suggest that she may be developing hypovolaemic shock, which requires immediate resuscitation (see Chapter 3). As sodium and potassium are lost from the circulation, toxic products of metabolism such as urea and creatinine are inadequately excreted by the kidney and so remain in the blood, as

The Case Scenario: Management and Care Issues

Mrs Brown has been stable overnight. She has received two injections of morphine for abdominal pain. However, as the morning progresses Mrs Brown's condition begins to deteriorate. She has been given a further injection of IM morphine to minimal effect and her pain is continuous and increasing in severity. Her observations and some blood results are compared to those taken on admission and the normal range below. Given this deterioration, Mrs Brown is planned for theatre within the hour.

	Normal range	On admission	12 hours later
Pulse (beats/min)	60–100	84	98
BP (mmHg)	100–140 systolic	150/80	115/75
Respirations (/min)	12–18	18	24
Temperature (°C)	35.6–37.8	36	37.5
SpO$_2$ (per cent)	95–99	97 on 40% oxygen	92–96 on 40% oxygen
Urine output	0.5 mL/kg/hr	Nil	100 mL
Sodium (mmol/L)	135–145	136	130
Potassium (mmol/L)	3.5–5.0	3.7	2.5
Chloride (mmol/L)	98–108	108	97
Urea (mmol/L)	2.2–7.7	7.2	12.4
Creatinine (µmol/L)	50–130	100	140
Leucocytes ($\times 10^9$/L)	3.5–9.0	5.4	9.0

Consider the following:

1. Explain the difference in blood results received over 12 hours.
2. What are the current treatment options for an obstructed bowel?
3. What factors might inform the choice of immediate surgical management?
4. What are Mrs Brown's main care issues?

reflected in Mrs Brown's blood results. The resultant hypoperfusion will stimulate an increase in respiratory rate in an effort to deliver more oxygen to the tissues; however, this may not be sustainable and an initial period of tachypnoea is often followed by a period of bradypnoea. Lastly, a rise in temperature and leucocyte count could indicate strangulation and/or peritonitis. Peritonitis is associated with a high mortality rate, particularly in the presence of hypovolaemic shock, and so the underlying cause requires immediate surgical intervention.

Surgical Management Strategies

Mrs Brown is likely to have an abdominal laparotomy, which will be guided by the radiological findings. Any adhesions that are likely to be responsible for her obstruction will be divided to relieve the obstruction. Should an obstructing lesion also be present, then this would be resected and the remaining small bowel rejoined in a 'primary re-anastamosis'. If a malignant lesion was responsible for the obstruction, then the bowel proximal to the obstruction may be brought to the surface of the abdomen in a stoma. If possible the malignancy would be removed; however, this may not always be the optimal course of action if the cancer has spread to secondary areas (metastasised), as a better quality of life may be achieved by not performing this surgery.

Mrs Brown should be aware from admission that she may ultimately need surgery to resolve her small bowel obstruction. Nevertheless she is likely to feel anxious, and should be reassured in a calm manner. The nurse can help by giving information about the procedure itself, what to expect in the anaesthetic room, details of the wound, the possibility of a stoma and/or drains, intravenous fluid lines and the patient controlled analgesia (PCA) she may have on return to the ward. The nurse is responsible for completing the theatre preparation checklist (Table 8.6) pertinent to Mrs Brown, ensuring that the safety checks in relation to patient identification and patient preparation have been made.

Mrs Brown's son should be contacted and fully informed and as the operation is a laparotomy Mrs Brown should be warned that she may have a temporary or permanent stoma formed. According to local policy, prophylactic antibiotics may be given to Mrs Brown on her induction in the anaesthetic room. This precaution is indicated due to the large number of bacteria present in the bowel, which could potentially move into the bloodstream during her surgery, though penicillin-based drugs would be avoided due to her allergy.

Mrs Brown has had previous abdominal surgery, which predisposes her to developing adhesions, which is one explanation for her obstruction. A second could be that the cancer that she was treated for five years ago has returned; this could be intrinsic or extrinsic to the bowel, but either way could result in an obstruction. Mrs Brown did in fact have adhesions that caused her small bowel obstruction, which were successfully divided, and a small portion of her bowel was resected. She made a good recovery and was discharged home eight days after her surgery.

Table 8.6 Theatre checklist

- Informed consent – gained by the surgeon and / or anaesthetist and documented in notes.
- Trend of vital signs observations clearly recorded and present.
- Medical notes, X-rays, prescription chart and supporting documentation.
- Weight (kg).
- Waterlow score (or similar pressure sore risk assessment).
- Pre-theatre oxygenation with 24% oxygen via a venturi mask to maintain oxygen saturation at more than 95%.
- Venous blood sample results received and documented clearly in the notes.
- Blood group, save and cross match ready for use in the blood bank.
- Check current drug therapy and ensure the patient has not been taking anticoagulant therapy. A clotting screen may be required.
- Intravenous access with IV 0.9% sodium chloride infusion.
- Empty urinary catheter and document on fluid balance chart.
- Pain assessment and relief.
- Pre-medication – might not be required if the patient has been receiving regular opiate pain relief.
- Prophylactic IV antibiotic cover may be administered at the surgeon's discretion.
- Nil by mouth: 4 hours is considered to be sufficient time to ensure that the stomach is emptied Nasogastric bag emptied and contents measured and documented if appropriate.
- Name bands on both wrists stating name, date of birth and hospital ID number.
- Allergy alert bands for penicillin on both wrists.
- Skin cleansing will be determined by local hospital policy and surgeon preference.
- Operation site clearly marked by the surgeon.
- MRSA screening: nasal, axilla and groin swabs sent for MC&S.
- MRSA prophylaxis: Octenesan® body wash and hair shampoo and Bactroban® ointments.
- Measure and fit TED stockings.
- Theatre gown and cap to cover hair to reduce risk of infection.
- Remove personal items such as jewellery (or cover band rings), contact lenses, dentures, hair pieces, hearing aids, body piercing (or cover), false nails. Safely store belongings as per local policy.

Recent Advances in Treatment

Adhesive small bowel obstruction can be relieved by laparoscopic surgery, a newly emerging technique in this area, although the number of patients who have undergone this procedure is rather small, which has given rise to relatively few evaluative studies. Often an additional surgical incision of up to 5 cm (laparoscopic assisted) is required to resect necrotic bowel, and in some patients a larger incision (laparoscopic converted) is necessary. The general conclusion, though, is that laparoscopy 'is associated with reduced hospital stay, early recovery and decreased morbidity, [and that] laparoscopy assisted and converted surgeries do not differ significantly from laparotomy in regard to patient outcome' (Khaikin et al., 2007, p. 742).

Summary

Small bowel obstruction is said to occur when the contents of the small bowel fail to move forward. Causes are either mechanical or paralytic and the most common cause in the developed world is adhesions associated with previous surgery or radiotherapy.

In 69 per cent of cases adhesive small bowel obstruction will resolve spontaneously, though some patients do need immediate surgery particularly if the blood supply to the bowel has been compromised, such as in strangulation. This is more often associated with a total rather than partial obstruction and thus current practice is to assess the completeness of the obstruction and whether the bowel circulation has been compromised (Williams et al., 2005). This chapter has discussed the pathophysiology of small bowel obstruction and identified how such changes can be identified from the signs and symptoms presented by patients such as Mrs Brown. Key aspects of patient management include nursing the patient 'nil by mouth', regular aspiration of a nasogastric tube, intravenous fluids to prevent hypovolaemia and strict fluid balance measurement. Increasing pain, further abdominal distension and signs of shock or peritonitis (suspected if increasing pain is less responsive to analgesia, guarding of the abdomen, raised white cell count and pyrexia) are all signs of deterioration that should prompt immediate surgical intervention. The management of a patient with small bowel obstruction is, as Williams et al. (2005, p. 1144) state, 'a fine balance between waiting for the obstruction to resolve with conservative therapy and rushing the patient off to the operating room'. The nurse has a crucial role in the assessment of this fine balance.

Further Reading

Kossi, J., P. Salminen, A. Rantala and M. Laato. 'Population Based Study of the Surgical Workload and Economic Impact of Bowel Obstruction Caused by Postoperative Adhesions', *British Journal of Surgery*, 90 (2003), 1441–4.

Maglinte, D. D. T., F. M. Kelvin, K. Sandresegaran, A. Nakeeb, S. Romano, J. C. Lappas and T. J. Howard. 'Radiology of Small Bowel Obstruction: Contemporary Approach and Controversies', *Abdominal Imaging*, 30 (2005), 160–78.

Martini, F. H. *Fundamentals of Anatomy and Physiology*, 8th edn (San Francisco: Pearson, Benjamin Cummings, 2009).

Miller, G., J. Boman, I. Shrier and P. H. Gordon. 'Natural History of Patients with Adhesive Small Bowel Obstruction', *British Journal of Surgery*, **87** (2000), 1240–7.

References

Bassett, C. and L. Makin. *Caring for the Seriously ill Patient* (London: Arnold, 2000).

Cox, M. R., I. F. Gunn, M. C. Eastman, R. F. Hunt and A.W. Heinz. 'The Safety and Duration of Non-operative Treatment for Adhesive Small Bowel Obstruction', *Australia and New Zealand Journal of Surgery*, **63** (1993), 367–71.

Desser, T. S. and M. Gross, 2008. 'Multidetector Row Computed Tomography of Small Bowel Obstruction'. *Seminars in Ultrasound CT and MRI*, **29** (2008), 308–21.

Diaz, J. J. et al. 'Guidelines for Management of Small Bowel Obstruction', *Journal of Trauma-Injury Infection and Critical Care*, **64**(6) (2008), 1651–64.

Doherty, G. M. and L. W. Way (eds). *Current Surgical Diagnosis and Treatment*, 12th edn (New York: McGraw-Hill, 2006).

EAST. *Practice Parameter Workgroup for Management of Small Bowel Obstruction* (Eastern Association for the Surgery of Trauma, 2007), http://www.east.org/portal/

Foster, N. M., M. McGory, D. Zingmond and C. Y. Ko. 'Small Bowel Obstruction: A Population Based Appraisal', *Journal of the American College of Surgeons*, **203** (2006), 170–6.

Furukawa, A., M. Yamasaki, M. Takahashi, N. Nitta, T. Tanaka, S. Kanasaki, K. Yokoyama, K. Murata and T. Sakamoto. 'CT Diagnosis of Small Bowel Obstruction: Scanning Technique, Interpretation and Role in the Diagnosis', *Seminars in Ultrasound, CT and MRI*, **24**(5) (2003), 336–52.

Garden, O. J., A. W. Bradbury, J. R. L. Forsythe and R. W. Parks. *Principles and Practice of Surgery*, 5th edn (Edinburgh: Churchill Livingstone, 2007).

Geerts, W. H., J. A. Heit, G. P. Clagett, G. F. Pineo, C. W. Colwell, F. A. Anderson and H. B. Wheeler. 'Prevention of Venous Thromboembolism', *Chest*, **119**(suppl.) (2001), 132–75.

Gil, J. M. G., C. M. L. Esturo and R. P. Ayala. 'Intestinal Obstruction due to Ascaris', *The Internet Journal of Surgery*, **8**(2) (2006).

Hayanga, A. J., K. Bass-Wilkins and G. B. Bulkley. 'Current Management of Small Bowel Obstruction', *Advances in Surgery*, **39** (2005), 1–33,

Khaikin, M., N. Schneidereit, S. Cera, D. Sands, J. Efron, E. G. Weiss, J. J. Nogueras, A. M. Vernava 3rd and S. D. Wexner. 'Laparoscopic vs. Open Surgery for Acute Adhesive Small Bowel Obstruction: Patients' Outcomes and Cost Effectiveness', *Surgical Endoscopy*, **21** (2007), 742–6.

Maglinte, D. D. T., D. E. Heilkamp, T. J. Howard, F. M. Kelvin and J. C. Lapass. 'Current Concepts in Imaging of Small Bowel Obstruction', *Radiologic Clinics of North America*, **41**(2) (2003), 263–83.

Maglinte, D. D. T., B. L. Reyes, B. H. Harman et al. 'Reliability and Role of Plain Film Radiography and CT in the Diagnosis of Small Bowel Obstruction', *American Journal of Roentgenology*, **167** (1996), 1451–5.

Martini, F. H. *Fundamentals of Anatomy and Physiology*, 8th edn (San Francisco: Pearson Benjamin Cummings, 2009).

Melander, S. D. *Case Studies in Critical Care Nursing. A Guide for Application and Review*, 3rd edn (Philadelphia: Saunders, 2004).

Mitchell, M. 'Nursing Intervention for Pre-operative Anxiety', *Nursing Standard*, **14**(37) (2000), 40–3.

NICE. *Venous Thromboembolism. Reducing the Risk of Venous Thromboembolism (Deep Vein Thrombosis and Pulmonary Embolism) in Inpatients Undergoing Surgery* (2007), http://guidance.nice.org.uk/CG46/Guidance/pdf/English

Randle, J., F. Coffey and M. Bradbury. *Oxford Handbook of Clinical Skills in Adult Nursing* (Oxford: Oxford University Press, 2009).

Royal College of Nursing. *Pressure Ulcer Risk Assessment and Prevention* (London: Royal College of Nursing, 2001).

Shelton, B. 'Intestinal Obstruction', *AACN Clinical Issues*, **10**(4) (1999), 478–91.

Sherwood, L. L. *Human Physiology from Cells to Systems*, 2nd edn (Minneapolis/St Paul: West Publishing, 1993).

Springhouse, Inc. (ed.). *Critical Care Nursing Made Incredibly Easy* (Philadelphia: Lippincott, Williams and Wilkins, 2004).

Suri. S., S. Gupta, P. J. Sudhakar et al. 'Comparative Evaluation of Plain Films, Ultrasound and CT in the Diagnosis of Small Bowel Obstruction', *Acta Radiologica*, **40** (1999), 422–8.

Urden, L. D., M. E. Lough and K. M. Stacy. *Priorities in Critical Care Nursing*, 2nd edn (St Louis: Mosby-Year Book, 1996).

Whiteing, N. and J. Hunter. 'Nursing Management of Patients Who Are Nil by Mouth', *Nursing Standard*, **22**(26) (2008), 40–5.

Williams, S. B., J. Greenspon, H. Young and B. Orkin. 'Small Bowel Obstruction: Conservative vs. Surgical Management', *Diseases of the Colon and Rectum*, **48** (2005), 1140–6.

9

Diabetic Ketoacidosis

Paula Holt

Introduction

Diabetes mellitus is a metabolic disorder that has multiple causes and is identified by the continued presence of a fasting plasma glucose level above 7 mmol/L with associated disturbances of carbohydrate, fat and protein metabolism. There are two distinct types of diabetes mellitus.

- Type 1 diabetes: reduced or absent insulin secretion caused by the autoimmune destruction of the pancreatic beta cells.
- Type 2: the action of the circulating insulin is reduced due to the presence of insulin resistance, which occurs with increased weight gain and inactivity.

Diabetes is an increasingly common, costly, serious, potentially debilitating and life-threatening condition. At present it affects 3.54 per cent of the UK population and a known 2.2 million people in the UK have been diagnosed with the condition; of these approximately 250,000 have type 1 diabetes and the remainder have type 2 (Diabetes UK, 2006). However, due to the insidious and hidden nature of diabetes it is estimated that there are a further 750,000 to 1,000,000 people living with type 2 diabetes in the UK who have not been diagnosed. Indeed, the incidence of both type 1 and type 2 diabetes is rising so rapidly that it is considered to have reached epidemic proportions due to the increasing levels of obesity as a result of sedentary lifestyles and high calorie, fat laden diets (Cowburn, 2004).

Chronic absence of or insufficient active circulating insulin causes blood glucose levels to rise, which over time will lead to the development of diabetes-related complications. In recognition of the severity of physical, psychological and socially debilitating factors associated with these complications, the Department of Health launched the National Service Framework

(NSF) for Diabetes Delivery Strategy (DH, 2003). The aim of this is to improve the care and management of people with diabetes with a vision to reduce and prevent the occurrence and development of diabetes-related complications. It also focuses on reducing the human and financial burden of diabetes in primary care, acute hospitals and community services.

While the long-term complications of diabetes resulting from poor blood glucose control have been recognised, sub-optimal blood glucose control in people with diabetes can also cause the acute complications of hypoglycaemia and hyperglycaemia. The seriousness of both conditions should not be underestimated as they can both be life threatening if not treated quickly and appropriately. A rapid escalation of blood glucose levels causing hyperglycaemia is responsible for the acute presentation of diabetic ketoacidosis (DKA). DKA is a life threatening complication that affects a significant number of people, leading to hospital admission each year. It is due to a relative or absolute deficiency of insulin and is the most common hyperglycaemic emergency in patients with diabetes (Umpierrez et al., 2004), with the person often requiring management in an intensive care unit due to the high level of monitoring required (Savage and Kilvert, 2006). DKA occurs predominantly in people who have type 1 diabetes but it can occur with type 2 diabetes, particularly in the presence of severe infection or episodes of metabolic stress. Therefore the focus of this chapter is the acute assessment and management of a young person presenting with DKA. The management strategies are based upon recommendations from the Joint Board of Diabetes Societies (2010), NICE (2004) and Diabetes NSF (DH, 2003).

Aim and Learning Outcomes

The Aim

The aim of this chapter is to provide the reader with a logical and comprehensive approach to the assessment and first line management of a person with diabetic ketoacidosis.

Learning Outcomes

At the end of this chapter the reader will be able to:

1. Identify and discuss the normal and altered pathophysiology of blood glucose control.
2. Differentiate between type 1 and type 2 diabetes.

3. Define and explain the pathophysiological changes that occur in the body as a result of hyperglycaemia.
4. Outline and describe the main causes of diabetic ketoacidosis.
5. Consider the assessment process and the investigations required to enable an accurate and timely diagnosis.
6. Using evidence-based practice, consider the immediate care and management that a person admitted to hospital with acute diabetic ketoacidosis will require.

The Case Scenario: The Presenting Complaint

Lucy is an 18-year-old who was diagnosed with Type 1 diabetes when she was six years old. Her diabetes is currently controlled with a basal/bolus insulin regimen. Lucy's insulin regimen comprises Lantus® (ultra-long acting peakless insulin) 22 units at bedtime to provide Lucy with her basal insulin requirements, supplemented by bolus administration of Novorapid® (rapid acting insulin) prior to each main meal to control the expected rise in post-prandial blood glucose level. The dose of the Novorapid® is determined by Lucy and is based upon the type and amount of food she is about to eat and her current blood glucose levels. On the day of admission Lucy had been shopping with her mother and friend. At lunchtime, having ordered a meal, Lucy realised that she did not have her Novorapid® insulin but, as she was hungry and her lunch had been served, she decided to eat and administer her insulin as soon as she returned home. Lucy was aware that this was not ideal but felt confident that her post-meal blood glucose levels would be partially maintained by the amount of walking around the shops she had done. Approximately two hours after lunch, Lucy complained of abdominal pain, leg cramps and nausea. She subsequently vomited, and appeared pale, sweaty and clammy and less alert than usual. Her mother and friend escorted her to the nearest accident and emergency unit. On admission Lucy is semi-conscious, her abdomen is tender and distended and she continues to vomit bile stained fluid. A provisional diagnosis of diabetic ketoacidosis is made.

Consider the following:

1. Describe the normal physiology of the pancreas, the production of insulin and the normal homeostatic control of blood glucose levels to maintain them between 4 and 7mmol/L.
2. Note the distinct features of type 1 and type 2 diabetes mellitus.
3. Consider the physiological changes in the body caused by diabetes that result in the development of hyperglycaemia.
4. What are the common pre-disposing factors, signs and symptoms of diabetic ketoacidosis?

Normal Blood Glucose Regulation

A good working knowledge of the normal physiological mechanism of blood glucose control is essential if healthcare practitioners are to fully understand, recognise and manage the implications of disordered blood glucose control.

Anatomy and Physiology in the Absence of Diabetes

The pancreas, a major organ in the body with endocrine and exocrine functions, plays a significant role in the normal homeostatic control of blood glucose. The endocrine pancreas consists of small clusters of cells called the islets of Langerhans, which are scattered among the exocrine cells and named after the German anatomist Paul Langerhans. There are approximately one million individual clusters of islet cells within the pancreas and each islet contains approximately 1,000 endocrine cells (Rorsman, 2005).

Within each islet of Langerhans there are four main types of cells. The alpha and beta cells are predominantly responsible for the regulation of blood glucose levels.

1. Alpha (α) cells make up approximately 20 per cent of all the cells in each islet. These secrete glucagon, which raises blood glucose levels.
2. Beta (β) cells account for approximately 75 per cent of all of the islet cells. These secrete insulin, which lowers blood glucose levels.
3. Delta (δ) cells are the majority of the remaining cells and they secrete somatostatin, which is a growth hormone inhibiting hormone.
4. F cells, also known as PP cells, are limited in number and are scattered sparsely throughout each islet of Langerhans. They secrete pancreatic polypeptide, which has a part to play in the exocrine function of the pancreas and is therefore not relevant to diabetes.

Normal Blood Glucose Homeostasis

At a cellular level, the availability of glucose is essential for normal energy production and cell function and the presence of insulin is required for the uptake of glucose into the cell. A range of mechanisms exist to control blood glucose levels and ensure adequate availability for the cells. The commonest source of glucose is from the ingestion of dietary simple sugars and/or complex carbohydrate foods such as pasta, potatoes, cakes and bread. The glucose from these foods is absorbed from the stomach and small intestine into the bloodstream, causing a direct rise in blood glucose

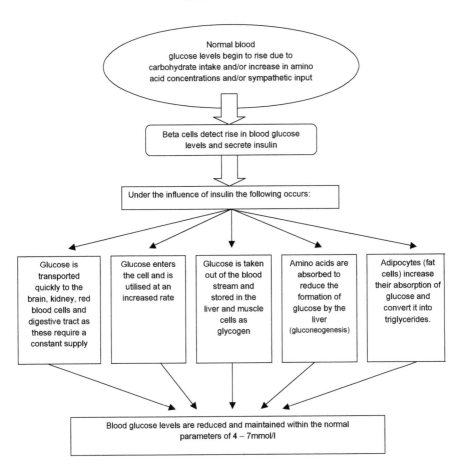

Figure 9.1   Action of insulin on target cells.

levels. The detection of a rise in glucose levels stimulates beta cells to secrete insulin and facilitate the uptake of glucose into the cell (Figure 9.1).

Glucagon Secretion

The secretion of glucagon from the pancreatic alpha cells is equally important as insulin in the maintenance of optimal blood glucose levels. In response to falling blood glucose levels glucagon is released, causing the conversion of glycogen into glucose within the liver. This process serves to raise blood glucose levels and prevent the person from experiencing hypoglycaemia (Figure 9.2). These homeostatic mechanisms are

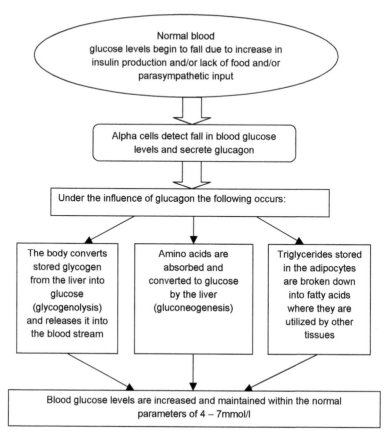

Figure 9.2   Action of glucagon on target cells.

designed to maintain blood glucose levels within the normal range of 4 to 7 mmol/L.

Amino acids, found in dietary protein as well as being synthesised by the body, also play a part in blood glucose control. In between meals or during a fast as blood glucose levels decrease amino acids are released from muscle cells into the bloodstream and transported to the liver. The liver converts amino acids into glucose via a process called 'gluconeogenesis'. This 'new' glucose is then transported back into the bloodstream, causing blood glucose levels to rise (Figure 9.2). This process is part of the body's compensatory mechanism to ensure that vital organs such as the kidneys and brain, which cannot store glucose, have a continuous supply regardless of whether the person has eaten or not.

The 'fight or flight' sympathetic mechanism, which is triggered when faced with a dangerous, difficult or frightening situation, can also enable an increase in blood glucose. Sympathetic stimulation of the anterior pituitary gland releases adreno-cortico-trophic hormone (ACTH), which stimulates the adrenal gland to release growth hormone, cortisol and adrenaline, which promote hepatic glucose release via the processes of gluconeogenesis and glycogenolysis. Simultaneously the pancreatic alpha cells secrete glucagon to provide the person with the extra energy that may be required to escape the dangerous situation. Each mechanism causes further increases in blood glucose levels (Figure 9.2). Once the fight or flight situation has abated, the parasympathetic nervous system triggers the release of insulin to reduce the elevated blood glucose levels back to within normal limits.

Once insulin has been secreted it is degraded and removed from the circulation by the liver and kidneys. This occurs quite rapidly after secretion, giving insulin an active biological half-life of only 6 to 10 minutes. It is expected that all insulin produced will be broken down within 12 to 20 minutes of secretion, thus preventing an abundance of circulating insulin, which could cause a decrease in blood glucose levels to below 4 mmol/L, leading to hypoglycaemia.

Diabetes Mellitus

Diabetes has been recognised as a disease since ancient times and was first described by Aretaeus of Cappadocia in the second century AD as a serious condition that involved the 'melting down of flesh and limbs into urine.' With greater insight into the causes and pathophysiology of diabetes it is now known that Aretaeus' description was not strictly accurate but it does illustrate some of the main physical changes that are witnessed in poorly controlled diabetes, such as weight loss and polyuria. It wasn't until 1889 that scientists discovered the link between the pancreas and the development of diabetes, and insulin as a treatment for diabetes was not developed until 1921 (Williams and Pickup, 2004).

Type 1 Diabetes

Type 1 diabetes is a chronic autoimmune disease in which the T lymphocytes progressively destroy the insulin-producing beta cells of the pancreas (Faideau et al., 2005), resulting in little or no production of insulin (Pozzilli and Mario, 2001). The rate of beta cell destruction varies quite considerably between people, but there is a tendency for it to be more rapid in infants and

Table 9.1   Signs and symptoms of diabetes

Type 1 diabetes	*Type 2 diabetes*
• Sudden/quick onset	• Gradual onset
	• May be no symptoms
• Polyuria	• Polyuria
• Thirst	• Thirst
• Glycosuria	• Glycosuria
• Weight loss	• Often no weight loss
	• Usually obese
• Tiredness and weakness	• Tiredness and weakness
• Ketosis	• No ketosis
• Blurring of vision	• Blurring of vision
• Skin infections	• Skin infections
• Genital soreness	• Genital soreness
• Absent C peptide	• C peptide detectable
• Islet cell antibodies present	• No markers of autoimmunity

Table 9.2   Predisposing factors for the development of diabetes

Type 1 diabetes	*Type 2 diabetes*
1. Familial or genetic link (Bonifacio 2004)	1. Ethnic group particularly Afro-Caribbean and South Asian people (Diabetes UK 2006)
2. Viral infections such as measles, mumps, rubella	2. Obesity
3. Early exposure to cow's milk (Akerblom 2002)	3. Reduced physical activity
4. Deficiency of vitamin D	4. Advancing age
5. Rapid growth and obesity in childhood	5. Smoking (Will et al. 2001)
6. Toxins such as Vacor and bafilomycins (Hettiarachichi et al. 2004)	6. Thrifty phenotype hypothesis (Hales et al. 2001)
	7. Psychological stress
	8. Exposure to pesticides (Kuehn 2008)
	9. Drinking fruit juice (Bazzano et al. 2008)
	10. IRS1 gene identified (Rung et al. 2009)

children and slower in adults. By the time Lucy exhibited classical signs and symptoms of diabetes (Table 9.1) it is thought that over 90 per cent of her beta cells would have been destroyed, causing a marked insulin deficiency, which is the hallmark of type 1 diabetes. Lucy was diagnosed as having type 1 diabetes when she was just six years old.

There are a number of factors that can increase the risk of developing diabetes (Table 9.2). Although Lucy does not report a history of diabetes in her family it is recognised that type 1 diabetes can be hereditary and there is a 23.3 per cent risk of developing multiple islet auto-antibodies if both parents have type 1 diabetes (Bonifacio et al., 2004).

Lucy will have developed auto-antibodies that will have progressively destroyed her beta cells. As she was quite young when this happened the onset of symptoms would have been rapid, probably spanning from a few days up to about a month in duration, when she would have presented at her general practitioner or accident and emergency unit. She would probably have been very unwell, with the typical signs and symptoms of ketoacidosis (Table 9.1). A diagnosis of type 1 diabetes means that Lucy would no longer have the beta cell capacity to produce insulin naturally and she would therefore rely upon artificially administered insulin, usually via the subcutaneous route, to control blood glucose levels for the rest of her life.

Type 2 Diabetes

The aetiology of type 2 diabetes is quite different from type 1 – so much so that they can almost be considered to be two different conditions. Type 2 diabetes accounts for 85 to 90 per cent of the total population who have diabetes and affects approximately 3 per cent of the total population of the UK (Diabetes UK, 2006). Unlike type 1 diabetes, type 2 diabetes is an insidious disease that can be present for up to 12 years before symptoms appear and a diagnosis is made. As a consequence, up to 50 per cent of people may have developed one or more of the complications of diabetes at the time of diagnosis (Table 9.3).

Type 2 diabetes is now a major healthcare concern and the association between obesity, sedentary lifestyles and diabetes is so close that in the 1970s the term 'diabesity' was coined (Haslam and James, 2005). The development of visceral abdominal fat found typically in 'apple shaped' people is the main link between obesity and diabetes. Visceral fat cells decrease the action of the circulating insulin, causing insulin resistance (Williams and Pickup, 2004). It is thought that currently up to 25 per cent of the population of the UK have a level of insulin resistance similar to that of people who have type 2 diabetes. In type 2 diabetes insulin is secreted but the presence

Table 9.3 Long-term complications of poorly controlled diabetes

---

- Diabetic retinopathy leading to blindness
- Peripheral neuropathy leading to loss of peripheral sensation and predisposing to the development of diabetic foot ulcer, which may necessitate limb amputation
- Ineffective immunity leading to poor healing and the potential for devastating infections requiring limb amputation
- Renal nephropathy leading to end stage renal disease (Happich et al. 2008)
- Peripheral and cardiovascular disease and stroke

---

of insulin resistance adversely affects the action and efficiency of the secreted insulin and therefore its ability to reduce blood glucose levels is impaired. The presence of insulin resistance also actively increases blood glucose levels further by stimulating the liver to form and release more glucose. This results in further rises in blood glucose levels and the development of symptoms of type 2 diabetes (Table 9.1). As a result, blood glucose levels continue to rise, signalling a need for further insulin to be secreted. The beta cells respond by producing more insulin, but over time they become exhausted and eventually the numbers of beta cells diminish. A state of hyperinsulinaemia exacerbates the insulin resistance further, creating other metabolic risk factors such as raised blood pressure and hyperlipidaemia (Broom, 2006). In turn, these metabolic risk factors increase the risk of developing cardiovascular disease, peripheral vascular disease and stroke (Table 9.3). Indeed, it is estimated that 70 to 80 per cent of people with type 2 diabetes will die prematurely (under the age of 65 years) of a myocardial infarction (Haffner et al., 1998). The link between chronic elevated blood glucose levels and the development of diabetes-related complications is evident in both type 1 and type 2 diabetes (DCCT, 1993). In type 2 diabetes careful dietary control may be sufficient to control blood glucose levels, but in many cases oral hypoglycaemic agents such as Glicazide® or Metformin® may be required. Careful blood glucose control in persons with type 1 and type 2 diabetes is the key ingredient to preventing acute hypoglycaemia and hyperglycaemia and delaying the progression of serious and life threatening complications of diabetes (DCCT, 1993; UKPDS, 1998). Further to this the National Institute for Health and Clinical Excellence (NICE) has published optimal target blood glucose levels that a person with diabetes is expected to achieve in order to significantly reduce their risk of complications. It also recommends close blood pressure and cholesterol monitoring and maintenance within set limits, given the strong link between diabetes and heart disease. Medical management strategies and patient education aimed at achieving these targets are also offered by NICE (NICE, 2004, 2008).

Hyperglycaemia and Diabetic Ketoacidosis

In Lucy's case the absence of insulin means that the normal homeostatic control of blood glucose does not occur: serum glucose levels rise yet cells are deprived of glucose for normal energy production and cellular function. Hyperglycaemia is the term used to describe a blood glucose level > 10 mmol/L. In response to the low intracellular glucose, accelerated hepatic glucose production is mediated by a range of compensatory mechanisms in a futile effort to enable cellular glucose uptake (Figure 9.3). Counter-regulatory hormones such as catecholamines, glucagon, growth hormone and cortisol are released to further increase the high blood glucose levels.

The lack of cellular glucose uptake leads to energy depletion and would cause Lucy to feel tired and lethargic. In a counter effort there will be an

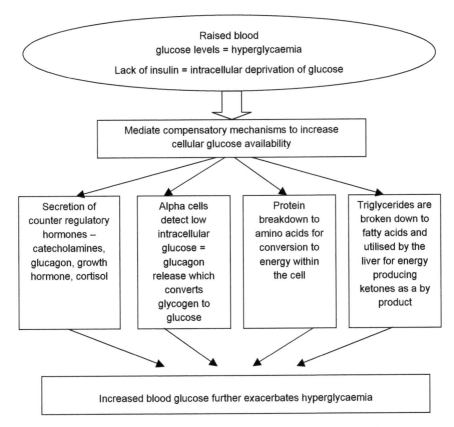

Figure 9.3 Compensatory mechanisms in response to hyperglycaemia and low intracellular glucose.

increase in the breakdown of proteins into constituent amino acids, which are subsequently converted by the body to energy. The liver will also increase absorption of the circulating amino acids and convert them to glucose, leading to a further increase in hyperglycaemia. The increased secretion of glucagon stimulates the liver to release stores of glycogen, which are also converted into glucose in a further misguided effort to increase blood glucose and intracellular levels of glucose. Once the liver's glycogen stores have been utilised, the breakdown of triglycerides into their constituent fatty acids will begin. These are converted by the liver into ketones in an attempt by the body to obtain further energy supplies. Ketones are then excreted via the kidneys and can be detected in the urine; however, when the production of ketone bodies exceeds the rate of excretion this can cause significant, life threatening acidosis (Kettyle and Arky, 1998). Circulating ketones are acidic and may lower the serum pH sufficiently to cause metabolic ketoacidosis. Hyperglycaemia leads to excessive diuresis and subsequent dehydration, and facilitates the movement of water and potassium out of the cells, which leads to intracellular dehydration, hypokalaemia, expansion of extracellular fluid and a loss of sodium (Kitabchi and Wall, 1999). Typically the signs and symptoms of hyperglycaemia such as polyuria, thirst and lethargy become evident when the blood glucose level rises to above 15 mmol/L. Thus, these mechanisms merely serve to increase blood glucose further; however, they do not facilitate cellular uptake and they do instigate a number of undesirable, life threatening side effects such as ketone production.

Assessment and Reaching a Diagnosis

The serious nature of DKA should not be underestimated because if there is underlying serious illness or if the DKA is misdiagnosed, left untreated or not treated sufficiently it can be life threatening (Ilag et al., 2003; Umpierrez et al., 2004). Lucy is acutely unwell and therefore requires a systematic and comprehensive assessment to provide a rapid, accurate diagnosis to inform immediate appropriate management and care. Her semi-conscious state should prompt an ABC approach.

Airway

Dehydration and metabolic acidosis can lead to altered conscious levels. Depending upon the stage of development of DKA, Lucy's level of consciousness may be anywhere along the conscious–unconscious continuum; however, true coma at admission is rare, being present in fewer than

The Case Scenario: The Immediate Assessment Priorities

Lucy is currently studying full time at school for her examinations, which she is finding quite stressful. She does not smoke, drink alcohol or take drugs and is of a slim build. She is an active member of the school swimming and netball teams. Both of her parents are alive and well and she has an older brother who is fit with no health concerns. There is no other history of diabetes in her immediate family. Further information gleaned from Lucy's mother confirms the omission of insulin with her lunch prior to admission. Lucy's mother also shares concerns regarding her daughter's general health and diabetes control recently and reports a three to four week history of increasing tiredness, lethargy, thirst, frequency of micturition (passing urine) and weight loss.

An immediate physiological assessment revealed the following:

Temperature: 36.8 °C
Pulse: 128 beats/min, regular
Respirations: 24/minute
Blood pressure: 104/64 mmHg
Capillary blood glucose level: 22.6 mmol/L
Potassium: 4.0 mmol/L
Venous blood ketones: 7.0 mmol/L
HbA1c: 9 per cent

Consider the following:

1. Explain the pathophysiological basis for Lucy's presenting signs and symptoms.
2. What are the common causes of diabetic ketoacidosis?
3. What are the immediate assessment priorities in this case and why?
4. Identify further clues in the information given by Lucy's mother that might be a cause for concern.

10 per cent of patients. Therefore airway assessment will be based upon individual circumstances. As Lucy is semi-conscious she will need to have her airway assessed at very regular intervals using the 'look, listen and feel' method of airway assessment (see Chapter 2) and the findings must be clearly reported and documented. It is good practice to include this assessment as part of the Glasgow Coma Score (GCS), which must be performed every thirty minutes initially due to Lucy's decreased level of consciousness (see Chapter 4). Altered consciousness levels should prompt an early assessment of capillary blood glucose via the finger prick method, particularly

when a history of diabetes is known. Lucy's capillary blood glucose was grossly raised above the normal levels of 4 to 7 mmol/L at 22.6 mmol/L and may explain her semi-conscious state.

Lucy presented with a history of nausea and vomiting, which presents a potential threat to airway patency. Nausea and vomiting may result from the compensatory breakdown of fats (lipolysis), initiated in an effort to release energy stores, leading to increased circulating fatty acids. Liver cells degrade fatty acids into fatty acyl-CoA, which can be converted by cell mitochondria into acetoacetate (ketone bodies). Excessive accumulation of ketones will increase blood acidity, lower the pH and lead to metabolic acidosis, which can present as nausea and vomiting. In some cases of decreased consciousness a nasogastric tube may be inserted as a precautionary measure to avoid the potential aspiration of gastric contents and therefore protect the airway. As Lucy's condition improves and she becomes fully alert and conscious and able to maintain her own airway, the frequency of assessment of her airway and GCS can be reduced.

Breathing

Lucy is tachypnoeic with a respiratory rate of 24 breaths per minute. She may begin to hyperventilate and develop Kussmaul respirations (Savage and Kilvert, 2006) in a compensatory effort to correct the metabolic acidosis. Chemoreceptors sense a fall in blood pH, which will activate the respiratory centre housed within the medulla, leading to an increased respiratory stimulus to 'blow off' carbon dioxide (CO_2). Carbon dioxide forms carbonic acid when dissolved in the bloodstream, further exacerbating acidity. Therefore increased excretion of CO_2 helps to reduce the acidity and increase the blood pH to a more normal level, which is slightly alkaline at 7.35 to 7.45. Excessive ketones may also appear on the breath, giving rise to a distinctive smell of acetone or pear drops. As the level of acidosis in Lucy's blood declines, a decrease in her respiratory rate back to within the normal parameters of 12 to 16 noiseless and effortless breaths per minute that do not have the characteristic ketotic acetone smell should be noted. Until this time Lucy will require her respiratory rate, depth, regularity, pattern and smell to be observed and recorded by the nurse for a minimum of 30 seconds every 30 minutes, and any negative changes reported to a senior nurse and the doctors responsible for her treatment. Lucy's oxygen saturation levels should be recorded via continuous non-invasive oxygen saturation monitoring and be maintained at > 95 per cent. A fall in oxygen saturation levels below 95 per cent will necessitate administration of 100 per cent oxygen via a mask.

Circulation

Compensatory increased excretion of adrenaline and stress hormones such as cortisol leads to increased blood glucose levels. Increased circulating adrenaline also has a direct effect upon the cardiac system, leading to increased heart rate, contractility and peripheral vasoconstriction. Lucy's heart rate may reflect this effect as it is above normal at 128 beats per minute, which is considered to be a tachycardia. As abnormal serum potassium levels can lead to potentially fatal cardiac arrhythmias, Lucy should be commenced on three or five lead cardiac monitoring to provide a continuous analysis of heart rate and rhythm, which should be documented every 30 minutes.

Currently Lucy's blood pressure is 104/64 mmHg, which may be normotensive for Lucy or could be lower than anticipated, but this will need to be monitored and charted every 30 minutes as a fall in BP could be indicative of impending dehydration. A rising blood glucose level > 15 mmol/L causes osmotic diuresis and polyuria, consequent thirst and lethargy. The subsequent loss of fluids and electrolytes leads to signs of dehydration. Hyperglycaemia facilitates water and potassium movement out of the cells, leading to intracellular dehydration and hypokalaemia and extracellular fluid accumulation. Strict monitoring of fluid input and output is essential to assess the degree of dehydration and rehydration. Lucy will also require observation for other signs of dehydration, such as turgor, thirst, dry mouth, muscle cramps and a decreased urine output, and a baseline measurement of these must be ascertained, from which improvement or deterioration can be determined. Low circulating volume results in a fall in stroke volume, cardiac output and consequent low BP, which will also initiate a range of compensatory mechanisms. A fall in BP causing less vessel wall stretch will be sensed by baroreceptors situated within the carotid sinus and aortic arch, which in turn stimulate the cardiac acceleratory centre housed within the medulla. Subsequent sympathetic nervous activation will lead to a further increase in heart rate and myocardial contraction in an effort to increase cardiac output and BP.

Excessive diuresis can lead to further depletion of potassium (K^+) levels and hypokalaemia. Lucy's potassium level is within normal limits but this does not give an accurate representation of the total body potassium levels, which will always be markedly depleted, with a deficit ranging from 3 to 12 mmol/kg (Page and Hall, 1999). This has the potential of causing fatal cardiac arrhythmias and consequently needs to be corrected immediately and carefully monitored. A 12 lead electrocardiograph should be performed, as T wave changes may indicate hypokalaemia. Lucy's serum potassium levels will be determined on admission and at one and two hours from commencement of treatment and then every two hours (Joint Board of Diabetes Societies (JBDS) Inpatient Care Group, 2010).

On admission venous blood will be tested for ketones using a hand-held blood ketone meter. This detects the presence of 3-beta-hydroxbutyrate, which is the dominating ketone body produced in the liver during periods of insulin deprivation and rising blood glucose levels. The measurement of blood ketones now represents best practice in monitoring the suppression of ketonaeamia compared to urinalysis and arterial blood measurements (JBDS Inpatient Care Group, 2010).

Lucy's medical and nursing assessment has revealed poor control of her blood glucose. This can be further substantiated from serum measurement of haemoglobin A1c (HbA1c) levels taken on admission. The HbA1c measures the amount of glucose in the blood that has bound irreversibly to a specific part of haemoglobin in red blood cells. HbA1c increases proportionately with increasing blood glucose concentration over prolonged periods. HbA1c circulates for the lifespan of the red blood cell, and so gives an indication of average blood glucose levels over the preceding two to three months. An unusually high blood glucose level for one or two days is unlikely to alter the HbA1c, but high blood glucose levels for longer periods of time will be reflected in a high HbA1c. The HbA1c target to be achieved in order to reduce the risk of long-term complications of diabetes is 6.5 to 7.5 per cent. Lucy's most recent HbA1c result of 9 per cent indicates that she has had poor blood glucose control for at least the past two to three months. This result suggests that her blood glucose levels have been higher than the normal limits of 4 to 7 mmol/L and as a consequence she is putting herself at an increased risk of developing serious acute and chronic diabetes-related complications. Previous HbA1c levels will help to identify a trend in Lucy's blood glucose control.

Specific questions may also reveal a more detailed history of Lucy's diabetes control. She has experienced increased levels of stress associated with examinations, which may have caused increased sympathetic mediated adrenaline release, leading to a physiological increase in blood glucose levels. In this situation Lucy should have been monitoring her blood glucose levels a minimum of four times per day, before breakfast and two hours after each of her main meals. The insulin regimen that Lucy is currently prescribed allows her the flexibility to give extra rapid acting insulin as a 'correction dose' to correct a high blood glucose level. In addition, if her pre-prandial blood glucose level is raised consistently in the morning then an increase in her basal insulin, Lantus®, may be required. Lucy and her family may require extra help and support from their healthcare team in managing fluctuating blood glucose levels during this stressful period.

On admission to the accident and emergency department Lucy's temperature is within normal limits, which at this stage of the assessment allows infection and/or sepsis to be ruled out as the potential cause of the DKA; however, it would be prudent for the doctor treating Lucy to take a blood sample for microscopy, culture and sensitivity (MC&S). In the immediate situation, if treatment for DKA is delayed or not sufficient the levels of acidosis will continue to rise and the body will eventually decompensate, causing the person to develop warm dry skin, hypothermia, hypoxia, a decreasing consciousness state and decreased renal, cardiac and respiratory output.

Reaching a Diagnosis: Specific Investigations

Rapid treatment of diabetic ketoacidosis is crucial and will impact on the potential survival of the patient (Savage and Kilvert, 2006). Therefore specific investigations need to be arranged immediately DKA is suspected in order to be able to confirm the diagnosis, determine a possible cause and commence treatment promptly.

Investigations will include:

- capillary blood glucose (tested at the bedside);
- venous blood glucose (laboratory test);
- blood 3-beta-hydroxybutyrate (blood ketones);
- urea and electrolytes;
- arterial blood gases;
- full blood count;
- electrocardiograph;
- chest X-ray;
- urinalysis;
- urine specimen for microscopy, culture and sensitivity;
- blood cultures;
- continuous cardiac monitoring;
- continuous pulse oximetry.

Causes of Hyperglycaemia and Diabetic Ketoacidosis

In Lucy's case, the main cause of DKA was having had lunch without a prior injection of insulin to counteract the expected rise in blood glucose levels. Other causes include:

- Insulin is leaking out of the injection site.
- Lipohypertrophy is caused by insulin being injected repeatedly into the same site, causing delayed and erratic absorption and action of insulin.

- The dose of insulin given is not enough for the amount and type of food eaten.
- In the event of planned exercise, the insulin dose is reduced to prevent possible hypoglycaemia, but the exercise is then cancelled or reduced in duration and/or intensity.
- Infection, injury, emotional stress and myocardial infarction cause the production of stress-responding hormones such as adrenaline and cortisol, which antagonise the effects of insulin and can result in hyperglycaemia and DKA (Kettyle and Arky, 1998).
- Menstruation causes a rise in blood glucose levels a few days before a menstrual period is due (Tamas et al., 1996).
- Steroids, thiazide diuretics and tricyclic antidepressants have been shown to increase blood glucose levels, which can lead to the development of DKA.

The Case Scenario: Medical Management and Care Issues

Within fifteen minutes of arriving in the accident and emergency department, Lucy has undergone a series of investigations and has given a detailed medical and social history. The results of the specific investigations are as follows:

Capillary blood glucose level: 22.6 mmol/L
Venous blood glucose level: 29.8 mmol/L
Blood 3-beta-hydroxybutyrate: 3.0 mmol/L
Sodium: 129 mmol/L
Potassium: 3.5 mmol/L
Bicarbonate: 11.0 mmol/L
pH: 7.28
Electrocardiograph: sinus tachycardia, 132 beats/min
Chest X-ray: no abnormalities detected
Urinalysis: ++++ glucose and ketones

A definitive diagnosis of diabetic ketoacidosis is reached and treatment is commenced immediately.

Consider the following:

1. With reference to the rationale consider what the immediate medical treatment would be.
2. What are Lucy's main care issues?

Management Strategies and the Role of the Nurse

Diabetic ketoacidosis is a medical emergency with a significant morbidity and mortality. It should be diagnosed quickly and managed intensively by the diabetes specialist team. Diagnosing diabetic ketoacidosis is not generally difficult but the combination of hyperglycaemia, acidosis and ketones must be found. A thorough and careful assessment is required however, to rule out the possibility of other conditions that can cause acidosis, such as salicylate overdose, sepsis or lactic acidosis.

The criteria to diagnose DKA are:

- raised blood glucose level > 11.1 mmol/L;
- blood ketones 3.0 mmol/L and over;
- significant acidosis measured as a serum venous bicarbonate level of < 15 mmol/L and/or arterial pH < 7.3.

The aim of treatment for DKA is threefold and may require slight modifications to suit the individual patient, so frequent reassessment is essential:

1. To correct the fluid and electrolyte disturbances.
2. To raise intracellular and lower extracellular levels of glucose.
3. To increase the blood pH.

Correct Fluid and Electrolyte Disturbances

Lucy will require good intravenous access via a large bore cannula into a peripheral vein. If this is not possible, or too difficult, then a central line will be inserted. Patients with DKA can typically have a 100 mL/kg of body weight water deficit and will require substantial amounts of intravenous fluids to reach an acceptable level of rehydration. Fluid replacement will be rapid initially and then be slowed down as Lucy's condition improves.

The JBDS Inpatient Care Group (2010) suggests giving a usually fit, healthy patient like Lucy:

- 1 L 0.9 per cent sodium chloride solution over the first hour;
- 1 L 0.9 per cent sodium chloride solution with potassium chloride over the next two hours and repeat;
- 1 L 0.9 per cent sodium chloride solution with potassium chloride over the next four hours and repeat;
- 1 L 0.9 per cent sodium chloride solution with potassium chloride over the next six hours.

Re-assessment of cardiovascular status is mandatory at 12 hours and further fluid may be required.

Potassium chloride (KCl) will be added to the intravenous fluids to correct hypokalaemia. The serum potassium level should be checked at 60 minutes and two hours and two-hourly thereafter. If the potassium level is outside the normal reference range, the appropriateness of potassium replacement should be re-assessed hourly. If the abnormal potassium level does not resolve quickly then senior medical advice should be sought (JBDS Inpatient Care Group, 2010). Once the ketoacidosis has resolved and the blood glucose and potassium levels are returned to within normal limits, the addition of KCl to the intravenous fluids can be discontinued.

Lucy also has a low sodium level, which is characteristic in DKA. Decreased levels of sodium in the gastrointestinal system may also exacerbate feelings of nausea and vomiting. The low sodium levels are compensated for with the infusion of 0.9 per cent sodium chloride, which is the recommended fluid of choice, and it is not usually necessary to give extra sodium as the blood sodium levels will correct themselves as the blood glucose levels return to normal.

An accurate fluid balance should be recorded to ensure that Lucy does not develop circulatory overload. The date and time of all intravenous and oral fluid intake and the amount of urine and other fluid losses such as vomit should be carefully recorded. If Lucy fails to pass a minimum urine output of 0.5 mL/kg/hr she will require a urinary catheter to be inserted using a strict aseptic technique (Savage and Kilvert, 2006). This will allow her kidney function to be monitored more closely and hourly urine measurements to be taken and recorded.

Raise Intracellular and Lower Extracellular Levels of Glucose

It is crucial that insulin therapy is instigated at the same time as the fluid replacement to prevent gluconeogenesis by the liver, which if allowed to develop and continue will serve to worsen the DKA and put Lucy's life in jeopardy. This should be done via a fixed-rate intravenous insulin infusion using Actrapid® at a dose of at least 0.1 unit/kg/hour (Kitabchi et al., 2009). This is preferred over a sliding scale regimen as it is able to accommodate obese or other insulin-resistant states such as pregnancy more effectively. However, the fixed rate may need to be adjusted in insulin-resistant people if the ketone concentration does not fall quickly enough (JBDS Inpatient Care Group, 2010). A stat dose of intramuscular insulin (0.1 unit/kg) should be given *only* if there is a delay in setting up the fixed rate insulin infusion. As Lucy normally takes Lantus® this should continue at the usual dose and usual time. The same principle applies if the patient is taking Levemir®.

Lucy's capillary blood glucose and blood ketone levels will need to be recorded hourly until the ketoacidosis has subsided and carefully entered on the appropriate chart. It is anticipated that the blood glucose should fall by 3 mmol/L/hour. If the blood glucose levels do not begin to fall with the administration of insulin the nurse should check that the syringe driver is turned on and working and the intravenous connections are connected and patent. Any problems found should be rectified and the insulin infusion recommenced at the set dose. While administering intravenous insulin it is important not to allow Lucy to become hypoglycaemic. Once the glucose level falls below 14 mmol/L a 10 per cent glucose infusion should be commenced at 125 mL/hour alongside the 0.9 per cent sodium chloride infusion. The fixed rate insulin infusion should be continued until Lucy has less than 0.3mmol/L of serum ketones and a venous pH over 7.3. It is important not to rely on the absence of urinary ketones in determining when to discontinue the insulin infusion, as urinary ketones will still be present for some time after the DKA has resolved.

To Increase the Blood pH

The administration of intravenous insulin is usually sufficient to increase the blood pH level and the level of ketones is a good indicator of the adequacy of the insulin regimen. The administration of bicarbonate has been associated with the development of potentially fatal cerebral oedema and hypokalaemia (Williams and Pickup, 2004) and should therefore be avoided as a treatment modality in DKA.

If Lucy's condition requires bed-rest with limited mobility for three or more days she will be prescribed twice daily, weight-adjusted subcutaneous injections of low molecular weight heparin as prophylaxis against the development of venous thromboembolism, as per NICE (2010) guidance. Once Lucy is rehydrated and her blood glucose levels have returned to within normal limits she should resume a normal diet and fluid intake and the insulin infusion can be discontinued. Once the intravenous insulin has been disconnected, within 10 to 15 minutes Lucy will no longer have any circulating active short-acting insulin. The Lantus® insulin injections should have been continued while she was receiving intravenous short-acting insulin, which means that when the insulin infusion is discontinued Lucy will not be completely insulin depleted and will have the required basal insulin still circulating in an effective form. She will therefore need to recommence her rapid-acting Novorapid® insulin, which should be given immediately prior to each of her meals or within 15 minutes of eating to avoid a recurrence of hyperglycaemia and potential ketoacidosis.

Following recovery from the acute event, care must focus upon returning Lucy to a well informed, healthy and happy lifestyle. The NSF (DH, 2003) identifies nine key areas in which diabetes care should be targeted, and sets out 12 standards for the prevention and management of diabetes. The Department of Health recognises that diabetes is a condition in which, with the right education, support and motivation, the individual can have almost total control. This requires healthcare professionals to ensure that all people with diabetes are encouraged and assisted to take an active role in their diabetes management. They also need to facilitate the patient's learning to enable them to develop the appropriate knowledge, skills and confidence to be able to make sometimes complex decisions regarding their blood glucose control. It is crucial that Lucy's lifestyle choices are incorporated into her blood glucose control regime. Although she altered her insulin dosage to suit her dietary intake she must also learn to be more vigilant with blood glucose monitoring and be prepared to alter her insulin regime to accommodate activities such as increased exercise or extreme changes to her normal pattern of daily activity.

Summary

This chapter has considered diabetic ketoacidosis, which is a potentially life threatening complication of diabetes. Following a brief outline of the anatomy and physiology of diabetes and the ways in which insulin and glucagon are secreted and broken down, the differences of type 1 and type 2 diabetes were highlighted. This information was then used to underpin the immediate assessment priorities and medical management of Lucy, a young person with diabetes, who presents at an accident and emergency unit with diabetic ketoacidosis. Within this, the physiology of hyperglycaemia and ensuing ketoacidosis is given, as well as the causes of high blood glucose levels. Information is given regarding the immediate assessment of Lucy and how the medical management and nursing care should be prioritised. Finally, the severity of ketoacidosis should not be underestimated. The high level of monitoring required during the acute event may necessitate transfer to an intensive care unit or high dependency unit for care by a specialist diabetes team until the condition becomes more stable.

Further Reading

Diabetes UK. *Guidelines for the Management of Diabetic Ketoacidosis in Children and Adolescents* (2001), www.diabetes.org.uk (accessed 22 July 2008).

Gillespie, G. L. and M. Campbell. 'Diabetic Ketoacidosis: Rapid Identification, Treatment, and Education Can Improve Survival Rates', *American Journal of Nursing*, **102** (2002), 13–16.

Hand, H. 'The Development of Diabetic Ketoacidosis', *Nursing Standard*, **15**(8) (2000), 47–55.

Holt, P. *Diabetes in Hospital: A Practical Approach for Healthcare Professionals* (Oxford: Wiley Blackwell, 2009).

Levy, D. *Practical Diabetes*, 2nd edn (Hertfordshire: Altman, 2006).

Rodacki, M., J. R. D. Pereira, A. M. N. De Oliveira et al. 'Ethnicity and Young Age Influence the Frequency of Diabetic Ketoacidosis at the Onset of Type 1 Diabetes', *Diabetes Research and Clinical Practice*, **78**(2) (2007), 259–62.

References

Akerblom, H. K., O. Vaarala, H. Hyoty, J. Ilanen and M. Knip. 'Environmental Factors in the Etiology of Type 1 Diabetes', *American Journal of Medical Genetics*, **115**(1) (2002), 18–29.

Bazzano, L. A., Li T. Y., K. J. Joshipura and F. B. Hu. 'Intake of Fruit, Vegetables and Fruit Juices and Riks of Diabetes in Women', *Diabetes Care*, **31** (2008), 1311–17.

Bonifacio, E., M. Hummel, M. Walter, S. Schmid and A. G. Ziegler. 'IDDM and Multiple Family History of Type 1 Diabetes Combine to Identify Neonates at High Risk for Type 1 Diabetes', *Diabetes Care*, **27** (2004), 2695–700.

Broom, I. 'Thinking about Abdominal Obesity and Cardiovascular Risk', *British Journal of Diabetes and Vascular Disease*, **6**(2) (2006), 58–61.

Cowburn, C. 'Preventing Type 2 Diabetes by Preventing Obesity: What Do Population-based Approaches Offer?', *Obesity in Practice*, **6**(1) (2004), 13–15.

Department of Health. *National Service Framework for Diabetes: Delivery Strategy* (London: Department of Health, 2003).

Diabetes Control and Complications Trial Research Group. 'The Effect of Intensive Treatment of Diabetes on the Development and Progression of Long-term Complications in Insulin-dependent Diabetes Mellitus', *New England Journal of Medicine*, **326** (1993), 683–9.

Diabetes UK. Reports and statistics (2006), http://www.diabetes.org.uk/Profesionals/ Information_resources/Reports/Diabetes_prevalence_2006/ (accessed 11 January 2009).

Faideau, B., E. Larger, F. Lepault, J. C. Carel and C. Boitard. 'Role of β-cells in Type 1 Diabetes Pathogenesis', *Diabetes*, **54** (2005), S87–S96.

Haffner, S. M., S. Lehto, T. Ronnemaa et al. 'Mortality from Coronary Heart Disease in Subjects with Type 2 Diabetes and in Nondiabetic Subjects with and without Prior Myocardial Infarction', *New England Journal of Medicine*, **339** (1998), 229–34.

Hales C. N. and D. J. P. Barker. 'The Thrifty Phenotype Hypothesis', *British Medical Bulletin*, **60**(1) (2001), 5–20.

Happich, M., R. Landfraf, W. Piehlmeier, P. Falkenstein and S. Stamentis. 'The Economic Burden of Nephropathy in Diabetic Patients in Germany 2002', *Diabetes Research in Clinical Practice*, doi:10.1016/j.diabres.2007.11.012 (2008).

Haslam, D. W. and W. P. T. James. 'Obesity', *The Lancet*, **366**(9492) (2005), 1197–209.

Hettiarachchi, K. D., P. Z. Zimmet and M. A. Myers. 'Transplacental Exposure to Bafilomycin Disrupts Pancreatic Islet Oranogenesis and Accelerates Diabetes Onset in NOD Mice', *Journal of Autoimmunity*, **22**(4) (2004), 287–96.

Ilag, L. L., S. Kronick, R. D. Ernst, L. Grondin, C. Alaniz, L. Liu and W. H. Herman. 'Impact of a Critical Pathway on Inpatient Management of Diabetic Ketoacidosis', *Diabetes Research and Clinical Practice*, **62**(1) (2003), 23–32.

Joint Board of Diabetes Societies Inpatient Care Group. 'The Management of Diabetic Ketoacidosis in Adults', *NHS Diabetes* (2010), www.nhs.uk/diabetes (accessed 23 March 2010).

Kettyle, W. M. and R. A. Arky. *Endocrine Pathophysiology* (Philadelphia: Lippincott Raven, 1998).

Keuhn, B. M. 'Pesticides–Diabetes Link', *Journal of the Americal Medical Association*, **300**(4) (2008), 386.

Kitabchi A. E., G. E. Umpierrez, J. M. Miles and J. N. Fisher. 'Hyperglycaemic Crises in Adult Patients with Diabetes: A Consensus Statement from the American Diabetes Association', *Diabetes Care*, **32** (2009), 1335.

Kitabchi, A. E. and Wall, B. M. 'Management of Diabetic Ketoacidosis', *American Family Physician*, **60** (1999), 455–64.

NICE. *Diagnosis and Management of Type 1 Diabetes in Children, Young People and Adults, Clinical Guideline 15* (London: National Institute for Health and Clinical Excellence, 2004), http://www.nice.org.uk/Guidance/CG15 (accessed 24 March 2009).

NICE. *Type 2 Diabetes. The Management of Type 2 diabetes. Clinical Guideline 66* (London: National Institute for Health and Clinical Excellence, 2008), http://www.nice.org.uk/guidance/index.jsp?action=downloadando=40754 (accessed 24 March 2009).

NICE. *Venous Thromboembolism: Reducing the Risk, Clinical Guidance 92* (London: National Institute for Health and Clinical Excellence, 2010), http://www.nice.org.uk/Guidance/CG92 (accessed 23 March 2010).

Page, S. R. Hall, G. M. *Diabetes Emergency and Hospital Management* (London: BMJ Books, 1999).

Pozzilli, P. and Mario, U. D. 'Autoimmune Diabetes not Requiring Insulin at Diagnosis (Latent Autoimmune Diabetes of the Adult)', *Diabetes Care*, **24** (2001), 1460–7.

Rorsman, P. 'Insulin Secretion: Function and Therapy of Pancreatic Beta-cells in Diabetes', *British Journal of Diabetes and Vascular Disease*, **5** (2005), 187–91.

Rung, J., S. Cauchi, A. Albrechtsen et al. 'Genetic Variant Near IRS1 Is Associated with Type 2 Diabetes, Insulin Resistance and Hyperinsulinaemia', *Nature Genetics*, **41** (2009), 1110–15.

Savage, M. W. and A. Kilvert. 'ABCD Guidelines for the Management of Hyperglycaemic Emergencies in Adults', *Practical Diabetes International*, **23**(5) (2006), 227–31.

Tamas, G., A. G. Tabak, P. Vargha and Z. Kerenyi. 'Effect of Menstrual Cycle on Insulin Demand in IDDM Women', *Diabetologia*, **39**(suppl. 1) (1996), A52 (abstract 188).

UK Prospective Diabetes Study (UKPDS) Group. 'Intensive Blood Glucose Control with Sulphonylureas or Insulin Compared with Conventional Treatment and Risk of Complications in Patients with Type 2 Diabetes (UKPDS 33)', *Lancet*, **352** (1998), 837–53.

Umpierrez, G. E., R. Cuervo, A. Karabell, K. Latif, A. X. Freire and A. E. Kitabchi. 'Treatment of Diabetic Ketoacidosis with Subcutaneous Insulin Aspart', *Diabetes Care*, **27** (2004), 1873–8.

Will J. C., D. A. Galuska, E. S. Ford, A. Mokdad and E. E. Calle. 'Cigarette Smoking and Diabetes Mellitus: Evidence of a Positive Association from a Large Prospective Cohort Study', *International Journal of Epidemiology*, **30**(3) (2001), 540–6.

Williams, G. and J. C. Pickup. *Handbook of Diabetes*, 3rd edn (Oxford: Blackwell, 2004).

10

Care and Management in Drug Misuse

Michelle Clayton and Bob McMaster

Introduction

Drugs misuse, whether deliberate or accidental, for recreational or self-harm purposes, is a growing concern for healthcare. The real and potential harms caused by drug misuse appear to be largely underestimated and misunderstood by many. This chapter seeks to address the challenges faced by healthcare professionals in assessing and managing some of the effects of two widely used drugs, paracetamol and cocaine.

Paracetamol

Paracetamol is a simple yet effective analgesic that until 1998 could be bought in large quantities from many retail outlets in the United Kingdom. It is the most commonly used substance for deliberate self-poisoning (Sheen et al., 2002). Hawton et al. (1995) reported that individuals who had taken an overdose knew that paracetamol was dangerous but there was a lack of knowledge about the specific effects that occurred and the timing of these side effects. Many individuals who have ingested excess paracetamol do not generally feel unwell in the first 24 to 48 hours despite the potential catastrophic harm to their liver that may occur during this period. Acute liver failure is a serious and life threatening event that may result from the toxic effects of excess paracetamol.

The British National Formulary (BNF) (2009) recommends between 0.5 and 1 g every four to six hours up to a maximum of 4 g in a 24-hour period for normal analgesic use in adults. This relatively narrow therapeutic range means that accidental as well as deliberate overdose is not difficult. A range of other over the counter medications also contain paracetamol, which may only be apparent on reading the product information. It is therefore important that individuals are cognisant of this to prevent an accidental overdose occurring. Due to its popularity as a drug of choice for deliberate self-poisoning the Medicines Control Agency (MCA) introduced legislation in 1998 to reduce the availability of paracetamol to 16 tablets (8 g) for non-pharmacy outlets and 32 (16 g) from pharmacies. Following the MCA legislation, the use of paracetamol products in suicide deaths has declined and reached an all time low of 242 deaths in 2007 (Information Centre for Health and Social Care, 2008).

Cocaine

Caring for patients suffering from the effects of recreational drug misuse is a relatively common activity for nurses working in emergency departments, acute medical and surgical wards and high dependency areas. The commonest drugs of misuse in the UK are cannabis, cocaine and heroin (Information Centre for Health and Social Care, 2008). Cannabis has a number of significant side effects with low frequency use, and the psychological consequences of long-term use are now recognised and are a cause for concern (Volkow, 2006). Heroin is well known for causing respiratory depression and its effects are well documented. Cocaine has a wide spectrum of effects across the dose range and on a number of body systems, including potentially life threatening effects that practitioners need to be aware of and be able to report early and manage.

The assessment and management of the acutely poisoned patient can pose a challenge by virtue of the diverse range of symptoms presented and the fact that some may be non-committal or unable to divulge what substances have been taken. Second, drugs affect different organs in different ways, resulting in a considerable number of possible differential diagnoses. Lastly, many ingested drugs have a serious but transient effect on individuals and will be excreted without serious harm; however, a number of drugs can invoke organ failure, leading to serious physical consequences and in some cases death. This chapter examines two case scenarios: one has engaged in deliberate self-harm with paracetamol poisoning and the second is suffering the effects of recreational drug misuse with cocaine.

Aim and Learning Outcomes

The Aim

This chapter aims to illustrate the physiological effects of poisoning and discuss the key issues in the assessment, care and management of two patients presenting with self-poisoning.

Learning Outcomes

At the end of this chapter the reader will be able to:

1. Appreciate the normal physiological effects of paracetamol and cocaine use.
2. With reference to the pathophysiological effect upon different organs, describe the common symptom presentation associated with paracetamol and cocaine misuse.
3. Identify the assessment and monitoring needs of the patient following drug misuse.
4. Consider the available treatment options following paracetamol overdose and cocaine misuse.

The Case Scenario: Paracetamol Overdose

Lucy is 17 years old and has been admitted to the accident and emergency department at 20.00 hours. She reports having taken 42 tablets of 500 mg paracetamol, which she found in the bathroom cupboard at home at 23.00 hours the previous evening following an argument with her boyfriend. She had cried herself to sleep and woke the next morning feeling a little nauseated and miserable but with no other symptoms. She regretted that she had taken the overdose of paracetamol and felt embarrassed by her actions and decided to forget about it. The nausea was sufficient to cause Lucy to phone in sick for work and return to bed for much of the day. At 17.00 hours her boyfriend phoned to apologise and agreed to meet Lucy. During the evening Lucy started to feel unwell, complaining of abdominal pain in her right upper quadrant, and so she confided in her boyfriend about the overdose of paracetamol. He escorted her to the A&E department of their local hospital. Lucy is now 21 hours post ingestion of excess paracetamol. On admission her observations were:

Conscious, alert and orientated: GCS = 15
Pulse: 98 beats/minute
BP: 140/92 mmHg
SpO_2: 98 per cent on air
Temperature: 37 °C

Consider the following:

1. What functions does the liver undertake?
2. What effects does paracetamol have on the body?
3. What assessment and investigations would be required? Consider the rationale for these investigations and relate them to the pathophysiology.

Liver Function

The liver is a complex organ with a multitude of important functions that exist to help maintain normal homeostasis (Table 10.1).

Many factors affect liver function, including congestion due to conges-tive cardiac failure, ascites, cirrhosis due to infections such as hepatitis or alcoholism, primary or secondary cancer and some drug toxicity, to name a

Table 10.1   Functions of the liver

The liver has more than 500 functions. Here are a few of the common ones.

1. Carbohydrate metabolism
    *   conversion of glucose to glycogen (glycogenesis)
    *   conversion of glycogen to glucose (glycogenolysis)
    *   conversion of amino acids to glucose (gluconeogenesis)
2. Fat meatbolism
    *   break down of fatty acid from acetyl coenzyme A (beta oxidation)
    *   break down of acetyl coenzyme A to ketones (ketogenesis)
    *   cholesterol and phospholipid synthesis
    *   synthesises lipoproteins to transport fatty acids, fats and cholesterol to and from cells
    *   cholesterol breakdown to bile salts
    *   fat storage
3. Protein metabolism
    *   deaminates amino acids for use as energy or conversion to carbohydrate or fats
    *   converts ammonia to less toxic urea for excretion
    *   synthesis of plasma proteins eg globulin, albumin, clotting factors – prothrombin and fibrinogen, anticlotting agents: heparin
4. Removal and detoxification of drugs and hormones from blood stream
    *   detoxification and excretion of drugs in bile salts, e.g. penicillin, steroid hormones: oestrogen, aldosterone, thyroxine
5. Excretion of bilirubin from red blood cell break down as bile
6. Synthesis of bile salts to aid emulsification and absorption of fats, cholesterol, phopholipid and lipoproteins
7. Storage for glucogen, vitamins A, B12, D, E, K, and minerals: iron, copper
8. Phagocytosis: Kupfer cells of liver phagocytose old red and white blood cells and some bacteria from the gut
9. Activation of vitamin D
10. Manufacture, break down and regulation of numerous hormones including sex hormones
11. Manufacture of enzymes and proteins which are responsible for most chemical reactions in the body, e.g. blood clotting and repair of damaged tissues

---

few. Disruption to normal liver function will affect several homeostatic mechanisms and a number of different organs, which will manifest in a wide variety of clinical features. Many patients with acute liver failure display signs of multiple organ dysfunction or failure.

Paracetamol Metabolism

A normal dose of paracetamol tablets taken for a headache would be metabolised via two pathways within the liver. One pathway involves the conjugation of approximately 90 to 95 per cent of the drug into inactive soluble metabolites, which are then excreted via the kidney. Conjugation is the combining of one substance with another substance to produce a different molecule. The remaining paracetamol is oxidised and converted into an unstable and toxic metabolite called N-acetyl-p-benzoquinonimine (NAPQI). This oxidation takes place in the cytochrome P-450 within the hepatocytes (liver cells). NAPQI is then normally rapidly combined with reduced glutathione S-transferases to render it harmless for excretion by the kidneys. Excess ingestion of paracetamol (commonly termed an overdose) quickly saturates the first pathway involving conjugation to non-toxic metabolites. Therefore more residual paracetamol relies upon the second pathway producing large quantities of NAPQI, which quickly depletes the available glutathione. Excess toxic NAPQI is therefore left to bind to liver cell membranes, causing necrosis. Intracellular glutathione is also an important mediator against oxygen free radicals, which are produced as a result of oxidative stress and are also toxic to normal cells; therefore, glutathione depletion leads to increased levels of oxygen free radicals (Aitio, 2006). At a cellular level the toxic metabolite NAPQI and oxygen free radicals bombard liver cells, causing substantial cell injury and death. Liver cell necrosis can occur with as little as 10 g (20 tablets) and death with 15 g, which is less than that taken by Lucy.

Within the first 12 to 24 hours post paracetamol overdose there may be no apparent clinical manifestations of liver damage or there may be signs of nausea, vomiting, diarrhoea or abdominal cramps. At this point, although individuals may regret their actions, the lack of severe symptoms may lull them into a false sense of security and deter them from seeking help. Some individuals will recover without intervention; however, by 48 hours some will develop liver cell injury and necrosis and between 72 and 96 hours acute liver failure and abnormal liver function will become apparent.

Assessment and Reaching a Diagnosis

On admission to the emergency department Lucy would be assessed using the ABCDE approach (see Chapter 2).

Airway and Breathing

It is quickly established that Lucy is self-ventilating on air with a SpO_2 of 98 per cent. Lucy's respiratory rate, depth and skin colour should be recorded every four hours unless there is an evident deterioration in her condition. Pulse oximetry provides continuous monitoring of her respiratory status.

Circulation

Lucy's pulse at 98 beats/minute and blood pressure (BP) (140/92 mmHg) were slightly elevated, though this may reflect some anxiety regarding her situation. Cardiac and BP monitoring will provide a continuous trace of rate, regularity, rhythm and changes in cardiac output as Lucy may be at risk from cardiac arrhythmias.

Disability

Lucy is currently alert and orientated. However, her level of consciousness should be assessed using APVU (see Chapter 2) or GCS (see Chapter 4) every 30 minutes if any changes are noted. Drowsiness, irritability or confusion from hepatic encephalopathy may signal liver failure.

Exposure

Additional four-hourly observations include temperature for pyrexia, capillary blood glucose for hypoglycaemia and signs of bleeding, as all could suggest deteriorating liver function. Assessment of renal function may reveal a decreasing urine output and a raised serum creatinine, and pain is not uncommon, either in the abdomen, particularly in the right upper quadrant, or in the back due to inflammation of the liver.

A careful history is taken from Lucy of the type, quantity and time since ingestion of the drugs. It is important to establish whether alcohol was also taken as it may potentiate the effects and contribute to altered behaviour. Vomiting since ingestion is noted, as this may reduce the amount of poison entering the bloodstream. Lucy will be asked for any history of previous deliberate self-harm episodes, and her intentions in taking the poison. A previous history of deliberate self-harm and suicidal ideation now would indicate a high risk for further attempts at suicide and referral for early mental health assessment and close observation would be required (Dolan and Holt, 2000). Lucy recounts her history as an impulsive deliberate self-harm act with no suicidal intent, and therefore the focus moves to investigating and treating her overdose.

Specific Investigations

A detailed clinical history and review of Lucy's past medical history, drug use (prescribed and recreational) and social and family history, and routine venous blood sampling for a range of further investigations, would be collected (Table 10.2). These would be repeated potentially on a number of occasions to allow for trends to be monitored.

Assessment of the liver enzymes alanine aminotransferase (ALT) or aspartate aminotransferase (AST) can be a useful indictor of the severity of liver cell damage but must be viewed with caution (Table 10.3). ALT is more liver specific than AST, which is expressed by a number of other tissues when damaged (Imperial and Keeffe, 2006). ALT levels can rise into the thousands following a paracetamol overdose. As ALT leaks out of damaged liver cells, serum levels rise and therefore offer some indication of the degree of liver cell damage. Once all liver cells are damaged ALT levels will start to fall. Therefore it is imperative that the ALT level is correlated with an indicator of synthetic function. Prothrombin time (PT) and international normalised ratio (INR) are measures of clotting time that rely upon the availability of clotting factors. An increase in PT and INR may suggest insufficient production of clotting factors and could therefore reflect acute cellular damage. It is not unusual for a PT to be in excess of 100 to 150 seconds and the INR to be between 8 and 12. This coagulopathy is an excellent indicator of the severity of liver cellular damage, and a continued increase in clotting time despite a falling ALT may be a poor prognostic sign. Other important blood tests include urea and electrolytes (U&Es) as a measure of renal function because excess paracetamol is toxic to kidney cells. Increased serum creatinine may indicate acute tubular necrosis. Blood glucose levels may reveal hypoglycaemia due to the liver's inability to convert stored glycogen to available glucose due to liver cell damage. Acid–base balance should be assessed by arterial blood gases (ABGs) and may reveal a metabolic acidosis due to hyperlactataemia. Damaged liver cells lose the ability to metabolise

Table 10.2   Routine venous blood sampling

- Full blood count (FBC): low Hb (anaemia), raised WBC (infection)
- Clotting screen: prothrombin time (PT) and international normalised ratio (INR) can provide a good guide to severity of disease
- Urea and electrolytes (U&E): electrolyte and renal function
- Serum paracetamol levels
- Liver function tests: particularly for ALT, AST, ALP, albumin, bilirubin, lactate
- Capillary blood glucose: for signs of hyperglycaemia (raised blood glucose) or hypoglycaemia (low)

Table 10.3 Liver function tests (LFTs): normal values

Test	Normal value
Alanine aminotransferase (ALT) – enzyme (also known as SGPT)	5–40 IU/L
Aspartate aminotransferase (AST) – enzyme (also known as SGOT)	5–60 IU/L
Alkaline phosphatase (ALP) – enzyme	30–130 IU/L
Gamma-glutamyl transferase (GGT or gamma GT) – enzyme	5–80 IU/L
Albumin – protein	3.9–5.0 g/dL
Globulin	20–30 g/L
Bilirubin – breakdown product of red cells	3–17 μmol/L
Lactate	0.5–2.2 mmol/L
Prothrombin time (PT)	12–16 seconds
International normalised ratio (INR)	1

Note: Normal values differ between men and women and local laboratory test procedures.

lactate, leading to raised levels, which can influence acid–base balance and precipitate acidosis (Table 10.3).

Immediate Management

Lucy should be admitted to an observation ward for continued monitoring of vital signs, evaluation of venous blood samples and administration of the antidote to paracetamol. Lucy's condition could be potentially life threatening and so she should be encouraged to inform her parents. They and her boyfriend will need clear, honest communication and a high level of emotional support during the next few hours.

Administration of the antidote N-acetylcysteine (Parvolex®) is currently dependent upon serum paracetamol levels, which are evaluated against the Rumack–Matthews nomogram. This is a graph that correlates the serum level of paracetamol against time since ingestion and states that levels above the curve require treatment with N-acetylcysteine (see the Emergency Treatment of Poisoning section of the British National Formulary, 2009). O'Grady (2005) suggests that Parvolex® should be administered intravenously as soon as possible while serum paracetamol levels are pending to prevent further damage to liver cells occurring. The dose of Parvolex® should be calculated on the basis of Lucy's weight and administered to a set regimen (Table 10.4). N-acetylcysteine assists in the production of cysteine, which acts as a glutathione donor to detoxify NAPQI. It also provides substances that bind directly to the reactive oxygen free radicals released (Jones, 2000). Side effects of N-acetylcysteine that should be watched for include rash, flushing and bronchospasm, which are more frequent in asthmatics (Schmidt and Dalhoff, 2001).

Table 10.4 Parvolex® administration regime – adult loading regime

150 mg/kg (Max 16.5 g) in 200 ml 5% dextrose over 15 minutes
50 mg/kg (max 5.5 g) in 500 ml 5% dextrose over 4 hours
100 mg/kg in 1000 ml (max 11 g) 5% dextrose over 16 hours
BNF in the Emergency Treatment of Poisoning section (BNF 2009)

Serum paracetamol levels are only effective in determining the overall risk of organ failure when measured four hours or longer after the initial overdose. Interpretation of serum paracetamol levels requires some caution in chronic alcoholics and in individuals taking enzyme inducing medication such as phenytoin, carbamazepine, rifampicin and isoniazid, as chronic alcohol consumption and some drugs induce the cytochrome P-450 pathway. Careful monitoring is especially required in individuals who are malnourished, as their intracellular levels of gluthatione may be diminished,

The Case Scenario: Medical Management and Care Issues

Lucy is admitted to the medical assessment unit where her condition continues to deteriorate. Despite commencing an intravenous infusion of Parvolex® Lucy is becoming more drowsy and difficult to rouse, her pupils are slightly dilated at 4 mm in diameter and their reaction to light remains brisk. Lucy's capillary blood glucose levels are recorded hourly, as they were 3.2 to 3.6 mmol/L despite an intravenous infusion of 10 per cent dextrose and she has not passed urine since admission.

Specific venous blood results revealed the following:

ALT levels: 2,592 IU/L (normal 5 to 35 IU/L)
PT: 59 seconds (normal 12 to 16 seconds)
INR: > 3.0
Blood glucose: 3.2 mmol/L (normal 4 to 7 mmol/L)
Creatinine: 340 µmol/L (normal 60 to 110 µmol/L)
Paracetamol levels: 0.3 mmol/L (or 45 mg/L) 24 hours post overdose
Arterial pH: 7.28

The nearest supraregional liver unit was contacted for advice and Lucy's parents and family were informed of her deteriorating condition and referral for specialist treatment.

Immediate Medical Management
1. What are the current treatment options for Lucy?
2. What factors might inform the choice of immediate management?
3. What are Lucy's main care issues?

those who have ingested other substances and patients with mental illness, who may not recount accurate information on the timing and amount of the overdose. They will also require treatment according to the high risk treatment line on the Rumack–Matthews nomogram.

Medical Management Strategies

Late presentation following paracetamol overdose as in Lucy's case is not uncommon but can often present additional healthcare challenges. Intravenous administration of N-acetylcysteine is recommended despite late presentation, as studies have shown that mortality was lower in groups that received N-acetylcysteine (Harrison et al., 1990). The improvement in survival is thought to relate to increases in cardiac output, oxygen extraction ratio and oxygen consumption (Harrison et al., 1991). Treatment will resolve the insult to the liver in the majority of cases; however, between 2 and 5 per cent will develop acute liver failure (O'Grady, 2006). Signs and symptoms of acute liver failure tend to develop over time post overdose (Table 10.5).

Table 10.5   Time frame and symptom presentation post paracetamol overdose

Stage	Time frame	Symptoms
1	12 to 24 hours	• Gastrointestinal cramping, nausea, vomiting or no clinical manifestations
2	24 to 48 hours	• Symptoms reduce but hepatoxocity and renal tubular necrosis developing.
		• Increased blood level of ALT/AST
		• Decreased production of clotting factors – increased bleeding risk Decreased ability to mobilise glucose – hypoglycaemia
		• Decreased urine output – oliguria
3	Days 3 to 5	• Peak hepatotoxic crisis.
		• Jaundice
		• Oliguria or anuria
		• Bruising and bleeding
		• Profound hypoglycaemia
		• Metabolic acidosis
4	Untreated or unsuccessful treatment	• Liver failure
		• Acute kidney injury (see Chapter 7)
		• Cerebral encephalopathy and oedema
		• Coma and death

Acute Liver Failure

Acute liver failure presents with a number of physiological manifestations that will require intensive care support. Hepatic encephalopathy is an altered neuropsychiatric state caused by failure of the liver to process toxins that have a deleterious effect upon cerebral function and may lead to cerebral oedema. Scales such as the West Haven Scale (Table 10.6) or the Glasgow Coma Score (See Chapter 4) or a narrative description of Lucy's temperament and manner may be used to assess the degree of hepatic encephalopathy. She is drowsy but must be observed for signs of deterioration such as irritability, confusion or coma.

The size of reaction to light of both pupils should be recorded hourly as increasing dilation and sluggish reaction may indicate an increasing intracranial pressure. The mechanism for cerebral oedema leading to raised intracranial pressure is poorly understood but it is thought to be due to raised levels of glutamine leading to an uptake of water in the astrocytes within the brain (Sargent and Fullwood, 2006). Suspected raised intracranial pressure may require invasive pressure monitoring and treatment with an intravenous infusion of mannitol (an intravascular osmotic agent that can draw fluid from brain), elective ventilation and expedient transfer to a supraregional liver centre. Failure to manage cerebral oedema

Table 10.6   West Haven criteria for semi-quantative grading of mental state

Grade	Symptoms
1	• Trivial lack of awareness • Euphoria or anxiety • Shortened attention span • Impaired performance of addition
2	• Lethargy or apathy • Minimal disorientation for time or place • Subtle personality change • Inappropriate behaviour • Impaired performance of subtraction
3	• Somnolence to semi-stupor, but responsive to verbal stimuli • Confusion • Gross disorientation
4	• Coma (unresponsive to verbal or noxious stimuli

Source: Adapted from Ferenci et al. (2002).

and lower the intracranial pressure will lead to brain stem herniation and death.

Hypoglycaemia is a common manifestation in acute liver failure due to the liver's inability to convert stored glycogen to available glucose. Blood glucose monitoring should be undertaken at least one- to two-hourly as profound hypoglycaemia may occur. Hypoglycaemia requires support with a range of intravenous dextrose products between 10 to 50 per cent to achieve normoglycaemia in the individual. Blood glucose monitoring should continue to occur until reliance on dextrose therapy is negated by restoration of native liver function.

Some degree of coagulopathy will occur and should not be prophylactically supported or corrected with blood products because PT and INR provide an excellent indictor of the liver's ability to make certain products, including clotting factors. Circulating levels of fibrinogen, prothrombin and factors V, VII, IX and X are reduced in acute liver failure (O'Grady, 2006). Administration of blood products such as fresh frozen plasma will mask the clotting results and hinder assessment of further liver deterioration. Management of risk is an important factor to ensure that Lucy remains safe and does not injure herself. Absorbent or alginate dressings should be applied to bleeding sites such as cannulae or wounds.

Hepatic lactic acid uptake and metabolism are directly affected by paracetamol overdose and will lead to a transient metabolic acidosis within 15 hours of overdose. Metabolic acidosis occurring after 15 hours is a poor prognostic indicator as it suggests a decrease in hepatic lactic acid clearance due to deteriorating liver function and an increase in peripheral lactic acid from profound tissue hypoxia (Makin and Williams, 1997). Metabolic acidosis of pH < 7.25 after fluid resuscitation and 24 hours after the overdose can be an indicator for admission onto the NHSBT supra urgent liver transplant waiting scheme (UK Transplant, 1999).

Acute liver failure creates a hyperdynamic circulation of high cardiac output, low mean arterial pressure (MAP) and low systemic vascular resistance (SVR) due to generalised vasodilation in the body from the release of cytokines and other vasoactive substances (Ellis and Wendon, 1996). Effective circulating volume is reduced and may need aggressive fluid resuscitation and vasopressors such as noradrenaline to support and improve the MAP and SVR. Hypovolaemia is also a potential side effect of IV mannitol administration; therefore accurate monitoring of Lucy's heart rate, BP, CVP, urine output and fluid intake every 30 minutes is imperative. Invasive cardiac output monitoring including arterial BP measurement may be necessary.

Lucy's renal function has also shown signs of deterioration, which is either due to the toxic effect of the excess paracetamol causing acute

Table 10.7   UK and Irish supraregional specialist liver centres

England
Addenbrookes Hospital, Cambridge
Freeman Hospital, Newcastle upon Tyne
King's College Hospital, London
Queen Elizabeth Hospital, Birmingham
Royal Free Hospital, London
St James's University Hospital, Leeds

Scotland
The Royal Infirmary of Edinburgh

Republic of Ireland
St Vincent's Hospital, Dublin

tubular necrosis or due to hypotension and volume depletion. Oliguria or anuria may follow, along with rises in serum creatinine and urea that may be severe enough to require haemodiafiltration.

The development of these symptoms should prompt immediate referral to a specialist supraregional liver centre that offers a liver transplantation service (Table 10.7). Early transfer of Lucy is important, as her condition can deteriorate rapidly (Polsen and Lee, 2005).

Acute liver failure has three possible treatment outcomes:

- restoration of native liver function with intensive therapy, including ventilation, monitoring of cerebral oedema, dialysis and care of the patient with multi-organ failure;
- liver transplantation due to the inability of the native liver to regenerate functional capacity;
- death.

Due to the immense physiological changes and rapid deterioration that occurs, Lucy and her family may not be aware of the seriousness of the situation. Clear information and explanation of the cause and speed of deterioration and the intensive therapy for multi-organ failure required is necessary. The possibility of liver transplantation, its potential risks and the lifestyle adaptation, including daily immunosuppressant medication, dietary restrictions in relation to unpasteurised products and shellfish, should be discussed. Liver transplantation is an effective treatment modality for patients with acute liver failure but a poor consent rate to donate organs by families continues to impact upon organ availability. Family refusal to donate organs is 39 per cent (Murphy and Hamilton, 2008), thus limiting the availability of organs for transplant, and the Organ Donation Taskforce has set a goal to increase organ donation by 50 per cent within five years (Department of Health, 2008).

Summary

Acute liver failure can have devastating effects on both the individual and their families due to the rapid deterioration that often occurs. The insult to the liver from excess paracetamol has consequences for all body systems and multi-organ failure is a common occurrence. Unfortunately individuals may be lulled into a false sense of security regarding the non-specific symptoms that present in the first instance after taking a paracetamol overdose; however, during this time major liver damage may develop. Lucy may have had a more uneventful recovery had she attended the emergency department earlier than 24 hours post ingestion. Her treatment would have commenced sooner and may have helped to prevent further liver damage and support liver function. Lucy like many others may have felt embarrassed that she had on impulse taken a significant amount of paracetamol in response to an argument with her boyfriend. The liver has a marvellous capacity to regenerate in some cases, but if native liver function cannot be supported and restored then liver transplantation is the only hope for survival. Early treatment and subsequent proactive referral to supraregional centres are key to survival. However, due to the shortage of donor organs, allocation of this scarce resource is required and patients must fulfil set criteria that grade the severity of their symptoms. Liver transplantation for acute liver failure has comparable survival results with other liver transplant categories and is a recognised treatment modality.

Useful Websites

British Liver Trust: http://www.britishlivertrust.org.uk/home.aspx

NHS Organ Donor Register on 0300 123 2323: http://www.uktransplant.org.uk

---

The discussion in this chapter now turns to an increasingly common self-poisoning problem witnessed in the emergency department. The second case focuses upon the assessment and management challenges presented by an individual who has engaged in recreational use of cocaine.

The Case Scenario: Cocaine Misuse

Stephen, a 32-year-old office worker, presents to the emergency department late in the evening complaining of chest pain, palpitations, dizziness and nausea. He is very talkative and sociable. A history reveals that Stephen has been drinking alcohol this evening and that he has 'snorted' (inhaled) two 'wraps' of cocaine about an hour ago. Stephen reports that he has used cocaine in the past and tends to take it at weekends to 'liven up his nights out'. On examination Stephen has a heart rate of 120 beats/minute, respirations of 24/minute, blood pressure of 185/100 mmHg, oxygen saturation of 99 per cent and a temperature of 37.8 °C. Glasgow Coma Score is 15/15 and his pupils are dilated and slow to react to light. There is an observable tremor in his hands and frequent generalised muscle twitching. Stephen is constantly wiping his nose. A provisional diagnosis of cocaine misuse is made.

Consider the following:

1. Compare Stephen's baseline observations to your understanding of normal ranges.
2. Identify any aspects of this brief initial assessment that would alert you to abnormal presenting signs or symptoms that would need to be closely monitored.
3. What are the common signs and symptoms associated with cocaine use?

Drug Misuse in the UK

The UK Perspective

Data from the NHS Information Centre for Health and Social Care (2008) reveals that drug misuse remains a significant problem in the UK, though there has been a slight decline in the overall use of drugs in the past five years. Data for 2006–7 show that 10 per cent of adults in England and Wales reported using one or more illicit drugs, and 3.4 per cent of adults admitted taking a class A drug (Table 10.8). Drug misuse and deaths associated with drug misuse are much more common in men than women, with 13.2 per cent of men reporting taking drugs compared with 6.9 per cent of women. Among young people aged 16 to 24 years, 24.1 per cent reported having tried illicit drugs, the commonest being cannabis and cocaine. A consequence of this has been a substantial rise in the number of patients admitted to hospital for the effects of drug poisoning, up from 7,057 patients in 1996 to 10,047 in 2006 (Information Centre for Health and Social Care, 2008).

Table 10.8 Classification of controlled drugs

It is an offence under the Misuse of Drugs Act 1971 to unlawfully manufacture, supply or possess drugs under the following classifications:

Class A – includes cocaine, alfentanyl, diamorphine (heroin), dipipanone, lysergide (LSD), methadone, methylenedioxymethamfetamine (MDMA, 'ecstasy'), morphine, opium, pethidine, phencyclidine, remifentanil and class B substances when prepared for injection

Class B – includes oral amphetamines, barbiturates, cannabis, cannabis resin, codeine, ethylmorphine, glutethimide, pentazocine, phenmetrazine and pholcodine

Class C – includes benzfetamine and chlorphentermine, buprenorphine, diethylpropion, mazindol, meprobamate, pemoline, pipradrol, most benzodiazepines, zolpidem, androgenic and anabolic steroids, clenbuterol, chorionic gonadotrophin (HCG), non-human chorionic gonadotrophin, somatotropin, somatrem, and somatropin

---

Cocaine Use

Cocaine is a natural extract of the leaves of the coca plant. It was used for many years as an appetite suppressant and a mood enhancing agent, and used medicinally as a local anaesthetic. However, its euphoric effect led to its misuse by the patients being treated and occasionally by health professionals, with the result that it was registered as a class A drug under the Misuse of Drugs Act in 1971. The misuse of cocaine increased steadily over a ten-year period, rising from 0.6 per cent of adults in 1996 to 2.6 per cent in 2006 (MacDonald, 2008), before declining slightly to 2.3 per cent of adults in 2008 (United Nations Office on Drugs and Crime (UNODC), 2009).

The drug can be taken into the body in a number of ways. The leaves can be eaten, dried and smoked, or processed into hydrochloride salt powder and inhaled nasally ('snorting') or dissolved and injected intravenously. Further processing can produce cocaine in its base form (crack cocaine), which readily vaporises when heated and can be inhaled ('freebasing'). Cocaine used at street level is frequently mixed with other products, usually to dilute the drug and increase the financial return, but sometimes also to modify the effect of the drug. Injecting cocaine mixed with heroin (called 'speedballing') reduces the irritability and agitation that users can experience when the effects of the cocaine begin to wear off. Taking alcohol with cocaine produces a new chemical in the body, cocaethylene, which has the same potency as cocaine but a prolonged action of up to six hours (National Highway Traffic Safety Administration (NHTSA), 2008).

The purity of street cocaine varies between 9 and 20 per cent (UNODC, 2009), with an average 'wrap' containing 20 to 120 mg of the drug (NHTSA, 2008). The euphoric effects that the user seeks are usually experienced at about 100 mg, though response is hugely variable between individuals, and repeated use can lead to both resistance to its effects and sensitivity to its side effects. The LD$_{50}$ (the dose that is fatal to 50 per cent of users) is 500 mg (NHTSA, 2008).

The onset and duration of action of cocaine is closely related to the method of intake. Eating cocaine is relatively inefficient, as oral and oesophageal blood vessels constrict on contact with the drug, and cocaine is neutralised by stomach acid. Thus absorption is slow, and peak effect occurs 60 minutes after ingestion, and can last for up to two hours. Nasal inhalation (or 'snorting') of cocaine results in nasal and sinus blood vessel constriction and thus a 57 per cent uptake of the drug, with peak effect at 15 minutes and lasting for 30 to 60 minutes. The fastest uptake of the drug occurs by intravenous injection or inhalation by smoking, after which the peak effect is achieved within three to five minutes and lasts for up to 15 minutes (Gerada and Ashworth, 1997).

Each method of intake is associated with side effects, the most significant of which accompany snorting, injection and inhalation. Cocaine has cardiovascular system effects, often producing chest pain and palpitations in patients, and can result in sudden cardiac death. It produces a feeling of intense euphoria with heightened sociability that rapidly descends into irritability, argumentativeness and depression. Injected cocaine is usually mixed with other products that cause thrombophlebitis and emboli. The prolonged vessel constriction that accompanies repeated snorting can cause ischaemia and necrosis of the nasal septum.

Cocaine is metabolised rapidly by the liver into harmless metabolites that are excreted in the urine. The average half-life of cocaine is 50 to 70 minutes (Couper and Logan, 2000), but the rate of excretion varies by dose and by method of intake, with measurable elimination half-lives of cocaine being shortest after smoking, then following intravenous use, and the longest time to elimination being associated with nasal inhalation. The metabolites of cocaine may remain measurable in the urine for up to three days after drug use (Cone et al., 2003).

It is important that the practitioner can identify behaviours and physiological signs that are the result of drug effect and side effect, and can anticipate the duration and severity of these in order to effectively monitor for and prevent potentially serious deterioration in Stephen's condition.

Patient Assessment and Immediate Management

Cardiovascular Effects

The first priority in Stephen's care is recognising and identifying potential life threatening effects from the cocaine and if present then the standard ABCDE approach should be implemented (Resuscitation Council UK, 2006) (see Chapter 2).

Airway and Breathing

Airway and breathing are not usually directly affected by cocaine, and in Stephen's case he is talking freely, indicating a patent airway. His respiratory rate is slightly elevated at 24 breaths/minute and his oxygen saturation is normal at 99 per cent. Checks of his respiratory function should be repeated at regular intervals of 30 minutes for up to six hours after cocaine use with alcohol, as a declining oxygen saturation and increasing respiratory rate may indicate respiratory impairment from myocardial depression.

Circulation

Stephen's observations of cardiac function showed his blood pressure to be 185/100 mmHg and his heart rate to be 120 beats/minute, both of which are raised above the normal measurements expected for someone of Stephen's age and can be directly attributed to cocaine use. The cardiovascular effects of cocaine are mediated by its ability to prevent re-uptake of noradrenaline (NA), to increase central sympathetic outflow and to interfere with sodium and potassium channels in cardiac conduction. The commonest manifestations are chest pain, tachycardia, conduction defects and an increased blood pressure (Knuepfer, 2003). These effects can be seen after single doses of cocaine, and would be much more likely with any dose greater than this.

The mechanism by which cocaine causes increased sympathetic outflow and release of adrenaline and noradrenaline is not completely understood. When combined with cocaine's ability to bind to noradrenaline transporter proteins the resulting high levels of noradrenaline in the synapse bind to adrenergic receptors in the body and cause prolonged vasoconstriction of central and peripheral blood vessels. This is seen in Stephen as hypertension (Knuepfer, 2003). Higher doses of cocaine can produce a significant hypertension that can result in coronary artery rupture or aortic dissection. Increased circulating catecholamines produce a tachycardia and systemic hypertension, both of which will increase myocardial workload and oxygen demand. At the same time, noradrenaline re-uptake blockade causes coronary vasoconstriction and a subsequent fall in myocardial oxygen supply. The outcome is myocardial ischaemia, and the user experiences flushing, chest pain and palpitations. Later, adrenaline and noradrenaline levels fall as the body experiences catecholamine depletion and blood pressure falls, causing fainting and light-headedness.

Cardiac monitoring should be commenced to observe the rate and rhythm of Stephen's heart. A 12-lead electrocardiograph (ECG) should be obtained as soon as possible to allow a close examination of his cardiac rhythm. Cocaine has an effect on cardiac rhythm by directly interfering with sodium channels and HERG-encoded potassium channels to produce delays in cardiac conduction, including prolongation of PR interval, QRS, QT and QTc (corrected QT at a rate of 60 beats/minute) (Figure 10.1). A prolonged QT interval can predispose life threatening tachyarrhythmias, including ventricular tachycardia (VT) and ventricular fibrillation (VF), and is associated with the drug at all doses; and higher doses cause myocardial depression (Knuepfer, 2003). Cocaine causes vasculitis in any vessel and accelerates atheroma formation. It increases platelet aggregation and thrombus formation and can lead to myocardial infarction (MI) (see Chapter 5). Cocaine use was found to be implicated in one in four myocardial infarctions in 18- to 45-year-old patients (Ghuran et al., 2001), and its cardiovascular effects account for most cocaine-related deaths (Kuczkowski 2006).The mild tachycardia that Stephen demonstrates requires observation only and will usually revert as the effects of the cocaine decline, usually over one to two hours, though the presence of alcohol may potentiate this for up to six hours. However, any chest pain or alteration in cardiac function should be reported to senior nursing and medical staff immediately. If a tachycardia other than VF or VT is present then treatment decisions should be based on the time since ingestion of the drug and the presence of haemodynamic compromise displayed as low blood pressure (systolic below 100 or diastolic below 50 mmHg), very fast heart rate (above 150 beats/minute) or patient discomfort from chest pain. Tachycardia occurring immediately after ingestion is likely to be the result of the action of cocaine on fast sodium channels in the myocardium, and as such may respond to intravenous sodium bicarbonate 1 mEq/kg given by intravenous bolus (Roldan and Hebal, 2008) or slow infusion of 50 mL of 8.4 per cent solution. Later onset tachycardia is usually due to myocardial ischaemia and can be treated with intravenous benzodiazepines such as Lorazepam 2 to 4 mg or intramuscularly given at 15 minute intervals to a maximum of 8 mg (Roldan and Hebal, 2008). The exact mechanism of action is not well understood and may be due to a reduction of the central effects of cocaine.

Careful interpretation of Stephen's ECG should be made to examine for

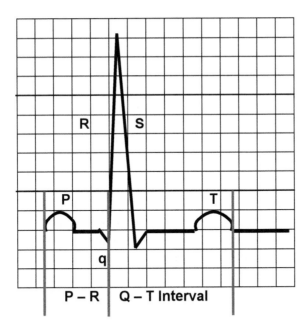

Figure 10.1   The normal PqRST complex.

myocardial ischaemia or infarction. Ischaemia may be seen by abnormal ST segment or T wave inversion (Figure 10.2 and also see Chapter 5). Initial treatment should be to provide supplemental oxygen, which may be enough to reverse the ischaemia. Oxygen should be given via nasal cannulae at a rate to maintain oxygen saturation at 94 to 98 per cent (British Thoracic Society, 2008). If ischaemia persists then intravenous benzodiazepines can be beneficial

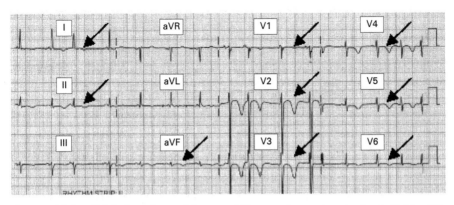

Figure 10.2   ECG showing widespread T wave inversion in leads I, II, aVF and V1 ToV6.

as described previously, or nitrates in the form of sublingual glyceryl trini-trate 2 mg can improve coronary perfusion (Bhangoo et al., 2006).

Signs of myocardial infarction (MI) should be treated with caution and wherever possible should be confirmed by changes to cardiac bio-markers such as troponin T or I (see Chapter 5). Stephen may be one of the many regular cocaine users to have a pre-existing abnormal ECG with ST elevation present due to early repolarisation of cardiac tissue. In these instances the positive predictive value of ECG is only 18 per cent (Hollander et al., 1994). Similarly, 50 per cent of cocaine users have an elevated creatinine phospho-kinase without infarction being present (McCord, 2008). In the absence of a convincing history and symptoms of cardiac chest pain and coronary risk factors care should be taken before considering reperfusion therapy such as thrombolysis or percutaneous coronary intervention (PCI) in a patient who may not require aggressive interventions that carry significant risks. If Stephen does have convincing signs of cocaine-induced MI then early access to percutaneous coronary reperfusion therapy offers the best outcome (McCord et al., 2008). If this is not immediately available then alternative therapies should focus on the administration of oxygen, benzodiazepines, nitrates and phentolamine (Knuepfer, 2003). Phentolamine is an α-receptor antagonist reported to reverse coronary vasoconstriction in cocaine-induced ischaemia and MI (Lange et al., 1989). Fibrinolytic therapy carries an increased risk of intracerebral haemorrhage in cocaine users, and a careful risk–benefit analysis should be performed prior to using this approach (Hollander et al., 1996).

There is little published evidence on how frequently observations should be repeated. However bearing in mind that the peak effects of cocaine occur within 45 to 90 minutes of nasal inhalation and the effects of cocaine with alcohol may last up to six hours (Roldan and Hebal, 2008) then repeated 30-minute observations of Stephen's hypertension should be sufficient to monitor its return to normal as the effects of the cocaine wear off. It will also highlight unrelenting hypertension and any sudden increases, in which case benzodiazepine therapy or nitrates will help to reverse the hypertension and minimise the risk of complications, particularly coronary artery rupture or aortic dissection. Any complaints from Stephen of sudden onset of worsening chest or abdominal pain radiating to the back should be reported immediately.

Stephen will require blood tests of urea and electrolytes to check that his renal function has not been affected by the central vasoconstriction effect of cocaine. An arterial blood gas will allow assessment of the blood pH, check-ing for metabolic acidosis (indicated by a pH below 7.34), which can result from the build-up of lactic acid from decreased tissue perfusion and increased cellular metabolism caused by cocaine (Hassan et al., 1996).

Stephen demonstrated a low grade hyperthermia of 37.8 °C, and an observable tremor and muscle twitching. The increase in catecholamine levels associated with cocaine use causes heat generation from increased muscular activity and tremor. The concurrent peripheral vasoconstriction limits heat loss through the skin, with the combined result of hyperthermia. Left untreated, severe hyperthermia will lead to muscle cell destruction, myoglobinuria and rhabdomyolysis, and may lead to eventual renal damage and failure (Craig et al., 2002) (see Chapter 7). In Stephen's case the low grade hyperthermia can be reduced by cold drinks or the use of intravenous fluids that are at below body temperature. Light coverings only should be used for bedding and any excess motor activity can be controlled with benzodiazepines (Craig et al., 2002).

Central Nervous System Effects

Cocaine has significant actions on neurotransmitters in the brain that result in changes in behaviour that can be observed and monitored. The primary attraction of cocaine for users is the intense euphoria and feeling of well-being that follows intake of the drug. Cocaine achieves this effect by blocking the reuptake of the monoamine neurotransmitters dopamine (DA) and serotonin (SER) in the brain.

In normal neurotransmission the generation of an action potential along a nerve cell causes dopamine release at the terminal button of the pre-synaptic neuron. The dopamine crosses the synapse to bind with receptors on the membrane of the post-synaptic cell and achieves cell excitation. Within the pleasure and reward centres of the brain (the nucleus accumbens, amygdala and hippocampus) the result is a feeling of happiness and well-being. As the action potential degrades then unused dopamine in the synapse is bound to dopamine transporter proteins (DAT) and moved back to the pre-synaptic neuron for storage and re-use, thus clearing the synapse ready for the next action potential and allowing the receptor cell to return to a normal relaxed state (Couper and Logan, 2000).

Cocaine acts by binding rapidly to the DAT and preventing 'mopping up' of unused dopamine and subsequent re-uptake at the pre-synaptic neurons. The dopamine remains in the synapse and continues to stimulate the receptor cells within the pleasure centres of the brain. The user experiences a sudden feeling of good-will, excitability and happiness, or 'rush', that lasts as long as sufficient cocaine is available to occupy the DAT, usually five to fifteen minutes (Couper and Logan, 2000). This effect can be enhanced and potentiated in the presence of alcohol, up to a period of six hours.

Stephen is very sociable and talkative during his assessment. His mood at this time should be documented, and checked and recorded at the same time as the vital signs observations are repeated. Observation should be maintained frequently for changes in Stephen's behaviour, and in particular if he starts to become withdrawn, irritable or aggressive. In response to the cocaine-related increase of dopamine in the synapse, the pre-synaptic terminals produce and store less dopamine. Thus as cocaine is removed from the synapse and excreted from the body, there is less neurotransmission at the receptor cells and the user experiences a 'crash'; that is, a period of low mood, irritability, and aggression. These changes may be masked as Stephen becomes tired and eventually goes to sleep. However, each waking to repeat observation of vital signs may be met by irritability and lack of cooperativeness. Persistence is required in order to maintain monitoring, coupled with understanding and reassurance and explanations to Stephen of how his behaviour and mood changes are related to the falling cocaine levels in his body (Couper and Logan, 2000). These mood changes will lessen as the cocaine is excreted. If Stephen exhibits paranoid thoughts or behaviour or discloses any thoughts of self harm then these should be reported immediately. Though unusual, extreme reactions to cocaine withdrawal can include paranoid psychosis, severe depression and suicide (Ovsiew and Munich, 2008).

Stephen should be encouraged to rest, eat and remain well hydrated during this withdrawal phase (Ovsiew and Munich 2008). The effects of cocaine are usually resolved within two to six hours, though if multiple doses have been taken then the effects can last for up to two days. Sudden withdrawal from the drug is not normally dangerous and may be restorative to body systems.

Stephen will most probably require transfer from the emergency department to an observation area or general medical ward as his need for ongoing monitoring will extend beyond the time frame of the four-hour emergency care standard. Consideration for discharge would be based on:

- a return to normal parameters for heart rate, blood pressure, respiratory rate, temperature and oxygen saturation;
- an absence of significant abnormality on ECG;
- an absence of new episodes of chest pain or headache;
- stable behaviour without reports of paranoia or plans for self harm.

The more prolonged effects of cocaine use that Stephen may experience after discharge are tremor and generalised muscle twitching lasting for a few days, and pronounced craving for the drug, which can last for several weeks (The Drugs Project, 2008). The desire for Stephen may then be to take the drug again to reverse the negative effects. However, the next dose of cocaine must be higher in order to achieve the same 'rush' and as doses increase then the

Table 10.9   Current services available for drug rehabilitation and support

---

- UK National Drugs helpline: 0800 77 66 00
- National Institute on Drug Abuse (available at http://www.nida.nih.gov/)
- We Do Recover: 0808 26 REHAB (73422)
- UK Drug Rehab Centres (available at http://www.uk-rehab.com)

'crashes' become more severe, causing depression and paranoia. At this point there is a risk that Stephen may enter a cycle of craving and withdrawal and may change from snorting cocaine to inhalation or intravenous injection in order to gain the maximum, most rapid response (Couper and Logan, 2000). Therefore the opportunity should be sought to offer Stephen an entry to a detoxification programme by providing information about and facilitating contact with locally available services. Their services may be advertised through mental health and drug service websites and the local social services directory (Table 10.9). Throughout his stay a positive approach should be utilised with Stephen, with an emphasis on providing clear information on the behavioural and physical effects of cocaine and their duration, and reassurance of their reduction as the drug is excreted from the body.

Summary

Stephen presented with signs of cocaine toxicity, which included central nervous system and cardiovascular system stimulation. A thorough assessment and ongoing monitoring of the physiological and behavioural effects helped to identify potentially life threatening complications. Interventions provided to Stephen were supportive in nature and based on apparent and emerging signs and symptoms. It is likely that Stephen would recover without serious physical sequelae. However, the longer-term psychological effects may be serious and Stephen should be offered the opportunity to enter detoxification for his cocaine misuse.

This chapter has discussed two very differing but also very common forms of self poisoning. In both cases, early recognition of the potential for serious harm and prompt assessment, diagnosis and treatment can minimise the likelihood of death from ingestion of these easily available poisons. However, as both case studies have highlighted, self poisoning brings about significant and harmful physiological changes, which can rapidly lead to loss of life. Skilled nursing assessment, intervention and ongoing monitoring can play a major role in caring for and supporting patients who self harm and their families, for whom the unexpected call to attend the emergency department is very distressing.

References

Paracetamol

Aitio, M. L. 'N-Acetylcysteine: Passe-Partout or Much Ado about Nothing?', *British Journal of Clinical Pharmacology*, **61**(1) (2006), 5–15.

Bhangoo, P., A. Parfitt and T. Wu. 'Best Evidence Topic Report. Cocaine Induced Myocardial Ischaemia: Nitrates versus Benzodiazepines', *Emergency Medicine Journal*, **23**(7) (2006), 568–9.

British Liver Trust. *A Brief Summary of the Liver's Function* (2009). Available from http://www.britishlivertrust.org.uk/home/the-liver/summary-of-the-livers-functions.aspx (accessed 9 July 2009).

British National Formulary. *BNF 57* (2009).

Cone, E. J., A. H. Sampson-Cone, W. D. Darwin, M. A. Huestis and J. M. Oyler. 'Urine Testing for Cocaine Abuse: Metabolic and Excretion Patterns Following Different Routes of Administration and Methods for Detection of False-negative Results', *Journal of Analytical Toxicology*, **27**(7) (2003), 386–401.

Department of Health. *Organs for Transplant: A Report from the Organ Donation Taskforce* (London: Department of Health, 2008).

Dolan, B. and L. Holt. *Accident and Emergency: From Theory to Practice* (London: Bailliere Tindall, 2000).

Ellis, A. and J. Wendon. 'Circulatory, Respiratory, Cerebral and Renal Derangements in Acute Liver Failure: Pathophysiology and Management', *Seminars in Liver Diseases*, **16** (1996), 379–88.

Ferenci, P., A. Lockwood, K. Mullen, R. Tarter, K. Weissenborn, A. T. Blei and Members of the Working Party. 'Hepatic Encephalopathy – Definition, Nomenclature, Diagnosis, and Quantification: Final Report of the Working Party at the 11th World Congresses of Gastroenterology, Vienna, 1998', *Hepathology*, **35** (2002), 716–21.

Gerada, C. and M. Ashworth. 'ABC of Mental Health. Addiction and Dependence I: Illicit Drugs', *British Medical Journal*, **315**(7103) (1997), 297–300.

Harrison, P., R. Keays, G. Bray et al. 'Improved Outcome of Paracetamol-induced Fulminant Hepatic Failure by Late Administration of Acetylcysteine', *Lancet*, **30** (1990), 1572–3.

Harrison, P., J. Wendon, A. Gimson et al. 'Improvement by Aceytlcysteine of Hemodynamics and Oxygen Transport in Fulminant Hepatic Failure', *New England Journal of Medicine*, **324** (1991), 1852–7.

Hawton, K., C, Ware, H. Mistry et al. 'Why Patients Choose Paracetamol for Self Poisoning and Their Knowledge of Its Dangers', *British Medical Journal*, **310** (1995), 164.

Imperial, J. and E. Keeffe. 'Laboratory Tests', in B. Bacon, J. O'Grady, A. Di Biscelgie and J. Lake (eds), *Comprehensive Clinical Hepatology*, 2nd edn (St Louis: Mosby, 2006).

Jones, A. Recent advances in the management of late paracetamol poisoning *Emergency Medicine*, **12** (2000), 14–21.

Makin, A. and R. Williams. 'Acetaminophen-induced Acute Liver Failure', in W. Lee and R. Williams (eds), *Acute Liver Failure* Cambridge: Cambridge University Press, 1997).

Murphy, C. and C. Hamilton. 'Potential Donor Audit – Summary Report for the 24 Month Period 1 April 2006–31 March 2008' (2008). Available from http://www.uktransplant.org.uk/ukt/statistics/potential_donor_audit/pdf/pda_ summary_report_2006-2008.pdf (accessed 9 July 2009).

National Statistics. *Drug Poisoning Deaths* (2008) Available from http://www. statistics.gov.uk/cci/nugget_print.asp?ID=806 (accessed 9 July 2009).

O'Grady, J. 'Acute Liver Failure', *Postgraduate Medical Journal*, **81** (2005), 148–54.

O'Grady, J. 'Acute Liver Failure', in B. Bacon, J. O'Grady, A. Di Biscelgie and J. Lake (eds), *Comprehensive Clinical Hepatology*, 2nd edn (St Louis: Mosby, 2006).

Polsen, J. and W. Lee. 'AASLD Position Paper: The Management of Acute Liver Failure', *Hepatology*, 41(5) (2005), 1179–97.

Sargent, S. and D. Fullwood. 'The Management of Hepatic Encephalopathy and Cerebral Oedema in Acute Liver Failure', *British Journal of Neuroscience Nursing*, **2**(9) (2006), 448–53.

Schmidt, L. E. and K. Dalhoff. 'Risk Factors in the Development of Adverse Reactions to N-acetylcysteine in Patients with Paracetamol Poisoning', *British Journal of Clinical Pharmacology*, **51** (2001), 87–91.

Sheen, C. L., J. F. Dillon, D. N. Bateman, K. J. Simpson and T. M. MacDonald. 'Paracetamol Toxicity: Epidemiology, Prevention and Costs to the Health-care System', *QJM: An International Journal of Medicine*, **95**(9) (2002), 609–19.

Sherlock, S. and J. Dooley. *Diseases of the Liver and Biliary System*, 11th edn (Oxford: Blackwell, 2002)

UK Transplant. *UK Transplant Organ Sharing Scheme Operating Principles for Liver Transplant Units in the UK and Republic of Ireland* (1999) Available from http://www.uktransplant.org.uk/ukt/about_transplants/organ_allocation/liver/ liver_organ_sharing_principles/liver_organ_sharing_principles.jsp#b1 (accessed 9 July 2009).

Cocaine Use

British Thoracic Society. 'Guideline for Emergency Oxygen Use in Adult Patients', *Thorax*, 63(suppl. IV) (2008).

Couper, F. and B. Logan. *Drug and Human Performance Fact Sheet D9: Cocaine*. National Highway Traffic Safety Administration (2000). Available at http://www.nhtsa.dot. gov/people/injury/research/job185drugs/cocain.htm (accessed on 13/6/2009).

Craig, G., C. G. Crandall, W. Vongpatanasin and R. G. Victor. 'Mechanisms of Cocaine-induced Hyperthermia in Humans', *Annals of Internal Medicine*, **136**(11) (2002), 785–91.

The Drugs Project. *Cocaine* (2008). Available at http://drugsproject.co.uk/cocaine/ (accessed 21 November 2008).

Ghuran, A., L. R. van der Wieken and J. Nolan. 'Cardiovascular Complications of Recreational Drugs', *British Medical Journal*, **323** (2001), 464–6.

Hassan, T. B., J. A. Pickett, S. Durham and P. Barker. 'Diagnostic Indicators in the Early Recognition of Severe Cocaine Intoxication', *Journal of Accident and Emergency Medicine*, **13** (1996), 261–3.

Hollander, J. E., R. S. Hoffman, P. Gennis, P. Fairweather, M. J. Disano, D. A. Schumb, J. A. Feldman, S. S. Fish, S. Dyer, P. Wax, C. Whelan and E. Schwartzwald.

'Prospective Multicenter Evaluation of Cocaine Associated Chest Pain. Cocaine Associated Chest Pain (COCHPA) Study Group', *Academic Emergency Medicine*, **1** (1994), 330–9.

Hollander, J. E., L. D. Wilson, P. J. Leo and R. D. Shih. 'Complications from the Use of Thrombolytic Agents in Patients with Cocaine Associated Chest Pain', *Journal of Emergency Medicine*, **14** (1996), 731–6.

Information Centre for Health and Social Care. *Statistics on Drug Misuse: England 2008* (London: Health and Social Care Information Centre, 2008).

Knuepfer, M. M. 'Cardiovascular Disorders Associated with Cocaine Use: Myths and Truths', *Pharmacology and Therapeutics*, **97** (2003), 181–222.

Kuczkowski, K. M. 'More on the Idiosyncratic Effects of Cocaine on the Heart', *Emergency Medicine Journal*, **24** (2007), 147.

Lange, R. A., R. G. Cigarroa, C. W. Yancy Jr, J. E. Willard, J. J. Popma, M. N. Sills, W. McBride, A. S. Kim and L. D. Hillis. 'Cocaine-induced Coronary-artery Vasoconstriction', *New England Journal of Medicine*, **321** (1989), 1557–62.

McCord, J., H. Neid, J. E. Hollander, J. A. de Lemos, B. Cercek, P. W. Hsue, B. Gibler, E. M. Ohman, B. Drew, G. Philippides and L. K. Newby. 'Management of Cocaine-associated Chest Pain and Myocardial Infarction: A Scientific Statement From the American Heart Association Acute Cardiac Care Committee of the Council on Clinical Cardiology', *Circulation*, **117** (2008), 1897–907.

MacDonald, H. 'Cocaine Use in England Rises as Cannabis Use Falls', *British Medical Journal*, **337** (2008), 1367.

McEvoy, A. W., N. D. Kitchen and D. G. T. Thomas. 'Intracerebral Haemorrhage in Young Adults: The Emerging Importance of Drug Misuse', *British Medical Journal*, **320** (2000), 1322–4.

National Highway Traffic Safety Administration. *Drug and Human Performance Factsheets: Cocaine* (2007). Available from http://www.nhtsa.dot.gov/people/injury/research/job185drugs/cocain.htm (accessed 21 November 2008).

Ovsiew, F. and R. Munich. *Principles of Inpatient Psychiatry* (London: Lippincott, Williams & Wilkins, 2008).

Resuscitation Council UK. *Advanced Life Support Guidelines* (London: Resuscitation Council UK, 2006).

Roldan, C. J. and R. Hebal. *Cocaine Toxicity* (Emedicine from Medscape, 2008). Available at http://emedicine.medscape.com/article/165716-overview (accessed 13 June 2009).

United Nations Office on Drugs and Crime. *World Drug Report* (Washington, DC: UNODC, 2009). Available at: http://www.unodc.org/unodc/en/data-and-analysis/WDR-2009.html (accessed 24 June 2009).

Volkow, N. D. *Research Report Series: Marijuana Abuse* (National Institute on Drug Abuse, 2006). Available at: http://www.nida.nih.gov/ResearchReports/Marijuana/default.html (accessed 21 November 2008).

11

Musculoskeletal Trauma

Julia Maz

Introduction

There is a wide spectrum of trauma and injuries that affect the musculoskeletal system in terms of cause, structural damage and outcome. In 2006, 28,673 people suffered serious injuries and a further 226,559 minor injuries on UK roads. This is in addition to the 3,172 people who were killed (DfT, 2007). Musculoskeletal problems account for an estimated 3.5 million emergency department attendances each year and are a significant cause of disability. Acute trauma is caused by a single, clear event and demonstrates a wide variety of injury patterns ranging from minor self-limiting sprains to fractures and/or dislocations of joints. Traumatic injury is a public health concern and the World Health Organisation estimates that injury is the leading cause of death worldwide among individuals between the ages of 1 and 44 years. Bone, soft tissue and associated neurovascular injuries are rarely emergencies unless accompanied by a life threatening haemorrhage as in certain amputations, pelvic and femoral fractures.

Trauma-associated deaths are known to occur in three so called 'peaks' (ATLS, 2004). The first peak of death occurs at the time of injury. It may be instantaneous or within a few minutes and is due to overwhelming primary injury to major organs or structures such as the brain, heart or great vessels. In most situations these injuries are irrecoverable, although rapid treatment and transfer may save some patients. Primary prevention has a major role in reducing the incidence of these injuries (Greaves, 2002; Driscoll, 2003; ATLS, 2004). The second peak lasts from the end of the first period to several hours after the injury has taken place. It is during this time that many causes of morbidity and mortality are preventable by avoidance of secondary injury due to hypoxia, haemorrhage or any process that leads to inadequate tissue perfusion. Reversible life threatening conditions may include major haemorrhage from viscera, bone and vessels or pneumothoraces. Most definitive care is directed at this period, as skilled assessment and management should reduce mortality and disability (ATLS, 2004). The third peak of death occurs days or weeks after the injury and usually happens in a high dependency or intensive therapy area where sepsis and multiple organ failure ensue (Mikhail, 1999). Advances in intensive care therapy may reduce these deaths but improvements in initial management on admission will also reduce morbidity and mortality during this period.

Trauma patients represent the highest challenges to the healthcare system because assessment and management require a multidisciplinary team effort. Seriously ill patients must be treated when histories, injuries and status are not well established. The focus of this chapter is on the management of an individual presenting with a traumatic long bone fracture (femur) and the management strategies offered take into account current evidence-based recommendations. Successful management of musculoskeletal injury is dependent upon the efficacy of early resuscitation, followed by detailed physical examination and diagnostic studies to establish the priorities for life-saving management, further treatment and rehabilitative care. Management generally occurs in four distinct phases:

1. Acute or resuscitation period (0 to 3 hours).
2. Primary or stabilisation period (3 to 72 hours).
3. Secondary or regeneration period (3 to 8 days).
4. Tertiary or rehabilitation period (beyond day 8).

This chapter is primarily concerned with phases 1 and 2.

Aim and Learning Outcomes

The Aim

The aim of this chapter is to explore the assessment and management of an individual presenting with a compound fracture of a major long bone with significant injury potential. A case scenario illustrates the key principles that underpin the assessment and management of such a fracture.

Learning Outcomes

At the end of this chapter the reader will be able to:

1. Discuss the normal anatomy of the musculoskeletal system.
2. Define and explain the resultant pathophysiological processes that occur following trauma.

3. Consider the initial assessment process and the immediate prioritisation of care following musculoskeletal trauma.
4. Explore the rationale for the management and care of a person with a long bone fracture.
5. Recognise the common complications associated with a long bone fracture.
6. Appreciate the value of multidisciplinary team work in the management of musculoskeletal trauma.

The Case Scenario: The Presenting Complaint

Paul is a fit, healthy 28-year-old salesman who normally drives to work by car, but today he decided to travel on his motorbike. He left home at 8.00 a.m wearing full protective clothing, including a helmet. Five minutes later a van pulled out of a junction without stopping and as Paul was travelling at 40 miles per hour he was unable to avoid the impact. An ambulance arrived at the scene 12 minutes later and made the following observations:

   Paul is alert and orientated to time and place with no reported loss of
      consciousness and no apparent neurological deficit.
   GCS score: 15 and both pupils are equal and react to light.
   Respiratory rate: 18 breaths per minute and SpO_2 is 99 per cent on air.
   Temperature: 36.3 °C.
   Pulse: 80 beats per minute.
   BP: 140/80 mmHg.

The paramedic crew apply a hard cervical collar and position Paul on a spinal board. An intravenous infusion of haemaccel 500 mL is commenced and IV morphine 2.5 mg administered for pain with IV Maxolon® 10 mg (anti-emetic). A single wound to the right middle thigh shows a bony protrusion, which is oozing blood. Paul denies any other injury and has no ongoing health problems, his lungs are clear and his abdomen is soft. He is haemodynamically stable en route to hospital according to the ambulance report.

   Consider the following:

1. Review the normal anatomy and physiology of the musculoskeletal system.
2. Understand the importance of mechanisms of injury.
3. Consider the physiological changes in the body caused by bony trauma.
4. What are the common clinical features of a fracture?

The Musculoskeletal System

The musculoskeletal system and related neurovascular structures consists of bones, joints, tendons, ligaments, muscles, blood vessels and nerves. The skeletal system contains 206 bones, which provide support, strength, movement and protection to the body and organs. Bones also store calcium and are involved in blood cell production.

Bones are characterised by shape as long (Figure 11.1), short, flat or irregular, with the shape of a particular bone suited for a unique function or purpose. The skeleton is composed of two types of bones: cancellous and cortical. Cancellous (spongy) bone is found in the skull, vertebrae, pelvis and end of long bones. Cortical (dense) bone is found in the long bones. Bones are supplied by blood vessels, nerves and lymphatic vessels that nourish bone tissue and allow the bone to repair injuries. The periosteum covers the bones and provides an additional blood supply. Bone is connected to other bone by stabilising bands of elastic, fibrous connective tissue called ligaments. Non-elastic fibrous cords that connect muscle to bone are tendons. Dense connective tissue found between the ribs, in the nasal septum, ear, larynx, trachea, bronchi, between vertebrae and on

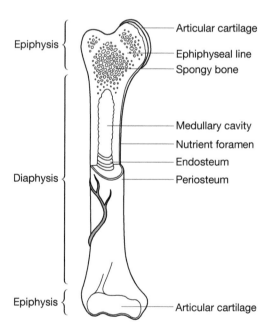

Figure 11.1   A long bone.

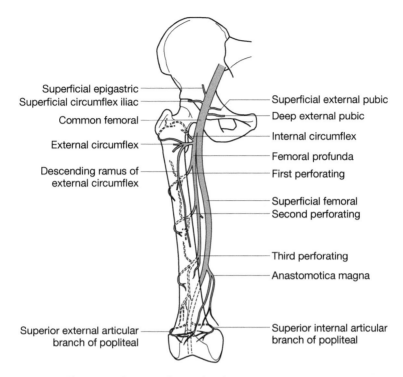

Figure 11.2   The vascular supply to the femur.

articulating surfaces is known as cartilage. Cartilage has a limited vascular supply, whereas bone tissue contains abundant blood vessels (Figure 11.2).

Joints are classified as non-synovial (such as the sacro-iliac) and synovial (for example, the shoulder). Synovial joints have two articulating surfaces covered with cartilage and surrounded by a two-layered synovial membrane sac to facilitate movement. The entire joint is then encapsulated by dense, ligamentous material. Joints provide mobility and stability, flexion and extension, medial and lateral rotation, and abduction and adduction. Joint movement is enhanced by muscles and ligaments that overlie the joint.

Nerves and arteries lie in close proximity to bones and muscle groups, with arterioles distributed throughout the periosteum to provide nutrients, and nerves to provide sensation and movement. Close proximity of arteries and nerves to bone structures increases the risk for injury with trauma to soft tissue, muscle, bone or joint. Bone is a living tissue with the same requirements as all living material, including respiration, assimilation, excretion, reproduction and response to stimulation (Table 11.1).

Table 11.1 Key requirements of bone

Respiration

The cells of bone require oxygen for metabolism and release carbon dioxide which must be removed from their environment. If either process ceases the cells of the bone tissue will die in the same way as any other living tissue.

Assimilation

Nutrition is necessary for growth and replacement of damaged cells; therefore protein, fat, carbohydrate, water, mineral salts and vitamins must reach the cells of bone in a steady consistent supply.

Excretion

Products of metabolism are produced continually and must be excreted from bone cells and tissues. These include such products as excess water, lactic acid and urea.

Reproduction

During the skeletal growth phase (16–18 years in most people), the bones are increasing in length and diameter. After growth has ceased new cells must still be produced to replace damaged or old ones. This requires a steady process of cell division and the production of new, fresh cells.

Response to stimulation

All tissues react to chemical, mechanical or nervous irritation and bone is no exception. It must repair itself when broken or damaged, respond to increased stresses by improving its strength in given areas, provide protrusions to which muscles are attached and react in general to the need for increased size and length.

The Femur

The femur is the longest, strongest, largest and heaviest tubular bone in the human body (Platzer, 2003; Whittle and Wood, 2003). It is capable of absorbing a huge amount of energy and resisting all but the greatest amount of trauma without damage. The femur can be divided into regions consisting of the head, neck, intertrochanteric, subtrochanteric (proximal), shaft and supracondylar and condylar regions (distal). In spite of the femur's strengths it is not immune to injury and when the femur is injured the situation may become life threatening. (See Dandy and Edwards (2009) for a detailed account of the anatomy of the femur.)

Long Bone Trauma: Mechanism of Injury

Musculoskeletal trauma is caused by either blunt or penetrating forces (Eckes-Roper, 2003). Blunt trauma to a femur is primarily associated with forces such as acceleration, deceleration, shearing and compression, which may result in injuries to other solid and hollow organs as well. Common causes of such injury are road traffic accidents, seat belt injuries, falls, sports injuries and explosions. Penetrating trauma is caused by an object penetrating the body, such as a gun shot wound, injuring skin, tissue, underlying organs, viscera and bone.

The mechanism of injury can be described as the effect of energy on human tissue. A clear history of the mechanism of injury is essential to make an accurate diagnosis in musculoskeletal trauma. Kinetic, thermal, electrical and radiation are examples of sources of energy that may cause injury. Paul has sustained injury (blunt trauma) resulting from kinetic energy, and it is imperative to determine how this energy was transmitted through the body and which organ systems were most likely to be affected. The most important concepts to consider when assessing the mechanism of injury are:

1. The anatomy of the area affected by trauma.
2. Newton's first law of motion, which states that an 'object at rest will remain at rest, and an object in motion will remain in motion until acted upon by an external force'.

Paul was travelling at approximately 40 miles per hour when his motorbike collided with the van. Paul's body would continue to move at 40 m.p.h. until it was acted upon by the 'external force' of the van, causing rapid deceleration to 0 m.p.h. Deceleration forces are transferred to the body at three different points of collision. The first collision occurs when the motorbike and vehicle strike and Paul continues to move forward. The second collision occurs when Paul hits the van and his body stops. The third collision point occurs when internal organs continue to move until they impact upon another organ, cavity wall or structure, or they are restrained suddenly by vasculature, muscles, ligaments or fascia. It is important to obtain information regarding potential patterns of injury relating to the energy and force of the accident as different damage occurs with each collision point and so each point must be considered separately to avoid missed injuries.

A fracture is defined as a disruption in the integrity of living bone, involving injury to the bone marrow, periosteum and adjacent soft tissue. The fracturing force can be direct or indirect (rotation, axial compression and bending without a direct impact). Fractures are divided into two general categories (Figure 11.3). Closed or simple fractures occur when the bone is broken but the skin is intact. Open or compound fractures, as in Paul's case, are characterised by bone protrusion puncture wounds where the bone punctures the skin or a foreign object penetrates the skin and bone, causing

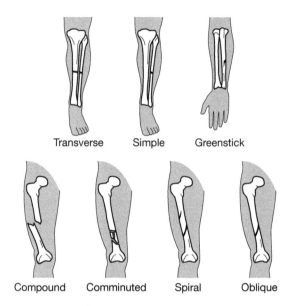

Figure 11.3   Long bone fractures.

a fracture. Examples of long bone fracture include fractures of the clavicle, the humerus, the radius and ulna, the metacarpals and phalanges, femoral shaft fractures, tibial fractures and metatarsal and phalangeal fractures. Fracture types are divided into oblique, transverse, spiral and comminuted (Figure 11.3). The clinical features of Paul's fracture include those outlined in Table 11.2.

An appreciation of high energy mechanisms of injury and an understanding of closed or open fractures can inform appropriate and timely management of pain control, swelling or possible contamination that could require multiple trips to operating theatres for wound irrigations and surgical debridement.

Table 11.2   Classic clinical features suggestive of a bone fracture

---

Pain throbbing and localised; often aggravated by active or passive movement

Swelling at the fracture site caused by oedema and/or haematoma formation which usually increases in the first 12 to 24 hours following injury

Deformity seen and felt, loss of function due to pain and the nature of the fracture

Bony tenderness and/or bruising at the fracture site

Crepitus (grating) heard or felt when the ends of the broken bone rub together

---

The Case Scenario: The Immediate Assessment Priorities

Paul arrives at the nearest accident and emergency department with the paramedic crew at 8.40 a.m. An immediate physiological assessment revealed the following:

Temperature: 36.2 °C
Pulse: 110 beats/min, regular
Respirations: 14 breaths per minute and SpO_2 = 99 per cent
Blood pressure: 100/60 mmHg
GCS: 15 and no apparent neurological deficits

Paul is assessed by a triage nurse, who notes that he continues to complain of severe pain, which he scores as 8 out of 10. Paul's right thigh is swollen, bruised and deformed and a compound comminuted fracture of the shaft of femur is suspected, with a 12 cm bony protrusion of the right mid thigh. He has a 2 litre intravenous infusion of 0.9 per cent sodium chloride and has received a further dose of IV morphine 2.5 mg for continued pain. He is receiving 15 litres of high flow oxygen via a non-rebreathe face mask.

Consider the following:

1. Explain the pathophysiology of trauma on the body.
2. What are the immediate assessment priorities in Paul's case and why?
3. Consider how you would carry out a more detailed assessment of Paul's condition. In particular, how would you check for any limb threatening conditions?

Assessment and Reaching a Diagnosis

Paul requires a systematic and comprehensive assessment to provide a rapid, accurate diagnosis to inform immediate appropriate management and care. The initial assessment and evaluation of Paul should always follow the principles of Advanced Trauma Life Support System (ATLS) (Committee ACoS, 2007), and includes the identification and treatment of life threatening injuries. The primary efforts in the initial phase are focused on life-saving procedures within the 'golden hour', which is known to be the time period in which life threatening conditions following major trauma may be cured by immediate therapeutic intervention (Magee, 2005; Stahal et al., 2005). The first step is evaluation of Paul's airway, breathing and circulation while maintaining spinal precautions until injury to the complete spine can be excluded clinically and radiographically (with X-rays or computed tomography (CT) scans). In practice these activities occur simultaneously but for the sake of narrative fluency each aspect will be discussed in turn. Rapid assessment identifies major injuries of head, cervical spine, chest and abdomen, and prioritises essential interventions.

Preliminary Assessment

Airway with Cervical Spine Protection

It is imperative that a clear and unobstructed airway is present. As Paul is speaking freely it is unlikely that there is any immediate threat to his airway. He is receiving high flow oxygen at 15 litres per minute via a non-rebreathe trauma mask with a reservoir bag so that high concentrations of O_2 can be delivered accurately. A vital nursing role is to ensure that the mask fits snugly over mouth and nose and that the flow rate is sufficient to keep the bag from collapsing during inspiration.

Given the high velocity injury Paul has sustained, a possible spinal injury should be considered. Careful removal of Paul's helmet is imperative for protection of the cervical spine (Table 11.3). Any patient with a possible cervical spine injury should have their neck immobilised in a neutral alignment to prevent further damage. Cervical spine damage is likely with deceleration injury as in Paul's case, hyperflexion or extension injury or any blunt injury above the clavicles. A fracture of the first rib seen on chest X-ray indicates high energy transfer and should always raise suspicion of cervical injury as well as intra-thoracic damage. When available a closely fitting firm cervical collar should be applied, secured with adhesive tape and sand bags placed on either side of the head to ensure immobility. Flexion of the cervical spine must be avoided to prevent airway compromise or aggravation of an existing spinal cord injury. This action has already been established by

Table 11.3 Helmet removal procedure

- An adequate airway can often be achieved with helmet in place especially when the potential exists for a complicating injury during a difficult helmet removal.
- Two people are needed to remove it – one person applies in-line immobilisation by placing hands on each side of helmet with fingers on the mandible, pulling carefully. N.B. cut or remove chin strap.
- A second person concurrently receives the weight of the patient's head by placing fingers of both hands on occipital region and thumbs at the angles of the mandible. The second person is now in control of the head and neck.
- The first person then removes the helmet by pulling laterally and carefully sliding it off.

Table 11.4   Clinical features of spinal cord trauma

Neck (cervical) and/or thoracic (chest)
Breathing difficulties (from paralysis of the breathing muscles) **and all** of list below

Lumbar and/or sacral (lower back)
- Loss of normal bowel and bladder control (may include constipation, incontinence, bladder spasms)
- Sensory changes: numbness, tingling sensation
- Motor changes: spasticity (increased muscle tone)
- Pain
- Weakness, paralysis

---

the paramedics on arrival at the accident scene. The front of the cervical collar is opened to inspect the neck for jugular vein distension and tracheal deviation and to palpate the carotid pulse and then securely closed. The cervical collar must fit properly to prevent flexion and extension of the cervical spine. A properly fitting collar has the following features:

1. The chin rests securely in the chin holder.
2. The collar does not cover the ears.
3. The bottom of the collar rests on the upper sternum (Licina and Nowitzke, 2005).

Clinical features of spinal cord injury (Table 11.4) can be quickly ascertained, such as numbness, tingling and inability to wriggle the toes and fingers. Full spinal immobilisation with the rigid cervical collar, a cervical immobilisation device (CID) and an immobilization board should be maintained throughout Paul's initial treatment. Should Paul vomit, he should be log-rolled as a unit with the equipment remaining intact, and then suctioning should be performed. Cervical spine X-rays from C1 to T1 may be obtained to determine the presence of spinal fractures. Providing Paul does not have radiological evidence of bony spine abnormalities, no abnormal neurological findings and no pain on palpation, the spinal immobilisation devices can be removed. Normal neurological findings include the absence of pain with a full range of cervical motion, though this is often difficult to assess in the presence of distracting injuries or head trauma. An MRI may be needed to evaluate the spine further.

Breathing

Respiration is assessed for rate, depth, pattern and noise every 30 minutes initially. Paul's deceleration injury may have caused rib fractures, which could affect his breathing. Signs of respiratory distress include rapid, shallow breaths, retraction of the intercostal muscles, nasal flaring and diminished or absent breath sounds. Paul's chest should be exposed and inspected for any surface trauma, penetrating wounds, paradoxical movements and flail segments. The rib cage and sternum are gently palpated for tenderness, crepitus and flail segments. A flail chest is defined as fractures in two or more adjacent ribs in two or more places or bilateral detachment of the sternum from the costal cartilage. The injury that Paul has sustained may have created a free-floating, unstable segment that moves in opposition to normal chest wall movement. Hence, a flail segment would move in when Paul breathes in and out with exhalation. A flail chest can cause hypoventilation of both lungs followed by atelectasis (alveolar collapse) and eventual hypoxia (Duggan and Kavanagh, 2005). Fortunately, Paul is not displaying these clinical features on initial assessment. Chest auscultation with a stethoscope may reveal normal air entry into both lungs, whereas unequal breath sounds on either side may indicate a collapsed lung due to a pneumothorax (air in pleural cavity) or a haemothorax (blood in pleural cavity).

Continuous pulse oximetry detects the percentage of arterial oxygen saturation in the blood and is a useful adjunct for determining adequacy of oxygenation; however, it must be remembered that the reading may not be accurate in a shocked trauma patient (Casey, 2001). (For further information refer to Elliott et al., 2006.) Arterial blood gas analysis should be performed in all patients with a potential chest injury since apparently minor chest wall injuries may cause significant hypoxaemia. The mechanics of breathing may be compromised by a disruption of the bony chest wall or diaphragm, accumulation of blood or air in the pleural cavities or haemorrhage and oedema in the lung itself, which reduces compliance. A neurological injury may alter the respiratory drive or pattern of breathing.

Circulation

Untreated fractures of the limbs can lead to significant blood loss, which may be external and obvious, or covert. The estimated blood loss for a closed fracture of the femur is 1,000 to 1,500 mL and this figure can be doubled if the fracture is compound, as in Paul's scenario, and should therefore be considered a potential cause of hypovolaemic shock (see Chapter 3). Paul's pulse rate, regularity, volume and blood pressure (BP) should be assessed and recorded initially every 30 minutes until a stable trend is established. His regular heart rate of 110 beats per minute suggests a sinus tachycardia, which may be caused by pain, anxiety or both, or may signal a compensatory sympathetic response to low BP caused by a fall in stroke volume and cardiac output (see Chapter 3). Paul's BP is initially within the normal range despite potential blood loss. This may be maintained by a series of compensatory mechanisms triggered in response to a fall in circulatory volume. A fall in stroke volume (SV), cardiac output (CO) and subsequent BP will trigger baroreceptors in the carotid sinus and aortic arch to stimulate the cardiac acceleratory centre within the medulla oblongata. This will excite sympathetic nervous activity, resulting in an increased heart rate, myocardial contractility, generalised vasoconstriction and arterial redistribution of blood flow to the vital organs. A subsequent fall in renal perfusion simultaneously stimulates the renin–angiotensin–aldosterone–ADH system to retain sodium (Na^+) and water (H_2O) and conserve circulating volume to maintain SV and CO and increase the BP (see Chapter 3). Blood pressure alone can therefore be extremely misleading and should be considered in conjunction with other parameters of circulatory assessment, including pulse rate, capillary refill, respiratory rate, conscious level and urine output.

Paul should have two large bore intravenous venflons (14 or 16 gauge) inserted into large veins, such as the antecubital fossa, to administer intravenous fluid such as 0.9 per cent sodium chloride, Haemaccel, 4 per cent albumin in 0.9 per cent saline or blood (see Chapter 3). The choice of fluid will depend on the degree of blood loss identified. As a guide, 0.9 per cent sodium chloride or Haemaccel could be used in Paul's situation, progressing to blood if more than three or four litres are required. A rule of thumb advocated by the British Trauma Society (2009) (www.trauma.org) for crystalloid solutions (e.g. 0.9 per cent saline, Hartman's solution) is that three times the blood volume loss will be required. Large transfusions (i.e. greater than one blood volume or five litres of blood in an adult) may require the administration of platelets and other coagulation factors (e.g. fresh frozen plasma). Careful monitoring of Paul's fluid input and output is essential to ensure that fluid resuscitation is optimised and that he is not volume overloaded.

A simple and important technique in reducing blood loss in Paul's situation involves immobilising the fracture with a long rigid splint such as an air splint. This helps to obviate bleeding and pain. In the case of untreated femoral shaft fractures, bony overlap and large open venous channels in muscle potentiate bleeding. Paul is not displaying any signs of arterial blood loss externally (bright red and pulsating) and oozing indicates that Paul is bleeding from the capillaries adjacent to the wound site (bright red). Direct pressure in the form of firm application of a sterile gauze pad for 10 to 15 minutes and elevation (if possible) should stop the bleeding. In the presence of compressible controllable bleeding (as in Paul's case) fluid resuscitation is designed to maintain normal pulse and blood pressure. However, in the presence of non-compressible or non-controllable bleeding (pelvic fractures

Table 11.5   SHOCK mnemonic

S	**Solutions** to add volume which will increase venous return. A combination of fluids, blood and plasma expanders (dextran, plasma and albumin are commonly used)
H	**Haemodynamics** is a way to measure potential hypovolaemic shock and evaluate interventions. Note the normal CVP= 5–15 cm/H2O
O	**Oxygen** will saturate RBCs and decrease tissue starvation
C	**Check** the skin (cold and clammy indicate the early stages of hypovolaemic shock)
K	**Kick** up the feet and legs (elevate if possible) and let gravity increase venous return

and bilateral limb fractures) or major bleeding elsewhere (abdomen and retroperitoneal bleeding), the object of resuscitation should be to maintain essential organ perfusion by maintaining a systolic blood pressure greater than 80 mmHg or restoring the radial pulse. Studies suggest that massive volume replacement without adequate haemorrhage control is associated with poor outcomes (Revell et al., 2003; Bozeman, 2008). The SHOCK mnemonic (Table 11.5) provides a simple but useful reminder of immediate considerations if hypovolaemic shock is suspected.

Disability

Paul may have sustained a head injury during the accident and therefore his neurological status should continue to be monitored every 30 minutes using the APVU and GCS scales until a stable trend is established (see Chapters 2 and 4). The trauma score (Table 11.6) is an objective method for determining injury severity that can be used as an adjunct to vital signs observation.

Table 11.6   Revised trauma score

Respiratory rate		Systolic BP		GCS	
10–29	4	>89	4	13–15	4
>29	3	76–89	3	9–12	3
6–9	2	50–75	2	6–8	2
1–5	1	1–49	1	4–5	1
0	0	0	0	<4	0

Source: trauma.org; Available: http://www.trauma.org/archive/scores/rts.html

Ideally trauma scores are calculated during three phases: in the pre-hospital setting; on arrival at the emergency department; and one hour later. Paul's trauma score is 12 so there is no need for immediate airway intervention, high flow oxygen via a face mask can be continued and a full clinical examination can be performed.

Exposure

While ensuring dignity and privacy, Paul's protective motorcycle garments must be carefully cut off using a pair of scissors to expose his entire body and allow inspection for ecchymosis (bruising), deformities, haemorrhage and skin colour. The nurse must listen for any abnormal sounds and carefully feel the movement of each bone, noting any movement that is unusual or provokes pain. Inspection, palpation, percussion and auscultation of the chest and abdomen will also be necessary to detect potential internal injuries. (See Epstein et al. (2008) for detailed clinical examination.) A warm environment should be maintained and prudent use of warmed blankets expedited.

Distal Limb Neurovascular Assessment

Once assured that no life threatening injury has been left unattended, the nurse needs to assess the femoral injury with particular emphasis upon neurovascular function of the distal limb and the open wound. Paul has a 'golden period' of six hours before potential ischaemia and myonecrosis (death of muscle tissue) are deemed irreversible. Assessment of the distal neurovascular function (nerve and circulatory status) of the affected limb should be checked initially every 5 to 15 minutes, documented and compared with the other limb and previous assessments throughout (Table 11.7).

Table 11.7 Neurovascular limb assessment

- Pulses distal to the injury and capillary refill distal to the injury
- Colour and temperature of the limb
- Pain and tenderness
- Soft tissue swelling or discolouration
- Limitation in range of movement
- Altered sensory perception
- Loss of function

Vascular Assessment

PULSES

The femoral, popliteal, posterior tibial and dorsalis pedis (pedal) pulses all require assessment for their presence and quality. To aid in future assessments, the location of the pulse may be marked with a magic marker. If a weak pulse or no pulse is found, the fracture may be putting pressure on the femoral artery or indeed the comminuted bone fragments may have damaged the artery and the orthopaedic team should be notified immediately. A weak pulse can be determined by comparing the pulse felt below the fracture with that of Paul's uninjured extremity. If there is any uncertainty as to the nature of the peripheral pulses below the fracture site, a Doppler ultrasound probe should be used to detect blood flow and, if located, the site marked on the skin. It is important to document the quality of the pulses and words such as weak, normal quality and bounding may be used. Paul's pulses appear present and of normal quality. Capillary refill time should also be assessed by depressing Paul's right toenail until blanching occurs. The nail is then released and the speed of colour refill is observed. Refill should occur in less than two seconds. The injured extremity should be compared with the unaffected limb.

COLOUR

The skin colour of Paul's leg gives a good indication of the adequacy of circulation and any potential problems (Table 11.8).

The skin distal to Paul's injury site should be palpated with the whole hand to assess temperature. The dorsum of the hand is more sensitive to temperature changes (Lumley, 2008). Paul's lower right extremity is warm to touch and pink in colour but should still be observed every 15 minutes. A cool or cold right foot indicates diminished arterial blood supply and may indicate the development of circulatory compromise, termed acute compartment syndrome. This develops when pressure in a fascial compartment increases and venous return is occluded (Brown and Sayers, 2007).

Table 11.8 Indication of circulatory problems

Colour	Circulatory problem
Pink or ruddy	Venous congestion
Mottled, dusky, pale	Inadequate arterial perfusion or arterial occlusion
Cyanotic	Inadequate arterial perfusion and/or insufficient venous return

Subsequently, although pulses may be present, perfusion is interrupted, muscle and nerve ischaemia ensues and, if untreated (usually via decompression fasciotomy), progresses to necrosis. Acute compartment syndrome is relatively infrequent in femoral fractures due to the capacity of the three compartments of the thigh to accommodate substantially higher blood volumes compared with those of the lower leg and the forearm. Severe bleeding into one or more compartments of the thigh is necessary to elevate the compartment pressure above the critical level (Brown and Sayers, 2007). That said, Paul is less than 35 years old and male, which have been identified as important indicators for the development of acute compartment syndrome (McQueen et al., 2000; Mithofer et al., 2004), and therefore prompt recognition of symptoms at this stage is imperative. Paul's right leg should be elevated unless there are signs of arterial compromise.

PAIN AND TENDERNESS

The exact area of pain should be assessed and excessive movement of Paul's injured limb minimised. It is important to determine if his pain is increasing despite analgesia, as severe pain is a cardinal feature of acute compartment syndrome. Alternatively, in the initial assessment severe pain on passive motion may be a sign of neurological compromise. A variety of data to assess Paul's pain, including his subjective reports, objective signs of distress (e.g. physiological signs, behavioural indicators) and pain assessment scales, should be used.

Neurological Assessment

SENSORY PERCEPTION

Paul's ability to detect pain, light touch, deep touch, heat, cold, vibratory sense, proprioception (spatial awareness) and two point discrimination should be assessed. Two point discrimination is assessed by having Paul close his eyes while the nurse lightly touches the area distal (furthest away) from the injury. Paul will be asked to discern the difference between two distinct points (for example, can he determine the difference between one or two fingers being applied to his right calf). If Paul can feel pressure but cannot differentiate between one or two digits, this is a sign of decreasing neurovascular function and requires immediate medical notification. Assessment for full sensation, abnormal sensation (paraesthesia), diminished sensation or numbness of Paul's right leg is tested using a sharp pointed object such as a sterile needle. It is vital that the sensory status of Paul's limb is established and Paul reports full sensation with no loss of two point discrimination. Sensory changes to Paul's right foot, for example, could indicate specific nerve injury or impending changes because of ischaemia. As Paul is able to determine the difference between light applications of one or two digits by the nurse this is a clear indicator that the femoral nerve arising from the lumbar plexus is intact.

MOTOR FUNCTION

Motor function is assessed by asking Paul to move his leg if possible through a range of motion. When checking the motor response, paralysis or inability to move the extremity distal to the injury may indicate a peripheral nerve injury or ischaemic changes resulting from oedema. If any part of this assessment provokes Paul's pain it must be stopped. Table 11.9 lists some suggested methods of testing specific nerves.

After initial evaluation the open wound on Paul's right thigh should be sealed with sterile dressings and the limb immobilised in an air splint. Debridement and irrigation with sterile saline solution in the emergency room should be avoided in case of inoculation of the deeper tissues with nosocomial organisms (Committee ACoS, 2007). Only easily accessible foreign bodies should be removed before the application of sterile dressings in Paul's case. Nevertheless, irrigation of the open wound in the emergency room is advocated by many clinicians in the case of heavily contaminated wounds. The practical value of obtaining specimen cultures from the open wound in the emergency room has been questioned since they usually isolate superficial contaminants or normal skin flora, while at the same time carry the risk of causing wound contamination (Committee ACoS, 2007).

At this stage Paul should have a range of continuous non-invasive monitoring, including ECG, automated sphygmomanometer, core temperature probe, urinary catheter and pulse oximeter, to aid frequent monitoring of vital physiological parameters. The core temperature probe will detect any potential for the development of hypothermia post trauma or pyrexia

Table 11.9 Testing specific nerve areas on the lower limb

Peroneal nerve
1. Sensory: touch lateral side of right great toe
2. Motor: ask Paul to wriggle the toes on his right foot

Femoral nerve
1. Sensory: touch anterior right thigh, medial aspect of right calf
2. Motor: loss of knee jerk

Tibial nerve
1. Sensory: touch each lateral and medial aspect on sole of foot
2. Motor: plantar flex ankle, flex great toe

---

suggesting infection. A urinary catheter will be inserted with a urometer to provide accurate measurement of Paul's urinary output on an hourly basis and to minimise movement where possible.

Specific Investigations

X-ray is an essential method of determining the exact nature of the fracture and assists with providing a clinical and radiological classification that can be used in communication across the entire multidisciplinary team. Table 11.10 lists a range of venous blood samples that will be taken during the acute assessment period and Table 11.11 includes the usual secondary assessment details, which will be collected over the following hours.

Simple, repetitive instruction and explanation may help to alleviate some of Paul's anxiety, fear and uncertainty regarding his condition during the assessment phase. Equally, adequate ongoing pain assessment and relief are important methods of ensuring his comfort, compliance, understanding and consensual participation throughout the process. Words of reassurance, praise and comfort can go far to help to reassure Paul.

Neurological and vascular injuries can occur in any fracture and are more likely in cases with increasing fracture deformity. Peripheral nerve injury would be suspected if Paul were to report experiencing motor or sensory deficiencies. Management of neurological injury involves immediate reduction of the fracture and possible nerve exploration, with subsequent follow up to assess whether or not neurological function returns.

Table 11.10 Routine venous blood sampling

1. Full blood count (FBC) – low Hb (anaemia), raised WBC (infection)
2. Clotting screen – if indicated by current medication, e.g. warfarin
3. Urea and electrolytes (U&E) – electrolyte balance and renal function
4. Capillary blood glucose if high or low glucose is suspected, e.g. diabetic patient
5. Blood group, save and cross match – for potential blood transfusion

Table 11.11 Secondary assessment

- Full clinical examination: peripheral pulses, jugular venous pressure (JVP), heart and lung sounds, ECG, systemic and musculo-skeletal examination
- Past medical history (PMH)
- Family (FH) and social history (SH)
- Systemic enquiry
- Drug history: prescribed, over-the-counter and recreational
- Chest/spinal/pelvic/limb X-ray

The Case Scenario: Medical Management and Care Issues

Within an hour of arriving in the accident and emergency department, a full primary assessment has revealed that Paul is currently haemodynamically stable, fully conscious and alert and apyrexial. A series of investigations including X-ray images of his right limb have confirmed that he has a displaced, compound, comminuted fracture of the right shaft of femur, classification 3A on the Gustilo and Anderson scale. There is also a bony protrusion at the right thigh, external rotation of the lower leg and multiple abrasions on both legs. The wound has been sealed with a transparent occlusive dressing. He is not displaying any evidence of neurovascular impairment to his right extremity. A detailed secondary assessment has also revealed the following:

Head: lower lip abrasion
Neck: no tenderness
Chest: tender and painful
Abdomen: no tenderness and pelvis stable
Past medical history: nil
Medications: nil
Haemoglobin: 12.7 g/dL (normal 12 to 18 g/dL)
Toxicology screening: negative
Electrocardiograph: normal sinus rhythm – rate 92 beats per minute
Chest/pelvic X-ray: no abnormalities detected
Urinalysis: no abnormalities detected

He has given a detailed medical and social history. A decision is reached to take Paul to the operating theatre for further surgical intervention.

Consider the following:

1. What are the immediate priorities in John's management and care?
2. What surgical intervention would be the most appropriate in Paul's case?

Medical Management Strategies

Paul's immediate medical priorities include the assessment and management of potential life threatening problems, limb threatening conditions and coexistent conditions resulting from his accident. This includes:

1. Ongoing observation of vital signs repeated every 30 minutes until a stable trend is established.
2. High flow oxygen therapy to maintain SpO_2 > 95 per cent.

3. IV access, fluid resuscitation and close fluid balance monitoring.
4. Regular pain assessment, analgesia and anti-emetic administration.
5. Entire body immobilisation until normal skull, spine and chest inspection is established.
6. Limb immobilisation.
7. Wound cleansing and occlusion.
8. Psychological support and reassurance.

Now that Paul's condition is stable, attention should be paid to the psychological aspects of management. Paul may feel threatened and liberal reassurance is needed because at this time Paul will not be able to evaluate the severity of his injury. Information and support for Paul and his family are important for their reassurance, cooperation and compliance in his management and care. The presence of familiar faces in an otherwise alien environment can help to orientate Paul and provide him with additional psychological support. Repeated simple explanations or instructions may become necessary if a deficit in recent memory is apparent.

Although he does not appear to have any immediate limb threatening neurovascular conditions, the open and complex nature of Paul's fracture will necessitate surgical intervention. His fracture can be classified as type 3A according to the Gustilo and Anderson score (Table 11.12).

The use of a classification system is important as it facilitates communication among medical and nursing clinicians regarding decision making, anticipating potential problems, suggesting treatment options and predicting patient and surgical outcomes (Ruedi et al., 2007). Various classification systems have been proposed in an effort to grade the extent of the initial musculoskeletal injury and to offer useful prognostic clues to help in deciding the optimal management (Sudkamp, 2000). The most widely used is that of Gustilo and Anderson (1984), which describes three groups of increasing severity based on the size of the open wound, the degree of its contamination and the extent of soft tissue injury (Table 11.12). Other classification systems include the Tscherne (Tscherne and Oestern, 1982) and Hanover

Table 11.12   Gustilo and Anderson classification of compound fractures

---

Type 1: low energy, wound < 1 cm
Type 2: wound > 1 cm with moderate soft tissue damage
Type 3: high energy wound > 1 cm with extensive soft tissue damage
   Type 3A: adequate soft tissue cover
   Type 3B: inadequate soft tissue cover
   Type 3C: associated with arterial injury

Table 11.13   The 5 Rs of fracture management

Resuscitation: shock may be related to pain and blood loss.

Reduction: realignment of fractured bone ends usually under general anaesthesia using an image intensifier.

Restriction: to prevent deformity and allow bone growth to proceed normally until bony union occurs. Methods used depend on bone affected and nature of injury, and include plaster cast, traction or internal or external fixation.

Restoration: limb immobilisation increases the risk of muscle and joint stiffness and loss of some function. Encourage to exercise all joints and muscles except those affected by the injury.

Rehabilitation: when the restriction is removed the limb must be exercised to restore normal ranges of movement.

Fracture Scales. However, the emphasis should be to appreciate the significance of the soft tissue injury more than committing to memory any of the scoring systems.

The five Rs summarise the main aims of fracture treatment and are summarised in Table 11.13.

The orthopaedic surgeon will manage the femoral fracture by inserting an intra-medullary nail into the femur shaft in an effort to promote healing by callus formation. This tends to promote more rapid bone healing than that achieved by external fixation, which relies upon primary healing and so enables a more rapid rehabilitation. With this type of surgery, bone fragments are repositioned and/or reduced into their normal alignment and then held together by the insertion of rods through the marrow space in the centre of the bone. The surgeon is therefore able to reposition the fracture fragments exactly.

Preparation for Theatre

Paul is likely to be placed on to the acute trauma list for intra-medullary nailing of the right femur as soon as an operating theatre, surgeon, anaesthetist and staff become available. This provides little time to ensure that the theatre preparation checklist (Chapter 8, Table 8.6) pertinent to Paul is completed.

The Case Scenario: Ongoing Care Issues

Paul is warded two hours later at 2 p.m. following wound debridement and reamed intra-medullary nailing of his right femoral fracture under general anaesthetic. The operating theatre notes record an uncomplicated procedure in the presence of continued physiological stability. An estimated blood loss of 1 litre is recorded. Paul received 3 litres of IV crystalloid and 4 units of blood. He is awake but drowsy and able to respond to verbal commands appropriately. A patient controlled analgesia (PCA) device of IV morphine 1 mg with a lockout dose of 10 minutes has been commenced. Paul has an IV infusion of Cephaloxin® and he has 100 per cent oxygen via venturi mask. Three small mepore dressings cover the wound at the intra-medullary nail insertion site and a medium sized mepore covers the wound following wound debridement. Both dressings are clean. A urinary catheter remains in situ. The post anaesthetic care unit records show an uneventful initial recovery.

Nursing Care Issues

1. Consider what the immediate post-operative care would be.
2. What are the nursing responsibilities and underpinning rationale with regard the PCA?
3. What potential complications may Paul develop following surgery with specific reference to the long bone surgery?

Ongoing Care Issues and the Role of the Nurse

Post-operative Observations

All patients require close observation of airway, breathing and circulation following a general anaesthetic. Assessment of vital signs should be clearly and accurately recorded every 30 minutes until a stable trend has been established and it is evident that potential complications have been avoided. Routine observations should include:

- Consciousness level: AVPU (see Chapter 2).
- Pulse: rate, regularity, depth.
- BP.
- Respiratory rate: rate, depth, noise.
- SpO_2.
- Skin colour.

- Urine output: the urinary catheter may have been removed; therefore note the first urine void (urine retention can occur post anaesthesia) and continue to record output.
- Temperature: four-hourly.
- IV cannula site and intravenous fluid infusion.
- Wound drainage.

Any changes or abnormal findings must be reported to senior nursing and medical staff immediately. Post-operative complications following internal fixation of a fractured femur are reasonably rare; nevertheless, the initial injury, anaesthesia and surgery may all pose some potential risk to Paul's well-being. It is beyond the scope of this chapter to engage with more detailed routine post-operative care and management; however, it is important to note the principles of orthopaedic nursing management (Kneale and Davis, 2005). Specific management issues pertaining to Paul will be outlined.

Post-operative Pain Management

It is accepted that pain represents the fifth vital sign requiring assessment post-operatively (Lorenz et al., 2009). The form of assessment tool used must reflect the fact that Paul is emerging from anaesthesia. The verbal rating scale (VRS) requires that Paul rate his perception of pain on a scale of 0 to 10, whereby 0 represents no pain and 10 the worst pain imaginable. This scale provides the nurse with an objective measure that may be re-evaluated as comfort measures are instituted. Paul is self reporting a score of 3 at this time. Management of Paul's acute pain begins with the affirmation that he should have access to the best level of pain relief that may be provided safely.

It is the nurse's responsibility to ensure that Paul is aware of and understands how to use the PCA for pain relief. He should be clear that when he experiences pain he can self administer a small bolus dose of morphine and that he should experience pain relief within a few minutes. PCA ensures that individuals can adjust the level of analgesic required according to the severity of pain. In theory, the plasma level of the analgesic will be relatively constant and side effects caused by fluctuations in plasma level will be eliminated.

Morphine is the most popular drug and will be considered here with reference to Paul. The ideal dose of morphine has been found to be 1 mg in a PCA device; however, regular review by the nurse is needed in every case to ensure that pain relief is adequate. The aim of the lock-out period is to prevent over-dosage occurring because of over-enthusiastic demands for more analgesia. The lock-out time should be long enough for the previous dose to have an effect. In practice, lockout times of between 5 and 10 minutes are enough for most opioids. A maximum dose can be programmed into most PCA devices to prevent overdose. In practice, it is more logical to accept that the analgesic requirements of patients will vary considerably and some patients may require large amounts to achieve adequate pain relief. Paul appears to be successfully titrating his analgesia to a point where he is comfortable rather than pain free, stating that he 'expects some pain after surgery'. It would be expected that Paul would progress on to oral analgesia the day following surgery. The nurse should take special notice of Paul developing pain that appears to be out of proportion to the injury and surgery and be suspicious of impending acute compartment syndrome. The orthopaedic medical team should be updated regarding pain control.

Neurovascular Limb Assessment

Neurovascular inspection of Paul's right limb should be performed in the same way as the pre-operative assessment. Additional observation of the site of surgery, the type of dressing, the presence of drains and/or drainage and the status of the distal extremities is equally important. Ongoing monitoring of extremity colour, capillary refill, sensation and mobility will be maintained every 15 minutes for the first 2 hours, every 30 minutes for the following 2 hours, hourly for the following 2 hours and thereafter every 2 hours for the following 18 hours. Acute compartment syndrome remains a potential complication in the post-operative phase (Weinstein and Buckwalter, 2005), and so neurovascular observation is aimed at recognising and addressing concerns early. Paul does not appear to have any unexpected changes in neurovascular status.

Monitor Wound Areas

Sutures or clips are usually used to close the wound and will be removed at approximately 10 days post-operation. The mepore dressings provide a sterile, self adhesive absorbent barrier and should be left intact unless the surgeon authorises otherwise. The nurse should maintain a high level of suspicion for infection given that Paul's injury was an open fracture. Prophylactic intravenous antibiotics may be used for longer durations with open fractures as compared to closed fractures (Buckholz et al., 2006). The nurse should assess for infection and report if pyrexia, increased pain, redness, swelling or discharge from the wound is noted and documented. Excessive blood loss should be measured and recorded on the fluid balance chart and in rare cases may necessitate a return to theatre for further explorararation. If a small drain is inserted near the wound site, blood loss should be recorded and the drain removed 24 to 48 hours later once bleeding has ceased. MRSA prophylaxis treatment will continue with antibacterial agents such as Octenidine® 0.3 per cent lotion applied to the body for three minutes every day and 2 per cent Mupirocin® nasal ointment three times a day for five days.

Monitor Potential Development of Complications

Deep vein thrombosis (DVT) and pulmonary embolism (PE) are important complications to recognise and prevent (Autar, 2007). DVT prophylaxis with subcutaneous injection of weight adjusted low molecular weight heparin (LMWH) should be medically prescribed once the post-operative bleeding risk is acceptable, usually 12 to 24 hours later (Rogers et al., 2002). Gentle distal limb movement to exercise limb muscles may also be encouraged and anti-embolic stockings (TEDs) measured and fitted to both limbs. Vigilant observation of all pressure areas and regular pressure relief is essential to prevent pressure sore development.

Emotional Support

Paul may experience many painful and frightening events before, during and after the operation. These experiences give rise to emotions that range from anxiety to sheer terror. Nurses can provide comfort and emotional support to the individual at this time of crisis. A calm, reassuring voice, clear explanation, time for listening and an approachable visibility can all provide Paul with some sense of security. Honesty with respect to pain, discomfort and issues related to enforced immobility should help. The acute care inpatient stay is brief, but it is the insightful nurse who can balance the issues discussed in this chapter with thoughtful consideration of the challenges ahead for Paul and his family. Family members should be encouraged to participate in Paul's care wherever possible.

Early Mobilisation

Paul will be able to get out of bed the following day once his observations are stable and the PCA has been removed. Physiotherapists will help Paul to learn to walk with the aid of crutches for the following five or six weeks. At this stage Paul should regain independence with his usual daily activities, including personal hygiene, and a healthy diet and fluid intake should have resumed.

Monitor Complications Specific to Intra-medullary Nailing

Early complications following operative fracture management include visceral injury, vascular injury, acute compartment syndrome and nerve injury. Fat embolism syndrome (FES) is a rare but recognised complication of long bone fractures, such as in Paul's case, with a reported incidence of 2 to 23 per cent in this patient group (Ganong, 1993). FES usually occurs 24 to 72 hours after a fracture or following surgery. Bone marrow from the fractured bone or other injured adipose tissue releases fatty globules that enter the bloodstream through torn veins at the injury site (Fort, 2002). Fatty globules may travel to the lungs, where they become entangled in the microvasculature of the lung to form an embolus with subsequent occlusion of the pulmonary circulation. They can also become trapped and cause occlusion of the small vessels of the brain and the kidneys. Lipase breaks down the trapped fat emboli into free fatty acids. Fat embolism can be prevented or reduced by moving the fractured extremity as little as possible prior to fixation, proper splinting and early surgical fixation of the fracture, which prevents the globules being released into the bone marrow. It is therefore imperative to monitor the patient's neurological and respiratory status carefully for any sign of confusion and hypoxaemia.

Summary

The importance of musculoskeletal trauma management cannot be overstated. A systematic approach to assessment and intervention improves patient outcomes through early recognition of potentially life threatening injuries and intervention for identified problems. Priorities in trauma management are to ensure adequate oxygenation and ventilation, control haemorrhage, and maintain tissue perfusion to vital organs. The management of any patient who has sustained a fracture must take into account not just the fracture but the whole patient. Patients require immediate assessment of their respiration, level of consciousness and circulation. Once care has been paid to these vital factors, nursing attention can be directed towards the injured limb, the vertebral column or the pelvis. The role of the nurse is of utmost importance and can have a profound impact on the patient's outcome.

This chapter has considered trauma of the femur, which is a potentially serious and life threatening event. It has provided insight into the importance of understanding the mechanism of injury, the extent of injury and one possible fixation technique. Potential complications and considerations have been outlined with a specific focus on priorities of assessment and management throughout the initial acute phase. The goal of treatment is alignment and function and the nursing role can significantly impact upon the quality of care and promote positive outcomes. By discussing the rationale for timely, appropriate interventions it has been shown that life and limb saving challenges can be overcome and a positive outcome attained.

Further Reading

Dandy, J. D. and D. J. Edwards. *Essential Orthopaedics and Trauma*, 5th edn (London: Churchill Livingstone, 2009).

Eliott, M., R. Tate and K. Page. 'Do Clinicians Know How to Use Pulse Oximetry? A Literature and Clinical Implications', *Australian Critical Care*, 19(4) (2006), 139–44.

Epstein, O., G. D. Perkin, J. Cookson, I. S. Watt, R. Rakhit, A. W. Robbins and G. A. W. Hornett. *Clinical Examination*, 4th edn (London: Mosby International Ltd, 2008).

O'Reilly, M. 'Major Trauma Management', in G. Jones (ed.), *Emergency Nursing Care: Principles and Practice* (London: Greenwich Medical Media, 2003).

References

ATLS. *American College of Surgeons: Committee on Trauma*, 7th edn (Chicago: American College of Surgeons, 2004).

Autar, R. 'NICE Guidelines on Reducing the Risk of Venous Thromboembolism (Deep Veined Thrombosis and Pulmonary Embolism) in Patients Undergoing Surgery, *Journal of Orthopaedic Nursing*, 11(3/4) (2007), 169–76.

Bozeman, W. P. *Shock, Haemorrhagic: Treatment and Medication* (2008). Available at http://emedicine.medscape.com (accessed 12 January 2009).

British Trauma Society (2009). Available at www.trauma.com (accessed 12 January 2009).

Brown, M. and R. Sayers. 'Compartment Syndromes', in R. Fitridge and M. Thompson (eds), *Mechanism of Vascular Disease: A Textbook for Vascular Surgeons* (Cambridge: Cambridge University Press, 2007).

Buckholz, R. W., J. D. Heckman, C. Court-Brown et al. *Rockwood and Green's Fractures in Adults*, 6th edn (Philadelphia: Lippincott Williams and Wilkins, 2006).

Casey, G. 'Oxygen Transport and the Use of Pulse Oximetry', *Nursing Standard*, 15(47) (2001), 46–53.

Committee ACoS. *Advanced Trauma Life Support (ATLS) for Doctors*, 8th edn (Chicago: Committee ACoS, 2007).

Department for Transport (DfT). *Highways Economics Notes No. 1: 2006* (London: Department for Transport, 2007), http://www.dft.gov.uk (accessed 1 April 2007).

Driscoll, P. *Trauma Resuscitation: The Team Approach* (Basingstoke: Macmillan, 2003).

Duggan, M. and B. P. Kavanagh. 'Pulmonary Atelectasis: A Pathogenic Perioperative Entity', *Anaesthesiology*, 102(4) (2005), 838–54.

Eckes-Roper, J. *Trauma Nursing Secrets* (Philadelphia: Hanley & Belfus Inc., 2003).

Elliott, M., R. Tate and K. Page. 'Do Clinicians Know How to Use Pulse Oximetry? A Literature and Clinical Implications', *Australian Critical Care*, 19(4) (2006), 139–44.

Fort, C. 'Getting a Fix on Long Bone Fracture', *Nursing*, 32(6) (2002), 32hn1–6.

Ganong, R. B. 'Fat Emboli in Isolated Fractures of the Tibia and Femur', *Clinical Orthopaedic Related Research*, 291 (1993), 208–14.

Greaves, I. *Trauma Care Manual* (London: Arnold, 2002).

Gustilo, R. B., R. M. Mendoza and D. N. Williams. 'Problems in the Management of Type III (Severe) Open Fractures: A New Classification of Type III Open Fractures', *Journal of Trauma*, 24 (1984), 742–6.

Kneale, D. and P. S. Davis. *Orthopaedic and Trauma Nursing*, 2nd edn (London: Churchill Livingstone, 2005).

Licina, P. and A. M. Nowitzke. 'Approach and Considerations Regarding the Patient with Spinal Injury', *International Journal of the Care of the Injured*, 36 (2005), SB 2–12.

Lorenz, K. A., C. D. Sherbourne and L. R. Shugarman. 'How Reliable Is Pain as the Fifth Vital Sign', *American Board of Family Medicine*, 22(3) (2009), 291–8.

Lumley, J. S. P. *Surface Anatomy: The Anatomical Basis Of Clinical Examination*, 4th edn (London: Churchill Livingstone, 2008).

McQueen, M. M., P. Gaston and C. M. Court-Brown. 'Acute Compartment Syndrome. Who Is at Risk?', *British Journal of Bone and Joint Surgery*, 82 (2000), 200–3.

Magee, D. J. *Orthopaedic Physical Assessment*, 4th edn (Philadelphia: Saunders Elsevier, 2005).

Mikhail, J. 'The Trauma Triad of Death: Hypothermia, Acidosis and Coagulopathy', *AACN Clinical Issues*, 10(1) (1999), 85–94.

Mithofer, K., D. W. Lhowe, M. S. Vrahas, D. T. Altman and G. T. Altman. 'Clinical Spectrum of Acute Compartment Syndrome of the Thigh and Its Relation to Associated Injuries', *Clinical Orthopaedic Related Research*, 425 (2004), 223–9.

Platzer, W. *Colour Atlas of Human Anatomy, Volume 1, Locomotor System*, 5th edn (Stuttgart: Thierne Verlag, 2003).

Revell, M., I. Greaves and K. Porter. 'Endpoints to Fluid Resuscitation in Haemorrhagic Shock', *Journal of Trauma-Injury, Infection and Critical Care*, 54(5) (2003), S563–7.

Rogers, F. B., M. D. Cipolle, G. Velmahos, G. Rozycki and F. A. Luchette. 'Practice Management Guidelines for the Prevention of Venous Thromboembolism in Trauma Patients', *Journal of trauma Injury, Infection and Critical Care*, 53 (2002), 142–64.

Ruedi, T. P., R. Buckley and C. Moran (eds). *AO Principles of Fracture Management* (New York: Thieme Medical Publishers, 2007).

Stahal, P. F., C. E. Hayde, W. Wyrwich and W. Ertal. 'Current Concepts of Polytrauma Management: from ATLS to "Damage Control"', *Orthopade*, 34 (2005), 823–36.

Sudkamp, N. 'Soft-tissue Injury: Pathophysiology and Its Influences on Fracture Management – Evaluation/Classification of Closed and Open Injuries', *AO Principles of Fracture Management* (Stuttgart: Thieme, 2000).

Tscherne, H. and H. J. Oestern. 'A New Classification of Soft-tissue Damage in Open and Closed Fractures', *Unfalheilkunde*, 85(3) (1982), 111–15.

Weinstein, S. L. and J. A. Buckwalter. *Turek's Orthopaedics Principles and Their Application*, 6th edn (Philadelphia: Lippincott, Williams and Wilkins, 2005).

Whittle, A. P. and G. W. Wood. 'Fractures of Lower Extremity', in T. S. Canale (ed.), *Campbell's Operative Orthopaedics, Volume 3*, 10th edn (London: Mosby, 2003).

Conclusion

The chapters in this book have provided a comprehensive review of the assessment and management required by acutely ill adults presenting with a range of common but serious acute illnesses. The primary purpose of the book is to identify and discuss the knowledge and skills required to recognise and respond in a timely and effective manner to the needs of the acutely ill adults. In these concluding pages the discussion briefly reviews issues that we consider will need to be addressed if healthcare professionals are to deliver the standard of care required by acutely ill adults.

The NPSA (2007) report, the NICE (2007) guideline (CG:50) and the Department of Health's (2008c) competencies all highlighted the importance of ensuring that nurses *in all* settings are able to recognise, interpret the significance of and act on data that indicates deterioration in at-risk patients and that requires urgent reassessment by specialist nursing or medical staff. Initial and continuing education plays an important role in ensuring that nurses have the competence to carry out these important activities in all settings (Manley and Hardy, 2006; Giddens, 2007). Knowledge and skill deficits are not confined to new graduates: nurses working outside of specialist critical and high dependency areas often do not systematically monitor at-risk patients; where they do, many of these nurses may not be able to interpret or appreciate the significance of the data obtained (NICE, 2007; Garside and Prescott, 2008).

Pre- and post-registration nurses have often developed a basic knowledge of the mechanisms of disease and have some competence in measuring vital signs and undertaking related assessments, including a primary survey and simple analyses of urine and blood (Garside and Prescott; 2008; Steen and Costello, 2008). However, many nurses have limited knowledge and understanding of normal physiological parameters. This means that, while most nurses can obtain and report on vital signs assessed, their ability to interpret and recognise the significance of these vital signs is frequently limited. In the absence of knowledge of normal parameters, abnormal assessment findings are unlikely to be recognised and acted upon. Different explanations for this situation have been identified; these include the lack of structured educational preparation and limited opportunities for learning within clinical placements, together with variable support from managers in provider organisations. However, in practice no single explanation can account for this observed deficit in knowledge and understanding (Chapple and Aston, 2004; Steen and Costello, 2008).

The NPSA (2007) report and NICE (2007) guidance identify the need for focused training and improved communication between healthcare professionals to achieve early recognition and appropriate response to acute illness in adults in hospital. In support of this the Department of Health (2008a, b) has defined programmes of training and specific competencies for two new roles: the assistant critical care practitioner (an advanced support worker role at level 4 on the NHS Career Framework) and advanced practitioners in critical care. Most registered nurses working in acute and critical care will function at a level in between these two important new roles but the competencies developed for patient assessment, monitoring vital signs and observation of the patient, together with basic airway management, may well inform and underpin future educational programmes in acute and critical care.

There is evidence that structured problem-oriented or problem-based learning approaches can increase nurses' engagement with learning, can develop critical thinking skills and can help to integrate knowledge and understanding of more complex concepts such as those required to be understood when working with pathophysiology and disease (Ehrenberg and Haggblom, 2007; Murray et al., 2008). The use of real and hypothetical case studies draws on the problem-based approach and has been used successfully in medicine and nursing to develop knowledge, understanding and clinical competence in acute and critical care settings (Cioffi, 2000; Alinier et al., 2006; Garside and Prescott, 2008). We advocate the use of case studies in learning about priorities in assessment and management of individuals requiring acute and critical care and have drawn upon this approach within the book to introduce and develop explanations of common signs, symptoms, responses and interventions in acute and critical illness. This approach can be used equally effectively in clinical practice settings and can contribute directly to helping nurses to apply knowledge directly to practice situations. In turn, patients and other health professionals will benefit as safe and appropriate care is provided.

References

Alinier, G., B. Hunt, R. Gordon and C. Harwood. 'Effectiveness of Intermediate-fidelity Simulation Training Technology in Undergraduate Nursing Education', *Journal of Advanced Nursing*, **54**(3) (2006), 359–69.

Chapple, M. and E. S. Aston. 'Practice Learning Teams: A Partnership Approach To Supporting Students' Clinical Learning', *Nurse Education in Practice*, **4**(2) (2004), 143–9.

Cioffi, J. 'Nurses' Experiences of Making Decisions to Call Emergency Assistance to Their Patients', *Journal of Advanced Nursing*, 32(1) (2000), 108–14.

Department of Health. *The National Education and Competence Framework for Advanced Critical Care Practitioners* (London: Department of Health, 2008a).

Department of Health. *The National Education and Competence Framework for Assistant Critical Care Practitioners* (London: Department of Health, 2008b).

Department of Health. *Recognising and Responding to Acutely Ill Patients in Hospital* (London: Department of Health, 2008c).

Ehrenberg, A. C. and M. Haggblom. 'Problem Based Learning in Clinical Nursing Education: Integrating Theory and Practice', *Nurse Education in Practice*, 7 (2006), 67–74.

Garside, J. and S. Prescott. 'Improving the Care of Acutely Ill Patients Outside ICU Settings', *Nursing Times*, 104(22) (2008), 25–6.

Giddens, J. F. 'A Survey of Physical Assessment Techniques Performed by RNs: Lessons for Nursing Education', *Journal of Nurse Education*, 46(2) (2007), 83–7.

Manley, K. and S. Hardy. *Improving Services to Patients through Ongoing Development of Critical Care Teams*. A report commissioned by the Department of Health (England). (London: Department of Health, 2006).

Murray, C., M. Grant, M. Howarth and J. Leigh. 'The Use of Simulation as a Teaching and Learning Approach to Support Practice Learning', *Nurse Education in Practice*, 8 (2008), 5–8.

National Institute for Health and Clinical Excellence. *Acutely Ill Patients in Hospital: Recognition of and Response to Acute Illness in Adults in Hospital*. NICE Clinical Guideline 50 (London: NICE, 2007).

National Patient Safety Agency. *Safer Care for the Acutely Ill Patient: Learning from Serious Incidents*. Fifth Report from the Patient Safety Observatory (London: NHS National Patient Safety Agency, 2007).

Steen, C. D. and J. Costello. 'Teaching Pre-registration Student Nurses to Assess Acutely Ill Patients: An Evaluation of Acute Illness Management Programme', *Nurse Education in Practice*, 8 (2008), 343–51.

Index